Breast Augmentation

Editor

BRADLEY P. BENGTSON

CLINICS IN
PLASTIC SURGERY

www.plasticsurgery.theclinics.com

October 2015 • Volume 42 • Number 4

ELSEVIER

1600 John F. Kennedy Boulevard • Suite 1800 • Philadelphia, Pennsylvania, 19103-2899

http://www.theclinics.com

CLINICS IN PLASTIC SURGERY Volume 42, Number 4
October 2015 ISSN 0094-1298, ISBN-13: 978-0-323-39113-9

Editor: Jessica McCool
Developmental Editor: Donald Mumford

Clinics in Plastic Surgery (ISSN 0094-1298) is published quarterly by Elsevier Inc., 360 Park Avenue South, New York, NY 10010-1710. Months of issue are January, April, July, and October. Business and Editorial Offices: 1600 John F. Kennedy Blvd., Suite 1800, Philadelphia, PA 19103-2899. Periodicals postage paid at New York, NY and additional mailing offices. Subscription prices are $490.00 per year for US individuals, $716.00 per year for US institutions, $240.00 per year for US students and residents, $555.00 per year for Canadian individuals, $853.00 per year for Canadian institutions, $630.00 per year for international individuals, $853.00 per year for international institutions, and $305.00 per year for Canadian and foreign students/residents. To receive student/resident rate, orders must be accompanied by name of affiliated institution, date of term, and the *signature* of program/residency coordinator on institution letterhead. Orders will be billed at individual rate until proof of status is received. Foreign air speed delivery is included in all *Clinics* subscription prices. All prices are subject to change without notice. **POSTMASTER:** Send address changes to *Clinics in Plastic Surgery*, Elsevier Health Sciences Division, Subscription Customer Service, 3251 Riverport Lane, Maryland Heights, MO 63043. **Customer Service: 1-800-654-2452 (US and Canada). From outside of the United States and Canada, call 314-447-8871. Fax: 314-447-8029. E-mail: JournalsCustomerService-usa@elsevier.com (for print support); JournalsOnlineSupport-usa@elsevier.com (for online support).**

Reprints. For copies of 100 or more of articles in this publication, please contact the Commercial Reprints Department, Elsevier Inc., 360 Park Avenue South, New York, New York 10010-1710. Tel.: +1-212-633-3874; Fax: +1-212-633-3820; E-mail: reprints@elsevier.com.

Clinics in Plastic Surgery is covered in *Current Contents, EMBASE/Excerpta Medica, Science Citation Index, MEDLINE/PubMed (Index Medicus), ASCA, and ISI/BIOMED.*

Contributors

EDITOR

BRADLEY P. BENGTSON, MD, FACS
Founder, Bengtson Center for Aesthetics and Plastic Surgery, Grand Rapids, Michigan; Associate Professor, Department of Surgery, School of Medicine, Michigan State University, East Lansing, Michigan

AUTHORS

WILLIAM P. ADAMS Jr, MD
Associate Clinical Professor, Department of Plastic Surgery, The University of Texas Southwestern Medical Center, University Park, Texas

BRADLEY P. BENGTSON, MD, FACS
Founder, Bengtson Center for Aesthetics and Plastic Surgery, Grand Rapids, Michigan; Associate Professor, Department of Surgery, School of Medicine, Michigan State University, East Lansing, Michigan

OLIVIER ALEXANDRE BRANFORD, MA, MBBS, PhD, MRCS, FRCS (Plast)
Department of Plastic Surgery, The Cadogan Clinic; Department of Plastic Surgery, The Royal Marsden, London, United Kingdom

MITCHELL H. BROWN, MD, MEd, FRCSC
Plastic and Reconstructive Surgeon, Associate Professor, Department of Surgery, University of Toronto, Toronto, Ontario, Canada

MICHAEL BRADLEY CALOBRACE, MD
Clinical Faculty, Division of Plastic Surgery, Department of Surgery, University of Louisville, Louisville; Clinical Faculty, Division of Plastic Surgery, Department of Surgery, University of Kentucky, Lexington, Kentucky

SIMON J. CHONG, BHB, MBChB, FRACS
Fellow, Department of Plastic, Reconstructive and Maxillofacial Surgery, Faculty of Medicine and Human Sciences, Macquarie University, Sydney, Australia

MARK W. CLEMENS, MD, FACS
Assistant Professor, Department of Plastic Surgery, The University of Texas MD Anderson Cancer Center, Houston, Texas

OLIVIER A. DEIGNI, MD, MPH
St Louis University, St Louis, Missouri

ANAND K. DEVA, BSc (Med), MBBS (Hons), MS, FRACS
Head, Department of Plastic, Reconstructive and Maxillofacial Surgery, Faculty of Medicine and Human Sciences, Macquarie University, Sydney, Australia

MARK D. EPSTEIN, MD, FACS
Assistant Professor of Surgery, Center for Aesthetic Surgery, Stony Brook, New York

SARAH E. FERENZ
Department of Biology, Cornell University, Ithaca, New York

ALLEN GABRIEL, MD, FACS
Clinical Associate Professor, Department of Plastic Surgery, Loma Linda University Medical Center, Loma Linda, California

ROLF GEMPERLI, MD, PhD
Plastic Surgeon, Department of Plastic Surgery, Hospital Albert Einstein; Chief, Department of Plastic Surgery, University of São Paulo School of Medicine, São Paulo, Brazil

CAROLINE A. GLICKSMAN, MD, FACS
Founder, Glicksman Plastic Surgery, Sea Girt, New Jersey; Associate Clinical Professor, Department of Surgery, Jersey Shore University Medical Center, Neptune, New Jersey

EMILY C. HARTMANN, MD, MS
Aesthetic Surgery Fellow, Marina Plastic Surgery, Marina del Rey, California; Keck School of Medicine of University of Southern California, Los Angeles, California

DAVID A. JANSSEN, MD, FACS
Fox Valley Plastic Surgery, Oshkosh, Wisconsin

MELVIN M. MACLIN II, MD
Parkcrest Plastic Surgery, St Louis, Missouri

PATRICK MALLUCCI, MBChB, MD, FRCS, FRCS (Plast)
Department of Plastic Surgery, The Cadogan Clinic; Department of Plastic Surgery, Royal Free Hampstead NHS Trust, London, United Kingdom

G. PATRICK MAXWELL, MD, FACS
Clinical Professor, Department of Plastic Surgery, Loma Linda University Medical Center, Loma Linda, California

ROBERTO N. MIRANDA, MD
Professor, Department of Hematopathology, The University of Texas MD Anderson Cancer Center, Houston, Texas

RYAN T.M. MITCHELL, MD, FRCSC
Bengtson Center for Aesthetics and Plastic Surgery, Grand Rapids, Michigan

ALEXANDRE MENDONÇA MUNHOZ, MD, PhD
Plastic Surgeon, Department of Plastic Surgery, Hospital Sírio-Libanês; Coordinator, Breast Plastic Surgery, Department of Plastic Surgery, University of São Paulo School of Medicine and Instituto do Câncer do Estado de São Paulo, São Paulo, Brazil

JOÃO CARLOS SAMPAIO GOES, MD, PhD
Plastic Surgeon, Department of Plastic Surgery, Hospital Albert Einstein; Chief, Breast Surgery and Plastic Surgery Department, Instituto Brasileiro do Controle do Câncer, São Paulo, Brazil

MICHAEL SCHEFLAN, MD
ISAPS Professor of Plastic Surgery, Scheflan Plastic Surgery, Tel Aviv, Israel

KEVIN H. SMALL, MD
Assistant Professor of Surgery, Plastic Surgery, Weill Cornell Medical College; Assistant Attending Surgeon, Plastic Surgery, New York Presbyterian Hospital, New York, New York

RON B. SOMOGYI, MD, MSc, FRCSC
Plastic and Reconstructive Surgeon, North York General Hospital, Toronto, Ontario, Canada

MICHELLE A. SPRING, MD, FACS
Marina Plastic Surgery Associates, Adjunct Clinical Assistant Professor of Surgery, Keck School of Medicine of University of Southern California, Los Angeles, California

W. GRANT STEVENS, MD, FACS
Marina Plastic Surgery Associates, Clinical Professor of Surgery, Keck School of Medicine of University of Southern California, Los Angeles, California

LOUIS L. STROCK, MD, FACS
Clinical Assistant Professor, Department of Plastic Surgery, The University of Texas Southwestern Medical Center, Dallas, Texas

WILLIAM F. WACHOLTZ, PhD
Department of Chemistry, University of Wisconsin, Oshkosh, Wisconsin

CHAD G. WENZEL, MD
Medical College of Wisconsin, Milwaukee, Wisconsin

Contents

CLINICS IN PLASTIC SURGERY

FORTHCOMING ISSUES

January 2016
Rhinoplasty: Multispecialty Approach
Babak Azizzadeh, *Editor*
Daniel Becker and Ronald P. Gruber, *Section Editors*

April 2016
Complications in Breast Reduction
Dennis C. Hammond, *Editor*

July 2016
Minimally Invasive Plastic Surgery for the Aging Face
Kenneth Rothaus, *Editor*

RECENT ISSUES

July 2015
Fat Grafting: Current Concept, Clinical Application, and Regenerative Potential, Part 2
Lee L.Q. Pu, Kotaro Yoshimura, and Sydney R. Coleman, *Editors*

April 2015
Fat Grafting: Current Concept, Clinical Application, and Regenerative Potential, Part 1
Lee L.Q. Pu, Kotaro Yoshimura, and Sydney R. Coleman, *Editors*

January 2015
Lower Lid and Midface: Multispecialty Approach
Babak Azizzadeh and Guy G. Massry, *Editors*

ISSUE OF RELATED INTEREST

Breast Cancer
Editor: Lisa Newman
Surgical Oncology Clinics of North America
July 2014. Volume 23, Issue 3
Available at: http://www.surgonc.theclinics.com/

Preface
Breast Augmentation

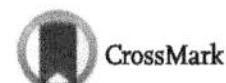

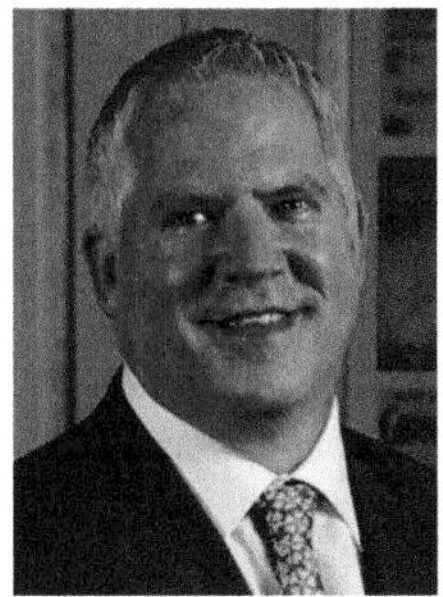

Bradley P. Bengtson, MD, FACS
Editor

It is an incredible honor and privilege to be asked to be the editor for this issue of *Clinics in Plastic Surgery* on breast augmentation. It certainly is humbling to be associated with my friends, colleagues, and teachers, Dr Pat Maxwell (October, 1988), Dr John Tebbetts (July, 2001), and Dr Scott Spear (January, 2009), who have previously edited these prior *Clinics in Plastic Surgery* on this important topic. It has been interesting to review these prior publications and see where we have been, where we are today in 2015, and perhaps take a small glimpse into the future.

Since Dr Spear's last *Clinics in Plastic Surgery* publication in 2009 on breast augmentation in which I contributed an article on "Complications, Reoperations, and Revisions in Breast Augmentation," we have unfortunately made very little headway into reducing complications or the number of breast revision surgeries. In fact, I believe on our current trajectory, within the next 10 years or possibly at the publication of the next breast augmentation issue of *Clinics in Plastic Surgery*, breast revision surgery may surpass primary augmentation. The technologies and techniques for breast revision are rapidly improving, although revision rates continue to remain high.

There is, however, a great deal about which to be excited and optimistic! There are a number of new products, devices, and techniques that all have the potential to decrease complications and significantly improve patient outcomes. Instead of focusing on standard approaches or classic textbook-related topics, I have decided instead to concentrate articles primarily on new technologies, devices, and approaches that have the potential to truly move the needle and improve patient experiences, improve patient outcomes, and decrease revision rates. Some of these topics we are reviewing that have personally transformed my practice include Standardization of the Bra Cup, Differences Between Saline and Silicone Implants, Improving Patient Education and Selection, Using 3D Imaging in Breast Augmentation Surgery, Delving Into the Etiology and Prevention of Capsular Contracture, Thoughts on Aesthetic Breast Ideals, Use and Patient Selection with Shaped Implants, Use of Fat Transfer in Breast Augmentation and Revision, and many others.

It is also very interesting to speculate on the future of breast augmentation. Will it include 3D Imaging with Holographic Projections or 3D Imaging Simulating Outcomes, Finally the

Clin Plastic Surg 42 (2015) xi–xii
http://dx.doi.org/10.1016/j.cps.2015.07.001
0094-1298/15/$ – see front matter

Definitive Etiology and Cure for Capsular Contracture, The True Significance and Etiology of ALCL and Determination of its Clinical Characteristics, The Ideal Internal Support of the Breast, New Implant Devices, Shells, Fills, and Shapes, and Improved Techniques and Technologies that Reduce Complications and Improve Outcomes?

In the meantime, I hope this issue dedicated to breast augmentation is helpful, is thought-provoking, and peaks your interest in areas where these experts are today, and most importantly, helps you improve your individual patient satisfaction and your surgical outcomes.

A special thanks to our authors for their time and expertise in contributing these articles, and to the editors at Elsevier.

Bradley P. Bengtson, MD, FACS
Bengtson Center for Aesthetics
and Plastic Surgery
555 MidTowne Street Northeast, Suite 110
Grand Rapids
MI 49503, USA

E-mail address:
drb@bengtsoncenter.com

The Evolution of Breast Implants

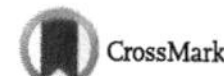

Allen Gabriel, MD*, G. Patrick Maxwell, MD

KEYWORDS

- Silicone breast implants • Textured implants • Round implants • Anatomic implants • Shaped implants • Highly cohesive implants

KEY POINTS

- Implant characteristics on the bench differ from implant performance within the body. Shape, feel, safety, and longevity of the implants remain important areas of research.
- The data provided by all 3 manufacturers show the safety and efficacy of these medical devices.
- Clinicians should strive to provide ongoing data and sound science to continue to improve clinical outcomes in the future.

INTRODUCTION

There has been a steady increase in breast augmentation surgery with the evolving importance of body image, changes in societal expectations, and the increasing acceptance of aesthetic surgery in the United States. Augmentation mammaplasty, performed 286,694 times in 2014, ranks as the most frequently performed cosmetic surgical procedure in women in the United States.[1]

The first report of successful breast augmentation appeared in 1895, in which Czerny[2] described transplanting a lipoma from the trunk to the breast in a patient deformed by a partial mastectomy. In 1954, Longacre[3] described a local dermal-fat flap for augmentation of the breast. Eventually, both adipose tissue and omentum were also used to augment the breast.

During the 1950s and 1960s, breast augmentation with solid alloplastic materials was performed using polyurethane, polytetrafluoroethylene (Teflon), and expanded polyvinyl alcohol formaldehyde (Ivalon sponge).[4] Ultimately, the use of these materials was discontinued after patients developed local tissue reactions, firmness, distortion of the breast, and significant discomfort.[5] Various other solid and semisolid materials have been injected directly into the breast parenchyma for augmentation, including epoxy resin, shellac, beeswax, paraffin, petroleum jelly, and liquid silicone.[6] In 1961, Uchida reported the injection of liquid silicone (polydimethylsiloxane) into the breast for breast augmentation.[5] This technique resulted in frequent complications, including recurrent infections, chronic inflammation, drainage, granuloma formation, and even necrosis.[7] Breast augmentation by injection of free liquid silicone and the various other solid and semisolid materials was abandoned in the United States in light of these complications.[8]

The evolution of the modern breast implant began with a 2-component prosthetic device manufactured with a less permeable silicone elastomer shell filled with a stable filling material, consisting of either saline solution or silicone gel. This shell and gel filler implant was originally developed by Cronin and Gerow in 1962 using silicone gel as the filling material contained within a thin, smooth silicone elastomer shell.[9] Since that time, both silicone gel and saline-filled implants have undergone several technical alterations and improvements.[10]

Disclosures: Drs G.P. Maxwell and A. Gabriel are consultants for Allergan and Dr G.P. Maxwell is a stockholder for Allergan and Mentor.

Department of Plastic Surgery, Loma Linda University Medical Center, 11175 Campus Street, Suite 21126, Loma Linda, CA 92350, USA
* Corresponding author.
E-mail address: gabrielallen@yahoo.com

Clin Plastic Surg 42 (2015) 399–404
http://dx.doi.org/10.1016/j.cps.2015.06.015
0094-1298/15/$ – see front matter

EVOLUTION OF SALINE IMPLANTS

The use of inflatable saline-filled breast implants was first reported in 1965 by Arion in France.[8] The saline-filled implant was developed in order to allow the noninflated implant to be introduced through a small incision, and then the implant was inflated in situ.[7]

Although these implants allow slight overfilling, aggressive overfilling may lead to a more spherical shape and scalloping along the implant edge, with knucklelike palpability and unnatural firmness. A disadvantage of saline-filled implants is that the consistency on palpation is similar to that of water instead of the more viscous feel of natural breast tissue.

EVOLUTION OF SILICONE IMPLANTS

The first-generation silicone gel–filled implant introduced in 1962 by Cronin and Gerow was manufactured by the Dow Corning Corporation.[9] The shell of the first-generation implant was constructed using a thick, smooth silicone elastomer as a 2-piece envelope with a seam along the periphery. The shell was filled with a moderately viscous silicone gel. The implant was anatomically shaped (teardrop) and had several Dacron fixation patches on the posterior aspect to help maintain the proper position of the implant. These early devices had a high contracture rate, caused by the quality of the shells and the lack of cohesivity of the gel, which then encouraged implant manufacturers to develop second-generation silicone gel–filled implants.[11]

In the 1970s, the second-generation silicone implants were developed in an effort to reduce the incidence of capsular contracture with a thinner, seamless shell and without Dacron patches incorporated into the shell. These implants were round and filled with a less viscous silicone gel to provide a more natural feel. However, the second-generation breast implants had problems with diffusion or bleed of microscopic silicone molecules into the periprosthetic intracapsular space because of their thin, permeable shells and low-viscosity silicone gel filler. This diffused silicone produced an oily, sticky residue surrounding the implant within the periprosthetic capsule, which was noticeable during explantation of older silicone-filled implants.[12]

The development of the third-generation silicone gel–filled implants in the 1980s focused on improving the strength and permeability of the shell in order to reduce silicone gel bleed from intact implants, and to reduce implant rupture and subsequent gel migration. The manufacturers designed new implant shells that consisted of multilayered silicone elastomer. These third-generation prostheses reduced gel bleed by introducing a barrier layer and a thicker shell, which significantly reduced the device shell failure rate.

After the US Food and Drug Administration (FDA) required the temporary restriction of third-generation silicone gel implants from the American market in 1992,[13–18] the fourth-generation and fifth-generation gel devices evolved. These silicone gel breast implants were designed under more stringent American Society for Testing Methodology[19] and FDA-influenced criteria for shell thickness and gel cohesiveness. Furthermore, they were manufactured with improved quality control,[20] and with a wider variety of surface textures and implant shapes. They are currently available from all 3 breast implant manufactures in the United States (Sientra, Allergan, and Mentor) (**Figs. 1–3**).[21–25]

During the same time the concept of anatomically shaped implants was introduced with the fifth-generation silicone gel implants.[26] In addition to having a textured surface, these anatomically shaped implants are filled with a more cohesive gel. The FDA approved fifth-generation implants from all of the US manufacturers in the following order: Sientra (2012), then Allergan and Mentor (both 2013). Each manufacturer was approved for a variety of shapes and styles, with Sientra offering 5 styles of the HSC+ line, 4 styles of the 410 implant from Allergan, and 1 CPG implant from Mentor.[22,27,28]

To further understand the evolution of silicone-filled implants, implant characteristics are further reviewed, because the resultant breast form not only depends on the soft tissue envelope (in augmentation and reconstruction) and the breast parenchyma (in augmentation) but also on the following implant characteristics: surface, filler, shell, and implant shape.

SURFACE

Surface characteristics have undergone changes and have evolved with all 3 manufacturers working

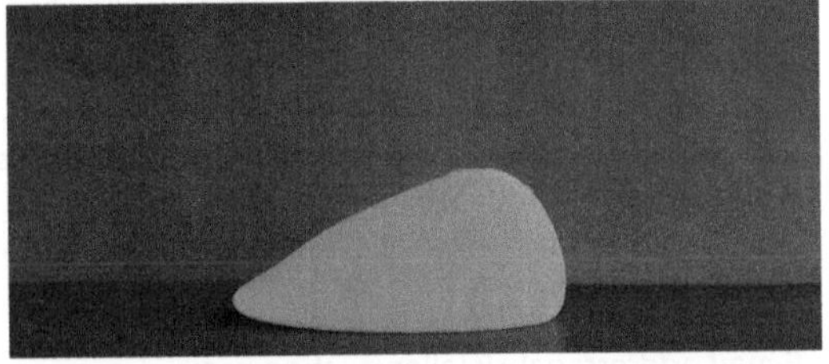

Fig. 1. Allergan's Natrelle 410 implant. (Allergan, Inc, Parsippany, NJ.)

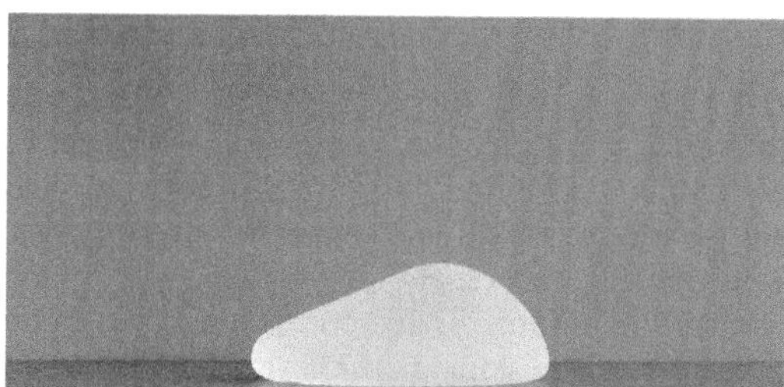

Fig. 2. Mentor's CPG implant. (Mentor Worldwide LLC, Santa Barbara, CA.)

toward the common goal of using texture to possibly minimize or even disrupt capsule formation.[29,30] The evolution of textured implants began with polyurethane-coated implants reportedly having lower capsular contracture rates.[31] These foam-coated implants were eventually removed voluntarily from the US market because of concern caused by difficulty in complete removal and theoretic concern of carcinogenic conversion of the coating. Polyurethane foams are thought to undergo partial chemical degradation under physiologic conditions, releasing compounds that could become carcinogens in animals but are not known human carcinogens.[32]

In the 1980s, manufacturers shifted their focus from foam-covered shells to textured silicone shells with different pore sizes. None of the textured surfaces are created in the same manner and each manufacturer has a proprietary process in place. One of the critical issues during the evolution of the texture is to find a way to stabilize the implant in the breast pocket. Studies have shown that the pore size is critical to allow for tissue adherence leading to the adhesive effect and implant stabilization.[33] However, it was not clear whether the pore size correlated with a reduction in capsular contracture, but did correlate with implant stabilization.[33] Danino and colleagues[33] compared the BIOCELL texture with pore diameter of 600 to 800 μm with a depth of 150 to 200 μm with Siltex with pore diameter of 70 to 150 μm. Siltex pores led to no adhesive effect.

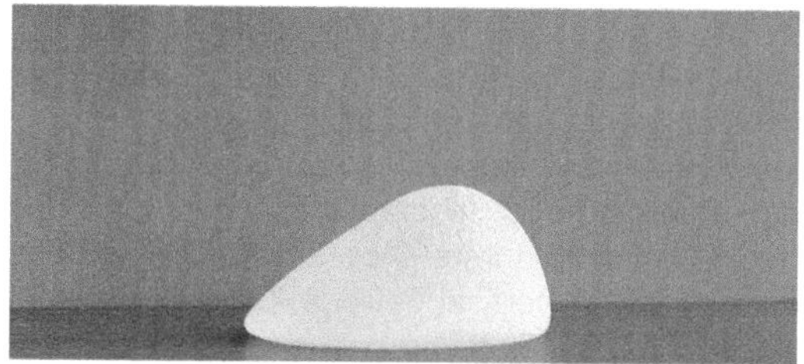

Fig. 3. Sientra's HSC+ implant. (Sientra, Inc, Santa Barbara, CA.)

The manufacturing process of textured surface implants can be complex, whereas smooth surface implants are made by dipping a mandrel into liquid silicone, creating multiple layers, followed by allowing the surface to cure in a laminar flow oven. Additional steps beyond creating smooth surface implants are involved in the creation of textured implants.[34] Sientra's Silimed implant (Sientra, Inc, Santa Barbara, CA), named as TRUE Texture, avoids the use of sodium chloride, sugar, soak/scrub, or pressure stamping.[28,35,36] Small, hollow pores are formed with minimal thin cell webbing that reduces particle formation. The BIOCELL (Allergan, Inc, Irvine, CA) texture is created using a loss-salt technique,[34] which includes a layer of salt crystals with a thin overcoat of silicone followed by curing in a laminar flow oven.[34] In contrast, the Siltex surface (Mentor Corp, Santa Barbara, CA) is created by imprint stamping,[34] which dips the chuck into uncured silicone, pushing it into polyurethane foam and finalizing the imprint with pressure.[34]

FILLER

Silicone is a mixture of semi-inorganic polymeric molecules composed of varying length chains of polydimethylsiloxane [$(CH_3)_2$-SiO] monomers. The physical properties of silicones are variable depending on the average polymer chain length and the degree of cross-linking between the polymer chains.[37] Liquid silicones are polymers with a short average length and very little cross-linking. They have the consistency of an oily fluid and are frequently used as lubricants in pharmaceuticals and medical devices. Silicone gels can be produced of varying viscosity by progressively increasing the length of the polymer chains or the degree of cross-linking.

When filler cross-linking is achieved to the degree that the silicone gel implant will maintain its dimensions and form (ie, gel distribution within the shell), the cohesive gel implant is considered to be form stable, although this terminology has recently been questioned because no gel implant on the market is truly form stable. Form stable may more appropriately refer to the ability of an implant to maintain shape. Technology exists to measure the cohesivity of the silicone gel of commercially available devices and was used to measure the stiffness of both Allergan and Mentor shaped and round implants. This study showed that the 410 implant (Allergan Inc) had the stiffest gel, representing the highest cohesivity versus the CPG implant (Mentor).[27] In a separate study, the Sientra form-stable implant was the least cohesive compared with both CPG and 410 implants. Note that cohesivity is only 1 implant characteristics and clinicians must take in to account various implant features in order to evaluate the implant as a whole.[27] In this same study, Allergan's round implants were the least cohesive compared with Mentor's round implants, and Sientra's implants were the most cohesive compared with both Allergan's and Mentor's round implants.

In the past, the effect of the filler material has been shown to have an effect on capsular contracture rates.[38–40] However, these studies compared the third-generation silicone implants with saline implants and therefore the current implants may have other outcomes since fourth-generation silicone breast implant safety and long-term outcomes have been described.[22,23,25,27,28,41]

SHELL

Extensive chemical cross-linking of the silicone gel polymer produces a solid form of silicone referred to as an elastomer, with a flexible, rubberlike quality. Silicone elastomers are used for the manufacture of facial implants, tissue expanders, and the outer shells of all breast prostheses.

Introducing shell modifications such as barrier layers and triple shell elastomer to protect the gel has led to safer implants.[22,23,27,28,42] The elastomeric shell characteristics also depend on the relationship of the gel and shell. Shell characteristics also depend on the thickness of each shell and how the internal gel is bonded to the shell, which leads to the stability of the final shape.

IMPLANT SHAPE

The maintenance of gel distribution within the shell helps to preserve the form stability.[42] The more cohesive the gel, the higher the gel/shell fill ratio, and the more enhanced bonding of the gel to the shell, which leads to more improved shape maintenance. The gel/shell fill ratio varies among the manufacturers and can produce visual clinical differences that may result in rippling and upper pole collapse if not used in the proper patients. Note that all types of implants in the round portfolio of United States manufacturers vary in the gel/shell fill ratio within the different profiles (ie, low, moderate, high). MRI study showed that shell rippling is still noted in a prone position in one of the most cohesive form-stable implants.[43] Changes in shape/form in different positions are generally not clinically significant but can be a patient concern.

DISCUSSION

The ideal size and shape of the female breast is inherently subjective and relates to both personal preference and to cultural norms. However, most surgeons agree that there are certain shared characteristics that represent the aesthetic ideal of the female breast form. These characteristics include a profile with a sloping or full upper pole and a gently curved lower pole with the nipple-areola complex at the point of maximal projection. The breast structure may be thought of as the breast parenchyma resting on the anterior chest wall surrounded by a soft tissue envelope made up of skin and subcutaneous adipose. The resulting form of the breast after augmentation mammaplasty is determined by the dynamic interaction of the breast implant, the parenchyma, and the soft tissue envelope.[44]

Silicone implants have undergone an evolution with the availability of both fourth-generation and fifth-generation devices from the 3 leading manufacturers in the United States. Concerns regarding autoimmune reaction against silicone implants remain among a small group of the population, despite the numerous studies showing the safety of the new implants.[22,23,25,27,28,41] Several clinical studies have shown no difference in the incidence of autoimmune diseases in patients receiving silicone gel implants after mastectomy compared with patients who had reconstruction with autogenous tissue.[45–51] Even meta-analysis research combining data from more than 87,000 women has revealed no association between silicone breast implants and connective tissue diseases.[52,53] Notably, virtually all industrialized nations in the world except the United States use silicone gel implants almost exclusively for breast augmentation.

There are important clinical differences in the use of the form-stable silicone implants compared with round devices. Careful dimensionally based patient analysis is crucial and implant selection should not exceed tissue characteristics and breast dimensions.[27]

SUMMARY

Implant characteristics on the bench differ from implant performance within the body. Shape, feel, safety, and longevity of the implants remain important areas of research. The data provided by all 3 manufacturers show the safety and efficacy of these medical devices. Clinicians should strive to provide ongoing data and sound science to continue to improve clinical outcomes in the future.

Editorial Comments by Bradley P. Bengtson, MD

The evolution of breast implants continues to add to the available options for patients and plastic surgeons, and has the potential to change outcomes. It is however a bit of a double-edged sword and adds to the challenges of the process as well by making proper implant and patient selection much more critical. Shaped implants as well as the new High Fill devices certainly add to our artists' palette of options. Dr Gabriel and Maxwell have given us an excellent review of the generational development of breast implants including changes and options in the shell, surface, fillers and shapes. Although we still remain limited in breast implant options available to plastic surgeons here in the United States verses Europe, Canada and the rest of the world, it is very encouraging the FDA has approved recent shaped devices along with higher cohesivity and fill devices that allow for less inherent visible implant wrinkling and rippling from lack of fill and shell dynamics. As presented the characteristics of breast implants Continue to evolve with the ultimate goal of maximizing patient outcomes and minimizing adverse events and revisions.

REFERENCES

1. Procedural statistics. 2014. Available at: http://www.surgery.org/media/statistics. Accessed March 2015.
2. Czerny V. Plastic replacement of the breast with a lipoma. Chir Kong Verhandl 1895;2:216.
3. Longacre JJ. Correction of the hypoplastic breast with special reference to reconstruction of the "nipple type breast" with local dermo-fat pedicle flaps. Plast Reconstr Surg (1946) 1954;14(6):431–41.
4. Edgerton MT, McClary AR. Augmentation mammaplasty; psychiatric implications and surgical indications; (with special reference to use of the polyvinyl alcohol sponge ivalon). Plast Reconstr Surg Transplant Bull 1958;21(4):279–305.
5. Maxwell GP, Gabriel A. Possible future development of implants and breast augmentation. Clin Plast Surg 2009;36(1):167–72, viii.
6. Clarkson P. Local mastectomy and augmentation mammaplasty for bilateral paraffinoma of breasts. Nurs Mirror Midwives J 1965;121(152):13–6.
7. Regnault P, Baker TJ, Gleason MC, et al. Clinical trial and evaluation of a proposed new inflatable mammary prosthesis. Plast Reconstr Surg 1972;50(3):220–6.
8. Maxwell GP, Gabriel A. The evolution of breast implants. Clin Plast Surg 2009;36(1):1–13, v.
9. Cronin TD, Brauer RO. Augmentation mammaplasty. Surg Clin North Am 1971;51(2):441–52.
10. Tanne JH. FDA approves silicone breast implants 14 years after their withdrawal. BMJ 2006;333(7579):1139.
11. Cronin TD, Greenberg RL. Our experiences with the Silastic gel breast prosthesis. Plast Reconstr Surg 1970;46(1):1–7.
12. Thomsen JL, Christensen L, Nielsen M, et al. Histologic changes and silicone concentrations in human breast tissue surrounding silicone breast prostheses. Plast Reconstr Surg 1990;85(1):38–41.
13. Cohen IK. Impact of the FDA ban on silicone breast implants. J Surg Oncol 1994;56(1):1.
14. Lundberg GD. The breast implant controversy. A clash of ethics and law. JAMA 1993;270(21):2608.
15. Kessler DA, Merkatz RB, Schapiro R. A call for higher standards for breast implants. JAMA 1993;270(21):2607–8.
16. Handel N, Wellisch D, Silverstein MJ, et al. Knowledge, concern, and satisfaction among augmentation mammaplasty patients. Ann Plast Surg 1993;30(1):13–20 [discussion: 20–2].
17. Stombler RE. Breast implants and the FDA: past, present, and future. Plast Surg Nurs 1993;13(4):185–7, 200.
18. Fisher JC. The silicone controversy–when will science prevail? N Engl J Med 1992;326(25):1696–8.
19. Guidoin R, Rolland C, Fleury D, et al. Physical characterization of unimplanted gel filled breast implants. Should old standards be revisited? ASAIO J 1994;40(4):943–58.
20. Sitbon E. Manufacturing of mammary implants: a manufacturing of high technology. Ann Chir Plast Esthet 2005;50(5):394–407 [in French].
21. Spear SL, Parikh PM, Goldstein JA. History of breast implants and the Food and Drug Administration. Clin Plast Surg 2009;36(1):15–21, v.
22. Cunningham B. The Mentor study on contour profile gel silicone MemoryGel breast implants. Plast Reconstr Surg 2007;120(7 Suppl 1):33S–9S.
23. Cunningham B. The mentor core study on silicone MemoryGel breast implants. Plast Reconstr Surg 2007;120(7 Suppl 1):19S–29S [discussion: 30S–2S].
24. Cunningham B, McCue J. Safety and effectiveness of Mentor's MemoryGel implants at 6 years. Aesthetic Plast Surg 2009;33(3):440–4.
25. Spear SL, Heden P. Allergan's silicone gel breast implants. Expert Rev Med Devices 2007;4(5):699–708.
26. Bengtson BP, Van Natta BW, Murphy DK, et al. Style 410 highly cohesive silicone breast implant core study results at 3 years. Plast Reconstr Surg 2007;120(7 Suppl 1):40S–8S.
27. Maxwell GP, Van Natta BW, Murphy DK, et al. Natrelle style 410 form-stable silicone breast implants: core study results at 6 years. Aesthet Surg J 2012;32(6):709–17.

28. Stevens WG, Harrington J, Alizadeh K, et al. Five-year follow-up data from the U.S. clinical trial for Sientra's U.S. Food and Drug Administration-approved Silimed® brand round and shaped implants with high-strength silicone gel. Plast Reconstr Surg 2012;130(5):973–81.
29. Brohim RM, Harrington J, Alizadeh K, et al. Early tissue reaction to textured breast implant surfaces. Ann Plast Surg 1992;28(4):354–62.
30. Abramo AC, De Oliveira VR, Ledo-Silva MC, et al. How texture-inducing contraction vectors affect the fibrous capsule shrinkage around breasts implants? Aesthetic Plast Surg 2010;34(5):555–60.
31. Handel N, Jensen JA, Black Q, et al. The fate of breast implants: a critical analysis of complications and outcomes. Plast Reconstr Surg 1995;96(7): 1521–33.
32. Daka JN, Chawla AS. Release of chemicals from polyurethane foam in the Meme breast implant. Biomater Artif Cells Immobilization Biotechnol 1993; 21(1):23–46.
33. Danino AM, Basmacioglu P, Saito S, et al. Comparison of the capsular response to the Biocell RTV and Mentor 1600 Siltex breast implant surface texturing: a scanning electron microscopic study. Plast Reconstr Surg 2001;108(7):2047–52.
34. Barr S, Hill E, Bayat A. Current implant surface technology: an examination of their nanostructure and their influence on fibroblast alignment and biocompatibility. Eplasty 2009;9:e22.
35. Stevens WG, Nahabedian MY, Calobrace MB, et al. Risk factor analysis for capsular contracture: a 5-year Sientra study analysis using round, smooth, and textured implants for breast augmentation. Plast Reconstr Surg 2013;132(5):1115–23.
36. Hammond DC, Perry LC, Maxwell GP, et al. Morphologic analysis of tissue-expander shape using a biomechanical model. Plast Reconstr Surg 1993; 92(2):255–9.
37. Brody GS. Silicone technology for the plastic surgeon. Clin Plast Surg 1988;15(4):517–20.
38. Asplund O. Capsular contracture in silicone gel and saline-filled breast implants after reconstruction. Plast Reconstr Surg 1984;73(2):270–5.
39. Burkhardt BR, Dempsey PD, Schnur PL, et al. Capsular contracture: a prospective study of the effect of local antibacterial agents. Plast Reconstr Surg 1986;77(6):919–32.
40. Gylbert L, Asplund O, Jurell G. Capsular contracture after breast reconstruction with silicone-gel and saline-filled implants: a 6-year follow-up. Plast Reconstr Surg 1990;85(3):373–7.
41. Spear SL, Murphy DK, Slicton A, et al. Inamed silicone breast implant core study results at 6 years. Plast Reconstr Surg 2007;120(7 Suppl 1):8S–16S [discussion: 17S–8S].
42. Brown MH, Shenker R, Silver SA. Cohesive silicone gel breast implants in aesthetic and reconstructive breast surgery. Plast Reconstr Surg 2005;116(3): 768–79 [discussion: 780–1].
43. Weum S, de Weerd L, Kristiansen B. Form stability of the Style 410 anatomically shaped cohesive silicone gel-filled breast implant in subglandular breast augmentation evaluated with magnetic resonance imaging. Plast Reconstr Surg 2011;127(1):409–13.
44. Tebbetts JB. Dual plane breast augmentation: optimizing implant-soft-tissue relationships in a wide range of breast types. Plast Reconstr Surg 2001; 107(5):1255–72.
45. Schusterman MA, Kroll SS, Reece GP, et al. Incidence of autoimmune disease in patients after breast reconstruction with silicone gel implants versus autogenous tissue: a preliminary report. Ann Plast Surg 1993;31(1):1–6.
46. Park AJ, Black RJ, Sarhadi NS, et al. Silicone gel-filled breast implants and connective tissue diseases. Plast Reconstr Surg 1998;101(2):261–8.
47. Edworthy SM, Martin L, Barr SG, et al. A clinical study of the relationship between silicone breast implants and connective tissue disease. J Rheumatol 1998;25(2):254–60.
48. Gabriel SE, O'Fallon WM, Kurland LT, et al. Risk of connective-tissue diseases and other disorders after breast implantation. N Engl J Med 1994;330(24): 1697–702.
49. Kaiser J. Panel discounts implant disease risk. Science 1999;284(5423):2065–6.
50. Nelson N. Institute of Medicine finds no link between breast implants and disease. J Natl Cancer Inst 1999;91(14):1191.
51. Nyren O, Yin L, Josefsson S, et al. Risk of connective tissue disease and related disorders among women with breast implants: a nation-wide retrospective cohort study in Sweden. BMJ 1998; 316(7129):417–22.
52. Sanchez-Guerrero J, Colditz GA, Karlson EW, et al. Silicone breast implants and the risk of connective-tissue diseases and symptoms. N Engl J Med 1995;332(25):1666–70.
53. Karlson EW, Hankinson SE, Liang MH, et al. Association of silicone breast implants with immunologic abnormalities: a prospective study. Am J Med 1999;106(1):11–9.

The Standardization of Bra Cup Measurements

Redefining Bra Sizing Language

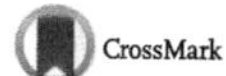

Bradley P. Bengtson, MD[a,b,*], Caroline A. Glicksman, MD[c,d]

KEYWORDS

- Breast augmentation • Bra cup sizing • Breast hemicircumference • Highly cohesive gel implant
- 3-D imaging • Sister sizes • Breast measurements • Tissue-based planning
- Biodimensional planning

KEY POINTS

- Patients and plastic surgeons communicate with “bra-cup sizing language.”
- There is no standard bra cup or sizing system, so no one is speaking the same language.
- Studying ~6000 patients, bra cup sizing may be standardized with one hemicircumference measurement only.
- We can all speak the same language and have a comparison among bra manufacturers.
- This bra cup sizing system will help set patient expectations preoperatively and postoperatively.

OVERVIEW

During the process of breast augmentation after discussing the safety of implants and cost, the discussion comes down to outcome and expectations. Every patient and her plastic surgeon may know there is no uniform bra cup sizing standard but we continue to speak using “bra cup” language. The standardization of bra cup sizing, although seemingly a simple and straightforward goal, has been elusive since the bra was designed and brought into a more modern style and design in the late 1800s.[1] There are many challenges in developing a standardized bra cup system. The first and most significant is that bra cup sizes are a continuum. Bra cups are categorized as if there is a specific or ideal bra cup size, when in reality women’s breasts occur as a fluid range of shapes, sizes, and volumes. A huge conundrum, however, is created because patients and plastic surgeons use and emphasize “bra cup size” language without any specific reference point.

In addition, within the process of breast augmentation, patient education, tissue-based planning, and implant selection are the most critical aspects of the process and outcome.[2] In any initial breast consultation the most frequently asked questions include: “Okay, so what size will I be after surgery?” or “What size will this implant make me?” Occasionally even more uneducated misconceptions arise: “My friend had 350’s and I want her cup size and to look like her.” Most patients have specific expectations regarding bra cup size, and failure to achieve real or unrealistic expectations remains the leading cause of patient dissatisfaction. In addition, implant size change remains one of the primary causes for breast revision in most studies, often exceeding actual surgical complications. Optimizing soft tissue coverage, while still achieving a patient’s postoperative goal, is perhaps the most significant factor in breast implant surgery if one is to produce stable

[a] Bengtson Center for Aesthetics and Plastic Surgery, 555 MidTowne Street, NE Suite 110, Grand Rapids, MI 49503, USA; [b] Department of Surgery, Michigan State University, 220 Trowbridge Road, East Lansing, MI 48824, USA; [c] Glicksman Plastic Surgery, 2164 State Highway 35, Building A, Sea Girt, NJ 08750, USA; [d] Department of Surgery, Jersey Shore University Medical Center, 1945 NJ-33, Neptune, NJ 07753, USA
* Corresponding author. Bengtson Center for Aesthetics and Plastic Surgery, 555 MidTowne Street, NE Suite 110, Grand Rapids, MI 49503.
E-mail address: drb@bengtsoncenter.com

Clin Plastic Surg 42 (2015) 405–411
http://dx.doi.org/10.1016/j.cps.2015.06.002
0094-1298/15/$ – see front matter

long-term results.[3] Hence the challenge: implant selection, which determines the eventual bra cup size, is critical in patient education and the management of patient expectations[4]; however, this is never truly achievable until all are speaking the same bra cup language. Patient and surgeon perceptions may never be exact, although there should be some overlap of a patient's goals and what range is best to maintain soft tissue support. This in no way, however, should minimize the importance or even dissuade from establishing some guidelines and standards that are useful in bridging this gap.

METHODS

The prospective data from more than 5993 patients enrolled and measured in the Allergan Medical silicone breast implant study (Allergan Style 410 Silicone Cohesive Breast Implant Study) undergoing primary breast augmentation were analyzed and also compared with a single-surgeon primary augmentation cohort of 450 patients. Data collected in this study included the breast hemicircumference (HC). This HC is measured as the medial breast inflection point, the most medial point of the breast, across the nipple areola level to the lateral breast inflection point. This HC is measured over the maximum apex of the breast. Data at 6 months and 1 year were recorded, with the reported measurements at 1 year used for this study. There were approximately 50 investigator surgeons in the overall study contributing these measurements. Measurements would be expected to vary a few millimeters from surgeon to surgeon, but should be consistent with their own measurements. In total, breast HC was recorded in 5993 patients and 11,986 breasts having primary breast augmentation. The breast HC data obtained preoperatively were then compared with the postoperative data collected at the 1-year follow-up visit. These data were collected from the national cohort and from the largest primary augmentation, single-surgeon cohort in the United States. Reported bra cup size from patients enrolled in the study was also detailed by size and bra manufacturer, preoperatively and postoperatively at 1 year. In addition, data were collected with regard to specific patient implant volume used in augmentation.

For the purpose of this study, most measurements were performed manually. However, more recently with the advent of three-dimensional (3-D) imaging systems, some measurements were performed and recorded by computer analysis with registered landmarks. Furthermore, we have confirmed and validated our 3-D data comparing the manual HC measurements with the Vectra 3-D computer-generated data (Canfield Scientific, Fairfield, NJ, USA). Manual HC measurements correlate to 0 to 1 mm from Vectra 3-D imaging HC measurements. Data among specific bra manufacturers were then compared to determine if there were any significant differences in bra cup sizing among manufacturers.

RESULTS

The patient's reported bra cup size and manufacturer were compared with the breast HC measured at 1 year in a large prospective study of primary breast augmentation patients. In addition, the data from the largest single-surgeon primary augmentation cohort in the United States were also evaluated separately in 450 patients to determine if there was any variability from a single surgeon verses multi-surgeon measurement methods. The data from both groups are shown (**Table 1**). For the national cohort, an average HC of 20.0 cm correlated to a reported bra cup size of a "B cup," 21.5 cm HC on average was a "C cup," 23.4 cm HC correlated to a "D cup," and 25.0 cm correlated to a "DD cup." In the single-surgeon cohort the data were similar with patients reporting "B cup" having a 19.3 cm HC, "C cup" 21.3 cm, "D cup" 23.5, and "DD cup" 25.3. The greatest degree of variability between the overall and single-surgeon cohorts was in the "B Cup" group, which varied by 7 mm. There was a 0- to 3-mm variance for the other cup sizes. There were a very limited number of "A Cup" patients within the large cohort, the average being 17.8 and the single-surgeon cohort 16.5 cm. The average postoperative bra cup measurements

Table 1
Postoperative hemicircumference measured across the maximum projection of the breast from the medial inflection point to the lateral inflection point where the breast creates a crease in the skin when the breast is displaced or pushed medially or laterally

	Post Hemicircumference	
Post Cup Size	Overall Data (cm)	Bengtson Cohort (cm)
B	20.0	19.3
C	21.5	21.3
D	23.4	23.5
DD	25.0	25.3

Overall data are collected, in addition to separate data from one surgeon site of the largest single-surgeon cohort.

between the single cohort and group cohort rounded to the nearest 0.5 cm are "B cup" 19.5 cm, "C cup" 21.5 cm, "D cup" 23.5 cm, and "DD cup" 25.0 cm (**Fig. 1**).

Within the main cohort, data from individual bra manufacturers were analyzed. The leading bra manufacturers reported by the patients in this study included Bali, Warners, Calvin Klein, Maidenform, and Victoria's Secret (**Table 2**). Victoria's Secret comprised the most, with 5328 of 6231 or 86% of the total of bras worn, thus the average HC is skewed toward the Victoria's Secret brand. However, some important information may be gleaned. Of the 187 patients wearing Bali, it took more volume and a greater HC to fill a reported cup on average: 4 mm more for size B, 3 mm size C, and 15 mm for size D. Calvin Klein, however, demonstrated a significantly smaller HC for each cup size. Of the 241 patients, the average cup size was 15 mm smaller for size A, 9 mm smaller for size B, 15 mm smaller for size C, and 18 mm smaller for D. The 424 patients who wore a Maidenform bra revealed a difference of 7 mm larger for size B but all other sizes essentially the same average. Warner bras required more breast to fill their bra cup: 6 mm for a "B," 5 mm for a "C," and 6 mm for "D" cup patients. Again, because Victoria's Secret was the dominant bra reported in close to 6000 patients, their sizes are essentially the same as the average recorded 1 to 2 mm different than the mean. Many patients rely on the information given to them at a retail store, so we further corroborated our findings by enlisting the services of an expert sizer from Victoria's Secret to confirm our measurements of a primary augmentation patient at a "C Cup," which we measured with a 21.5-cm HC in the middle of our C range. It is also very important to note that these measurement data and bra cup manufacturer data were collected during the years 2001 to 2008. Measurement systems, particularly Victoria's Secret, have changed as they have moved to more of a lingerie line, and in 2015 the system used for measurement will undersize patients one to two bra cup sizes, whereas other manufacturers have remained relatively in line with their measurements. Finally, the average volume in milliliters to bring a patient up one cup size from a B to a C or C to a D using our measurement techniques with shaped highly cohesive gel implants, and based on our data, was 205 mL.

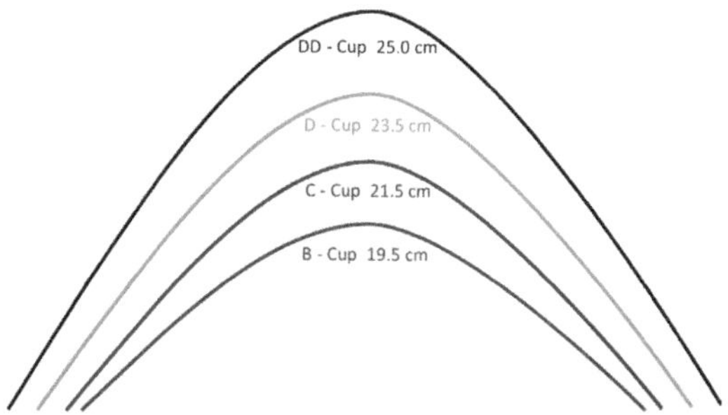

Fig. 1. Standardization of the bra cup can be based on one measurement, the breast hemicircumference. It is based on measuring the medial to lateral breast inflection points, which represent the take-offs points where the breast attaches to the chest wall. The average bra cup size measurement between the largest single-surgeon cohort and total group cohort is shown here.

DISCUSSION

Life is all about expectations. Patient and plastic surgeon understand there is no standard bra cup size; however, preoperative and postoperative bra cup size remains the primary terminology and language used to determine expected breast size postoperatively. Most breast patients have specific expectations with regards to bra cup size, and achieving real or unrealistic expectations with regard to cup size postoperatively is a leading cause of patient dissatisfaction and occasionally litigation. In addition breast implant size change remains a primary driver for breast revision.[5] Every plastic surgeon has heard: "I would just like to be a full "C," or "My plastic surgeon said I was going to be a "C" cup, and I'm only a "B." Bra sizes clearly vary among manufacturers and additional factors, such as demi and full cup coverage, specific fabrics, padding, and elastics, can all affect the fit of a bra. In addition, most bra cups are measured with a bra on, which can also affect the measurements.

There are multiple ways to try and skirt this cup size challenge, but all fall short and are mainly unhelpful. Surgeons have tried placing implants in bras, but breasts appear smaller when the implant is placed inside the body, so placing implants inside a bra or on the chest under a tight spandex shirt does not give a truly accurate visual of the postoperative result. The patient's individual breast tissue and shape also contribute significantly to their individual outcome. Patient education often relies on the use of before and after images, but searching for prior augmentation patients with a similar breast shape and preoperative volume is time consuming, often frustrating, and again does not answer the question of an actual postoperative bra cup size range. A patient's preoperative shape, soft tissue coverage, skin envelope, and existing volume remain a determinant of the outcome. The advent of 3-D imaging and

Table 2
Breast hemicircumference measurements from the medial and lateral breast inflection points across the maximum projection of the breast for the most commonly reported bra manufacturers in our study

	Post Hemicircumference				
Post Cup Size	Victoria's Secret (cm)	Calvin Klein (cm)	Maidenform (cm)	Bali (cm)	Warners (cm)
B	20.0	19.1	20.7	20.4	20.6
C	21.5	20.0	21.4	21.8	22.1
D	23.4	21.7	23.4	24.5	24.0
DD	25.0	23.0	25.0	26.0	25.5

As an example, Calvin Klein bras require less breast tissue to fill a designated bra cup size.

simulation continues to transform practices in many ways. In 2008, 3-D imaging was initiated and used for the HC measurements as a new method to confirm manual measurements recorded by the plastic surgeon (**Fig. 2**). Simulations can vastly improve the patient's preoperative educational experience, allowing patients to visualize and understand their breasts in ways previously unmatched.[6] Validated measurements are easily integrated visually into the new bra cup measurement system (**Fig. 1**). In addition, we continue to use our bra cup sizing system, which has been confirmed in more than 2000 additional breast patients measured. It is a significant benefit for the surgeon and particularly the patient to visualize their range of outcomes before surgery. An even greater benefit will be to claim the bra cup size range for what the patient is viewing.

Because this system is based on the HC alone, bra bandwidth must also be measured to obtain a properly fitted bra. Many women seek out the expertise of bra shop fitters, who in turn each have their own techniques for sizing and fitting their customers for their specific brands. For many patients, confusion exists when patients either underestimate or overestimate their thoracic circumference or band size. Also, few understand the concept of sister sizes, for example a patient wearing a 34C may also fit into a 36B bra. In the United States, the US Standard Clothing Size sets modest guidelines, but no formal standard inch-based brassiere sizing system currently exists.[7] Complicating the sizing process even further, a woman's breast size may vary on a monthly basis because of her menstrual cycle and weight gain and loss. Thus, establishment of an accurate band size is important, as is recognition that cup sizes are a range and ever changing.

From the purely medical standpoint, there are few published reports that describe a method for

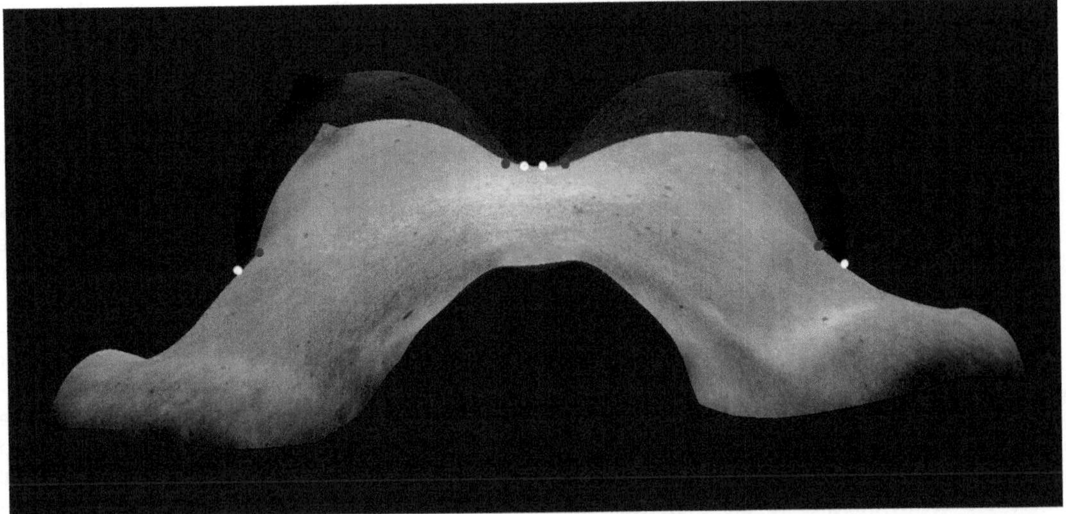

Fig. 2. The breast hemicircumference is shown here measured from the medial and lateral breast inflection points where the breast attaches to the chest. Shown here is a Canfield Vectra simulation of a breast augmentation identifying the measurement markings.

accurately predicting postoperative bra cup size after primary breast augmentation. The first published effort to develop standardized breast measurements in aesthetic breast surgery is credited to Maliniac in 1937.[8] He has also been credited for describing the vast differences that exist in women's breast size and shape. Smith and colleagues[9] published a connection between bra cup size and anthropomorphic measurements of the breast in 1986. They provided average values of 55 consecutive female volunteers without aesthetic evaluation. In 1998, Pechter[10] published an excellent review citing the origins of the modern bralike devices and was the first to develop a system that used the circumference of the breast as a predictor of bra cup size. In the direct breast measurement system Pechter proposed, he derived the following scale: A = 7 inches, B = 8 inches, C = 9 inches, D = 10 inches, with each 1-inch increment determining bra cup size up or down. His direct measurement system measured the HC of "small breasted" women while standing, and "full breasted" women while lying down. He determined that his new method corresponded to the stated cup size in 84% of the women evaluated. In a retrospective telephone survey Young and colleagues[11] followed 112 women who underwent a breast augmentation between 1980 and 1992. Based on the patient's recollection of preoperative and postoperative bra size, they concluded that the average breast augmentation caused a two-cup bra cup size increase. The authors also reported complication rates of 21%, including high capsular contracture rates, and concluded that capsular contracture distorts the breast into a more spherical shape and altered the volume to surface area relationship.

In a follow-up article to his previous work on breast augmentation and bra cup sizing, Pechter[12] studied the relationship between breast widths and underbust circumference and their correlation to bra cup size in 1000 women over 5 years. These combined measurements were then used to select an implant that would achieve the patient's desired postoperative bra cup size.[12] Pechter's article did not describe a specific volume required to increase or decrease a breast by one cup size. He defines the correlation between the breast width and underbust circumference to bra size. His system correlates every increase in 1 inch of breast width equals an increase in one cup size. He also never correlated these measurements to specific manufacturers. In addition, Pechter's measurements slightly overestimate our reported cup sizes by about 1 to 1.5 cm or about one-half of one bra cup; however, he has done the most recent formal study advancing this topic forward.

In their 1997 study, Qiao and coworkers[13] used the difference between the circumference at the level of the axilla and across the nipples to determine breast volume. These measurements in particular are most often used by bra manufacturers when determining the correct bra size for women. Since Maliniac's classic book was published in 1950,[14] there have been relatively few published studies that have gone on to further develop a standardized system to measure women's breasts.[15–17] The incorporation of tissue-based planning and anthropomorphic measurements into the preoperative evaluation of breast augmentation patients has been shown to improve patient understanding and accountability, and improve surgical outcomes.[4] They have not, however, helped significantly in fully setting patient expectations with respect to bra cup sizing.

In reviewing specific implant volumes required to achieve specific bra cup size changes, for instance from a reported A > C or B > C, our data show that approximately 205 mL increases a bra cup size by one cup with shaped breast implants. Prior literature has suggested that 100 mL would increase cup size by one cup, and thus, 225 mL would increase breast size by two cup sizes, with a range in the literature from 100 to 275 mL.[18,19]

Valid concerns have been raised concerning the data from this study, such as the implants studied were all shaped cohesive devices with most in the submuscular orretropectoral position. Although it is true shaped devices may revolumize the breast slightly differently than round or elliptical devices and affect the overall fill of the upper pole of the breast, the measurements of the breast HC are performed across the maximum projection of the breast, with the breast supported if any laxity or stretch is present. The device augments and elevates the breast volume on top of the implant and the final overall volume includes both implant and breast. The final HC should be very close regardless of the device shape, certainly not enough to vary a cup size significantly. However, it is important to confirm these data with round devices in the future. Again retrospectively the HC measurement correlates to reported bra cup sizes well regardless of implant shape.

There have been no studies to date that correlate standardized breast measurements with reported bra sizes specific to a manufacturer, preoperatively and postoperatively in primary breast augmentation from a large prospective clinical trial, or those that specifically correlate size change to a specific augmented volume. Our results parallel and confirm Pechter's work in a larger scale in correlating a breast HC measurement only used in determining a patient's bra cup size. By implementing our data showing an HC of 19.3 cm correlates to a reported bra cup size of a "B Cup," 21.5 cm HC on average was a "C Cup," 23.4 cm HC correlated to a "D Cup," and 25.0 cm a "DD Cup." This is the next step toward the standardization of bra cup sizing based on one measurement only (HC). We have also used this bra cup measurement data to retrospectively ask patients following surgery what is the most common bra cup they wear. With the exclusion now of Victoria's Secret, which currently tends to oversize cup sizes by one to two bra cup sizes, more than 80% of the last 2000 breast augmentations fall within half of a bra cup size based on our reported single HC measurement. The single-surgeon cohort data along with Pechter's bra cup measurement data are further supportive.

SUMMARY

Plastic surgeons and their patients continue to primarily use bra cup language in discussing augmentation, revision, and reconstruction outcomes; however, without a standardized system, no one is speaking the same language. Using the data collected in this large study, bra cup sizes may now be standardized along with a starting point for comparing all bra manufacturers with this standard with a simple conversion applied. This is a major advancement in that patients and plastic surgeons may now be speaking the same language. From a patient standpoint, this new method will help streamline bra cup sizing postoperatively, pointing them in the right bra cup direction depending on manufacturer, providing a more accurate and at least a common starting point for the patient and the surgeon.

By applying actual cup size language to specific visual outcomes, we hope to improve patient education and the management of expectations. The incorporation of visual tools including 3-D imaging provides patients the opportunity to visualize their range of outcomes and assign a specific cup size measurement; adding a specific bra manufacturer matched to their result will help further to meet expectations and improve surgeon-patient communication (**Fig. 1**). Sister size confusion may be eliminated because the HC measurement is independent of the band width that requires a separate independent measurement. To further improve the informed consent process, patients can sign off on their range of expected outcomes. This new standard should decrease the incidence of revisions for size change, which currently represents one of the leading reasons for revision. The future should be interesting and show new advancements in 3-D imaging and simulation. Will the addition of 3-D printing allow patients to visually evaluate their simulated size, or will we be able to holographically project the simulation onto the patient's body? Bra cups are indeed a conundrum and a continuum; however, our new objective bra cup sizing system based on one quick measurement is the beginning of a new era in developing an innovative bra cup sizing system and language that will yield significant benefits to the patient and the plastic surgeon.

Editorial Comments by Bradley P. Bengtson, MD

The universal language of breast size uses "bra-cup" language. We speak to our patients and other plastic surgeons using "bra cup language," when in fact without a standard, no one actually knows what the other person is talking about. Studying over 6000 patients and now also confirming a patient's bra cup measurement postoperatively in over an additional 3000 patients, this system is fast, easy and reproducible. It is independent of the band width which is measured separately. This system helps to set patient expectations, helps to limit unmet or unrealistic expectations, decreases potential litigation and assists getting plastic surgeons and their patients on the same page both preoperatively and postoperatively. A good simple starting point is a "C-cup" measured at 21.5 cm, increasing or decreasing 2–2.5 cm per cup. This technology may also be applied to 3-D imaging and simulation as well.

ACKNOWLEDGMENTS

The authors thank the 50 clinical investors who contributed to the collection of the data in the Allergan 410 Silicone Filled Breast Implant Study.

REFERENCES

1. Available at: http://en.wikipedia.org/wiki/Brassiere. Accessed April 1, 2015.
2. Adams WP. The process of breast augmentation: four sequential steps for optimizing outcomes for patients. Plast Reconstr Surg 2008;122:1892–900.
3. Tebbetts JB. Augmentation mammaplasty; tissue assessment and planning. In: Spear S, editor. Surgery of the breast, principles and art. 2nd edition. Philadelphia: Lippincott Williams & Wilkins; 2005. p. 1261.
4. Tebbetts JB. An approach that integrates patient education and informed consent in breast augmentation. Plast Reconstr Surg 2002;110(3):971–8.

5. Maxwell GP, Van Natta BW, Murphy DK, et al. Natrelle style 410 form-stable silicone breast implants: core study results at 6 years. Aesthet Surg J 2012; 32(6):709–17.
6. Glicksman C. Patient education in breast augmentation. In: Spear SL, editor. Surgery of the breast. 3rd edition. Baltimore (MD): Lippincott Williams & Wilkins; 2011. p. 1261.
7. US standard clothing sizes-definition for the clothing industry. Available at: http://www.apparelsearch.com/Definitions/Miscellaneous/US_standard_clothing_sizes.htm. Accessed April 1, 2015.
8. Maliniac JW. Sculpture in the living. New York: Lancet Press; 1934. p. 112.
9. Smith DJ, Palin WE, Katch VL, et al. Breast volume and anthropomorphic measurements: normal values. Plast Reconstr Surg 1986;78:331.
10. Pechter EA. A new method for determining bra size and predicting post- augmentation breast size. Plast Reconstr Surg 1998;102(4):1259–65.
11. Young L, Nemecek JR, Nemecek DA. The efficacy of breast augmentation: breast size increase, patient satisfaction, and psychological effects. Plast Reconstr Surg 1994;94:958.
12. Pechter E. Determining bra size for breast augmentation an improved technique for determining bra size with applicability to breast surgery. Plast Reconstr Surg 2008;121(5):348e–50e.
13. Qiao Q, Zhou G, Ling Y. Breast volume measurement in young Chinese women and clinical applications. Aesthetic Plast Surg 1997;21(5):362–8.
14. Maliniac JW. Breast deformities and their repair. 1st edition. New York: Grune & Stratton; 1950.
15. Penn J. Breast reduction. Br J Plast Surg 1955;7: 357.
16. Westreich M. Anthropomorphic breast measurement: protocol and results in 50 women with aesthetically perfect breasts and clinical application. Plast Reconstr Surg 1997;100(2):468–79.
17. Brown TP, Ringrose C, Hyland RE, et al. A method of assessing female breast morphometry and its clinical application. Br J Plast Surg 1999;52(5):355–9.
18. Karabulut AB, Ozden BC, Arcini AA. A nomogram for predicting the degree of breast augmentation according to implant size. Aesthetic Plast Surg 2008; 32:298–300.
19. Regnault P, Baker TJ, Gleason MC, et al. Clinical trial and evaluation of a proposed new inflatable mammary prosthesis. Plast Reconstr Surg 1972;50:220.

The Process of Breast Augmentation with Special Focus on Patient Education, Patient Selection and Implant Selection

William P. Adams Jr, MD[a,*], Kevin H. Small, MD[b,c]

KEYWORDS

- Breast augmentation • Patient education • Tissue-based planning • Patient selection
- Implant selection

KEY POINTS

- Breast augmentation is not simply a surgical procedure but a process of 4 steps: (1) comprehensive patient education and informed consent, (2) tissue-based preoperative planning, (3) refined surgical technique with rapid recovery, and (4) detailed postoperative education.
- The nonsurgical steps, patient education and tissue-based planning, are essential to optimizing postoperative outcomes and reducing reoperation rates.
- The surgeon and the patient must assume a mutual responsibility that the implant has been selected based on breast dimensions and soft tissue limitations.
- Dedicated education, comprehensive patient/surgeon consultation, analytical documentation, and 3-dimensional imaging should be coupled with tissue-based planning to optimize results.

INTRODUCTION

The critical analysis of breast augmentation and its associated complications has driven our surgical practice to redefine our approach. We have scrutinized factors that influence patient outcomes and have acknowledged key characteristics that shape the successes of this common surgical procedure. This assessment has redirected breast augmentation from a surgical procedure into a surgical process.[1] Four key components have been outlined in this surgical approach:

1. Comprehensive patient education and informed consent
2. Tissue-based preoperative planning
3. Refined surgical technique with rapid recovery
4. Detailed postoperative education

These 4 steps to breast augmentation have been integrated into our surgical practice and have improved the patient experience, the reoperation rate, the postoperative outcome, and overall patient/surgeon satisfaction.[1] Even though these 4 steps can exist independently, the integration of all 4 steps in a patient's surgical experience work synergistically to optimize esthetic outcomes. Our refined process was developed in part from published concepts[2] and other plastic surgical practices have adopted this same protocol with

[a] Department of Plastic Surgery, The University of Texas Southwestern Medical Center, 6901 Snider Plaza, Suite 120, University Park, TX 75205, USA; [b] Plastic Surgery, Weill Cornell Medical College, New York, NY, USA; [c] Plastic Surgery, New York Presbyterian Hospital, 156 William Street, 12th Floor, New York, NY 10038, USA
* Corresponding author.
E-mail address: wpajrmd@dr-adams.com

Clin Plastic Surg 42 (2015) 413–426
http://dx.doi.org/10.1016/j.cps.2015.06.001
0094-1298/15/$ – see front matter

plasticsurgery.theclinics.com

equally positive conclusions; thus, this breast augmentation 4-step process is both transferable and reproducible. This article focuses on the first 2 steps of this comprehensive 4-step process of breast augmentation.

PATIENT EDUCATION AND INFORMED CONSENT

Team Approach to Education

The first step in the process of breast augmentation is the educational component; this step is the most critical aspect of the process and is frequently neglected by plastic surgeons. This approach solidifies a surgeon/patient partnership before surgical intervention, because this process requires not only the surgeon but also the entire staff of the clinical practice to be an integral participant in the subprocess of patient education. Thus, the surgical team has a responsibility to introduce the patient to the philosophy of the surgical practice. Instructional material and promotional multimedia may serve as an adjunct to the standards of the practice and influence patient education.

The patient and practice must create a partnership for implant selection and postoperative care. Together, they develop a mutual understanding that the implant will not only be selected based on patient preference, but also must incorporate breast dimensions and tissue characteristics. The patient must understand the limitations of her breast envelope and the implications of implant selection based on breast topography. Together, they will review patient images and physical attributes to delineate breast asymmetry and anatomic boundaries that impact implant selection. Furthermore, the practice patient educator and surgeon have a responsibility to discuss various implant options (eg, silicone vs saline, anatomic vs round, textured vs smooth) and how the selected implant is influenced by patient characteristics. This partnership in implant selection and postoperative care has been proven to enhance patient satisfaction and overall esthetic outcomes.[1] Recently, in our practice, 3-dimensional imaging has significantly revolutionized this partnership by allowing patients to visualize how an implant "fits their breasts," as well as potential differences between shaped and round implants.

The informed consent process is integrated into the educational process[3]; the risks should be discussed including, but not limited to, bleeding, infection, capsular contracture, implant malposition, rippling, and need for reoperation. A preoperative understanding of the complication profile will empower the patient to assume responsibility for the final decision. A new development that deserves attention during the patient consultation is the association of anaplastic large cell lymphoma (ALCL) and breast augmentation. Current evidence suggests the risk of developing ALCL is 0.1% to 0.3% per 100,000; in relative terms, a patient is approximately 2 times more likely to be struck by an asteroid than to develop ALCL.[4] Patients typically present with a delayed seroma after 1 year. The clinical course is indolent, and effective treatment includes removal of the implant and capsulectomy. Adjuvant therapy is rarely recommended. Fewer than 50 cases have been reported in the medical literature, but patients should be aware of this recent finding. Initial studies have suggested a correlation of ALCL with textured implants and/or certain bacteria, but more investigations need to be undertaken for any definitive conclusions.[4]

Determine Patient Knowledge/Patient Desires

The process of patient education and informed consent requires a multimodality approach. More often than not, patients have a misconstrued perception of breast augmentation based on previous experiences or multimedia influence. The surgeon and practice have a responsibility to dismantle any misconceived notions and educate patients on the relationship of breast tissue and implant selection. Our practice requires each patient to complete documents before an education consultation by our patient education specialist (**Fig. 1**). This consultation, in person or over the phone, typically lasts 45 to 60 minutes and discusses concepts, issues, and limitations related to the process of breast augmentation. This consultation is able to decontaminate any misinformation and convey the importance of tissue-based planning and implant selection. For example, the coordinator can dispel the inaccurate association of cup size and breast augmentation; most women wear inappropriate bras for their cup size and cup size is nonstandardized within the industry. At this time, the patient educator also can determine if the patient desires a "natural-look" or an "augmented-look" for her breast augmentation; this mentality will directly impact the rest of the consultation and implant selection. Again, 3-dimensional imaging can be an integral component of this discussion; patients can project various "looks" and can even overlay a bra or camisole on these simulations to optimize visualization. Thus, patients and surgeons can select the implant based on the breast envelope and implant characteristics rather than improper misconceptions.

The education coordinator initially performs the consultation with the patient, typically done in

Patient Concerns

____
____
____
____
____
____
____
____
____
____
____
____

Additional Questions for Dr. Adams

____
____
____
____
____
____
____
____
____
____
____
____

Have you had any type of Plastic Surgery before?
☐ **Are you happy with your results?**
☐ **My role in your care**
☐ **Our commitment to patient education**
☐ **What we'll talk about today**
☐ **Have you read the information we provided you?**
☐ **Clinical evaluation sheet medical history and patient preferences**
☐ **Brief history of augmentation**
☐ **Alternatives versus a single approach**
☐ **Do implants cause disease? The research and sources**
☐ **Breast implants and breast cancer**
☐ **Breast implants and mammography**
All implants interfere with mammograms
☐ **Breast implant technology**
☐ Constantly changing alternatives- current alternatives
☐ Limitations of implants- no implant is without tradeoffs
☐ **Summarizing the alternatives**
☐ Incision alternatives- inframammary, axillary, periareolar
☐ Implant pocket locations- retromammary, retropectoral, dual plane, totally submuscular
☐ Current implant choices (all saline)- Smooth round, textured round, textured shaped or anatomic-types and manufacturers
☐ Fitting the procedure and implant to your tissues to minimize long-term risks and compromises
☐ **Determining the best size**
☐ If you could just pick a size, what would it be?
☐ Which is more important, size or problems long-term?
☐ Common misconceptions
☐ How implant size affects your tissues- now and later
☐ Bra cup sizing-we can't guarantee cup size
☐ Balancing your breast with your figure
☐ Measuring your breast, understanding your tissues
☐ Concentrating on shape, fill, dimensions
☐ Photos and planning the operation
☐ **The operation- what's it like**
☐ Day surgery routine
☐ The facility and facility personnel
☐ Anesthesia
Safety of anesthesia, misconceptions, risks
Local versus general anesthesia
Our anesthesia personnel
☐ **During surgery**
☐ What will occur, expected time frame
☐ **After surgery**
☐ Waking in recovery, then to stepdown with caregiver
☐ **Detailed instructions will be given to you**
Tells you and your caregiver what to expect and do
What we do simplifies your instructions
☐ **Recovery and activity**
☐ Importance of resuming normal activity
☐ What we do and what we need you to do
☐ No bandages, bras, straps, drains or special

☐ **Risks of augmentation**
☐ This is a totally elective operation with risks and uncontrollable factors
☐ Bleeding
☐ Infection
☐ Sensation compromise
☐ Capsular contracture
☐ Unsatisfactory aesthetic results or scarring
☐ Interference with cancer detection
☐ Complications may require additional surgery, longer recovery, additional costs
☐ Reviewed risks on consent forms & documents
☐ **Capsular contracture and breast firmness**
☐ What is it?
☐ How a capsule forms
☐ Controlling the capsule
☐ How often does it occur?
☐ Correcting the hard breast
☐ **Factors that the surgeon cannot predict or control**
☐ Capsular contracture
☐ Different degrees, if severe, requires reoperation
☐ Surgeon alone makes final decisions re: reoperation
☐ All costs are patient's responsibility, no insurance
☐ Tissue stretch problems- increase with implant size
o Stretch allowing implant shift downward or outward
☐ Stretch allowing implant rotation
☐ Traction rippling
☐ Your request for a different size implant after surgery
☐ **All costs for any surgery relating to factors the surgeon cannot predict or control are the patient's responsibility (surgeon fees, facility fees, anesthesia, lab, time off work)- includes capsular contracture, stretch deformities, implant size changes.**
☐ **Importance of communicating with us**
We want to do what you want
You must be honest with us at all times
The surgeon cannot read your mind
☐ **What you can expect from Dr. Adams**
Type of care. Written materials. Photos. The operation. Your care.
☐ **Dr. Adams' Qualifications**
Surgical training, board certification, professional affiliations, scientific publications, other.
☐ **Patient has read all information material provided (Yes/No) _____Pt. Initial.**
☐ **Discussed any significant other's involvement, gave patient copy of Will There Be Anyone Else Involved.**
☐ **Written information provided patient was discussed in detail with patient, answered patient's questions to patient's satisfaction.**
☐ **All informed consent documents discussed in detail with patient, answered patient's questions.**

_______Pt. Initial _______Pt. Educator Initial

Fig. 1. Our breast augmentation patient educator consultation checklist.

person or on the phone, as a separate consult that precedes the surgeon consultation. During the surgeon consultation, the surgeon can objectively review the breast dimensions, confirm the patient's goals, and formulate a surgical plan. In the patient-surgeon interaction, asymmetries are identified and directly addressed using an image analysis sheet (**Fig. 2**). Patients must have realistic expectations on intermammary distance, cleavage, implant characteristics, and implant palpability. By dispelling any misconceived notions, the surgeon and the patient can synergistically select the appropriate implant based on individualized tissue. Additionally, with joint preoperative

Patient: «Person_First_Name» «Person_Last_Name»

Date: ____________

❒ L/R breast larger- breasts will **never match!!!**
❒ L/R nipple-areola higher on chest- will not be totally corrected
❒ L/R fold beneath breast higher on chest- will not be totally corrected
❒ Nipple position on the breast mounds is different on the two sides and cannot be totally corrected
❒ Gap between breasts can only be narrowed somewhat- a gap of at least _____cm. will likely remain
❒ Chest wall asymmetries exist that cannot be corrected and will affect breast shape
❒ The position of the entire breast on the chest wall will not change. If one fold beneath the breast is lower than the other, it will also be lower after your augmentation.
❒ The basic shape and configuration of the breasts will be similar to their current appearance and not change drastically, but will be larger
❒ Thinner tissue inferior and lateral can result in implant palpability

❒ Other: ____

❒ Other: ____

❒ Other: ____

❒ Other: ____

Patient Please Initial below to document your understanding and acceptance of the above.

_____ Dr. Adams has reviewed my patient images with me in detail. I have seen, understand, and accept each of the factors listed above that will not change or may be only partially improved following my augmentation. I totally understand and accept that my breasts or components of my breasts will never match on the two sides, and that perfection is not an option, only improvement in the size of my breasts.

Fig. 2. Our breast augmentation patient image analysis checklist.

planning and implant selection, patients will accept their postoperative results and rarely present for size-exchange procedures. Approximately 20% of patients in our practice may question their size postoperatively, but they are reminded of the preoperative planning with the associated photographs, which usually reaffirms implant size selection and patient satisfaction.[5]

IMPLANT CHARACTERISTICS/SURGICAL APPROACH

Shaped Versus Round

Breast implants can be either round or anatomically shaped. Of note, round implants are used in 95% of primary breast augmentations in the United States.[4] Within both subsets, there are a wide variety of widths, heights, and projections. Anatomic implants may even have more variability because of their naturally asymmetric shape. Plastic surgeons should vary implant selection to optimally "best fit" a breast envelope. However, surgeons may use only one implant style because of their training or comfort. Our practice believes some situations dictate a certain implant based on patient preference or breast anatomy.[5] Superseding all of these sentiments is the concept that the best patient for an anatomic implant is the patient who "wants it." Indications for both round implants and anatomic implants are outlined as follows:

Round implants
1. Desired augmented look
2. Good soft tissue coverage/good basic breast shape
3. Revision surgery (change of implants, capsular contraction, implant rupture, rotation)
4. Recurrent implant rotation/concerned about rotation

Anatomic implants
1. Desiring a natural look with minimal or no breast tissue
2. Shapeless breast or breast with poor soft tissue coverage
3. Constricted lower pole or tuberous breast deformity
4. Simple or complex asymmetry
5. Ptosis or lower pole laxity (poor tissue may limit placement)

Smooth Versus Textured

Textured devices were initially created to mimic the external shell of polyurethane implants; these implants had a coarse porous exterior with very low capsular contracture rates.[6] Recent Level 1 trials have not demonstrated lower capsular contracture rates in textured implants in the subpectoral pocket; however, some clinical studies have suggested reduced capsular contracture rates using textured implants in the subglandular space.[6] Most likely, the low capsular contracture rates seen in polyurethane implants were related to a biochemical reaction and not the texturing of the device.[6] Of note, smooth implants are currently used in approximately 90% of patients receiving primary breast augmentation in the United States.[4] Our practice uses texturing only for anatomic implants.

Saline Versus Silicone

A patient's anatomy or personal preference may dictate saline or silicone filler; however, the fillers have distinct properties that should be discussed during the initial patient consultation. Advantages of saline implants include smaller incisions from a remote location, less required monitoring, and decreased costs. Disadvantages of saline implants include increased risk of wrinkling and palpability, less natural touch, more tissue effects over time, and spontaneous deflation. Advantages of silicone implants include less wrinkling and palpability, no risk of sudden deflation, and a more natural touch. Disadvantages of silicone implants include MRI monitoring, "silent rupture," increased costs, and a slightly longer incision. The implant choice in our practice is typically selected by patient preferences and breast anatomy.

Pocket Plane

Implants can be placed in the subpectoral, subglandular, subfascial, or dual-plane pocket. Advantages of the subpectoral position include improved upper pole contour, decreased incidence of capsular contracture, and better breast tissue visualization during mammography. Disadvantages include increased discomfort from submuscular dissection and potential rare occurrence of implant distortion by pectoralis contraction, although a proper dual-plane pocket negates all these disadvantages.

Subglandular placement of implants may be appealing because of misconceptions of decreased postoperative pain and ease of dissection; however, the disadvantages of subglandular positioning typically outweigh these positives, including poor superior pole esthetics and rippling, increased capsular contracture, and difficult mammography imaging.

Subfascial placement has been suggested by various investigators to offer the same protection as submuscular placement against capsular contracture with less postoperative pain; however, the pectoralis fascia layer is typically thin and requires a tedious dissection. Our practice has found minimal clinical indications for subfascial placement.

The dual-plane technique places the implant partially subglandular and submuscularly. Incremental and planned release of the submuscular fibers at the muscle-gland interface allows the surgeon to vary the muscle coverage of the implant leading to optimal implant–breast parenchyma dynamics.[7,8] Dual-plane position eliminates virtually all of the disadvantages of the traditional submuscular approach while maintaining the benefits of muscle coverage.[9] All implants placed in our practice are dual-plane with the exception of true body builders.

Incision Selection

Popular available incisions for breast augmentations include inframammary, peri-areolar, axillary, and peri-umbilical. Certain patient anatomy or implant choice may suggest an incisional approach; however, often the chosen incision is patient/surgeon preference. The inframammary approach continues to be the most popular access for breast augmentation, as it provides the best control. This approach offers visualization of the subpectoral plane without violating the breast parenchyma. Indications for this incision include small areolar diameter, large form-stabled implants, glandular ptosis, and large-volume implants (>400 mL). The real challenge/key point of the inframammary approach is placement of the incision at the postoperative inframammary crease (the new inframammary fold [IMF] incision). If the placement is miscalculated and the inframammary crease is repositioned intraoperatively, the scar will not be in the optimal location and poor quality. Furthermore, a malpositioned IMF would alter the postoperative nipple-to-IMF distance and inherently distort overall breast esthetics. The inframammary approach has evolved as the preferred surgical access of our practice; this incision is predictable and reproducible when implant-specific tissue-based principles are followed and provides the most control. We place the calculated postoperative fold starting 1 cm medial to the areola, then extending a length laterally that will accommodate the size of the implant (typically 4–5 cm).

The peri-areolar incision hemi-circumnavigates the areola, usually hidden with an inconspicuous scar at the pigment of the areola and native breast skin; however, recent studies have shown an increase in bacterial load, and subsequently, increased capsular contracture with this incision.[10–12] Thus, we typically avoid this access choice in our practice.

Axillary access for breast augmentation is an intriguing approach because many surgeons market this access as scarless. Indications for axillary breast augmentation include small areola diameter and small silicone implants or saline implants. The patient also must have appropriate breast anatomy: adequate breast tissue, normal body habitus, and ideal shape. This incisional approach can be either blunt dissection or endoscopic assisted. Of note, blunt dissection is technically easier but requires experience, and the endoscopic approach necessitates complex technical equipment. Both axillary techniques have an increased risk of superior implant malposition because of the poor visualization of the inframammary crease. Furthermore, this procedure may be more painful, and revisional surgery normally requires an additional remote incision. Surgeons must avoid the axillary fat during this dissection to prevent lymphatic trauma and associated sequelae. Some science has demonstrated a higher capsular contracture rate with the trans-axillary incision as well,[4,5] although some proponents of the incision have documented similar rates.[13]

The peri-umbilical approach (trans-umbilical breast augmentation) has been discussed in the literature for saline devices. This approach requires an extensive blunt dissection in the subscarpal plane to access the subpectoral pocket and is typically reserved only for surgeon preference.[4] The approach has many drawbacks and does not execute breast augmentation at the highest level.

During the education and surgeon consult, patients who desire various incisions are presented these data points, and in the past 5 years, all have requested the new IMF incision.

Limitations Patients Should Understand

There are certain patient anatomic variations that may influence implant selection and deserve mentioning. For example, plastic surgeons and patients must recognize chest wall morphologies, which can affect the orientation of the breasts, and thus, the positioning of the implants. A round chest wall lateralizes the breasts; and alternatively, a rectangular chest wall medializes the breasts. Patients are counseled that the position and morphology of the breast on the chest wall cannot be altered with breast augmentation. Furthermore, hemithorax asymmetry or scoliosis may require different implants despite equivalent breast volumes to recreate symmetric chest topographies.[4]

A separate unique patient population is the postpartum breast augmentations. After pregnancy, the breast tissue atrophies with poor skin elasticity. This skin/soft tissue transformation may accentuate implant visualization and migration. Silicone implants with conservative volumes may decrease postoperative rippling and bottoming out. Furthermore, these patients may have nipple hypertrophy and nipple/breast ptosis. Concurrent nipple correction or mastopexy may augment the overall cosmesis.[4]

PREOPERATIVE ASSESSMENT/CONSULT KEY POINTS

Patient History

Psychosocial elements may impact the surgical course; for example, the patient and surgeon must discuss the motivations behind surgery. Does the patient hope to achieve a "natural" or "obvious" breast augmentation? We generally assimilate all of this information in the education portion of the consult.

Physical Examination/Measurements Key Points

Basic measurements are needed to assess tissue coverage before implant selection, including breast base width, skin stretch, and nipple-to-IMF distance on stretch. The combination of these breast measurements and breast type are essential for implant-specific tissue-based planning. In breast augmentation surgery, neither the artist (no measurements) nor the engineer (only measurements) is ideal, but our group has proven that scientific measurements create surgical boundaries for an artist to optimally function.[14]

Breast base width

The breast base width (BBW) is the actual width of the pocket in which the implant will be placed. The BBW is inherently smaller than the actual width of the breast. The BBW is the linear measurement across the widest transverse portion of breast (usually at the nipple) from the medial border of the breast mound to the lateral border of the breast mound (**Fig. 3**).

Skin stretch

The skin stretch (SS) is measured by grasping the skin of the medial areola and pulling the breast maximally anteriorly. The SS distance correlates to the anterior-posterior excursion measured with a caliper (**Fig. 4**).

Nipple-inframammary fold on stretch

The nipple-inframammary (N:IMF) fold measurement is obtained by using flexible tape from the midpoint of the nipple under maximal stretch to the IMF (**Fig. 5**).

Breast type (implant-specific planning)

The breast type has evolved from the High-5 System to measure the contribution of the patient's existing parenchyma for implant-specific tissue-based planning. We have determined 5 breast types and these are subdivided based on envelope quality and N:IMF on stretch (**Fig. 6**).

Breast Type I (very tight) SS <1.5 cm
Breast Type II (tight) SS 1.5–2 cm
Breast Type III (average) SS 2–3 cm
Breast Type IV (loose) SS 3–4 cm with N:IMF <9 cm
Breast Type V (very loose) SS 3–4 cm with N:IMF >9 cm

Fig. 7 represents the integration of BBW, SS, N:IMF, and breast type to create a blueprint for implant selection for implant-specific tissue-based planning.

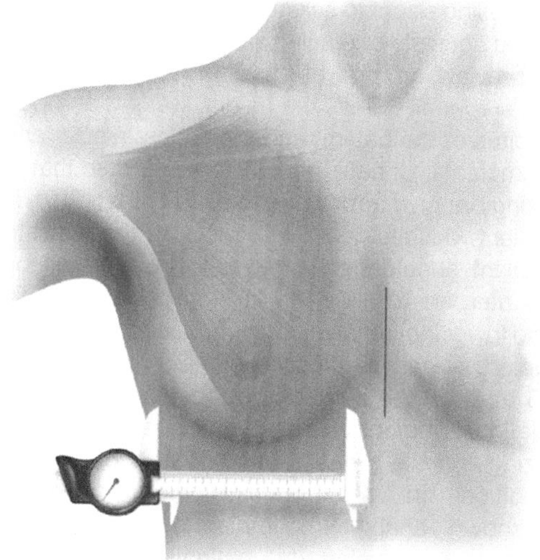

Fig. 3. The BBW measurement.

Photography

An instrumental part of the breast examination and patient education is patient photography. Together, the surgeon and patient can identify any asymmetries; in addition, this discussion allows the surgeon to reiterate that postoperative breasts will not be identical. Furthermore, by using photographs, the surgeon can outline important concepts, including likelihood of implant palpability, rationale for implant pocket dissection and incision choice, the expectations of cleavage and IMF, and the ideal implant. A useful adjunct to this discussion is a "breast-augmentation image analysis form" that guides the surgeon through the necessary points[1] (see **Fig. 2**).

Recently, 3-dimensional imaging has become an integral part of our consultation and patient education.[15] The various viewpoints from a 3-dimensional model exponentially surpass the information from a 2-dimensional photograph; thus, the patient and surgeon have visual data to augment tissue-based implant selection. Furthermore, simulated 3-dimensional images allow the patient to see a "natural" versus "augmented" look and can thus make an informed decision for implant selection.

IMPLANT SELECTION: TISSUE-BASED CLINICAL ANALYSIS AND PLANNING

Selecting the appropriate implant for breast augmentation remains a challenge for many plastic surgeons. Patients typically discuss magazine photographs, cup sizes, and friends' experiences when suggesting implants for their respective surgery. However, these subjective anecdotes have little value in selecting the proper implant for particular breast morphology. Recent premarket approval studies have documented elevated reoperation rates after breast augmentation from 15% to 24% in 6 years. With recent scientific studies,

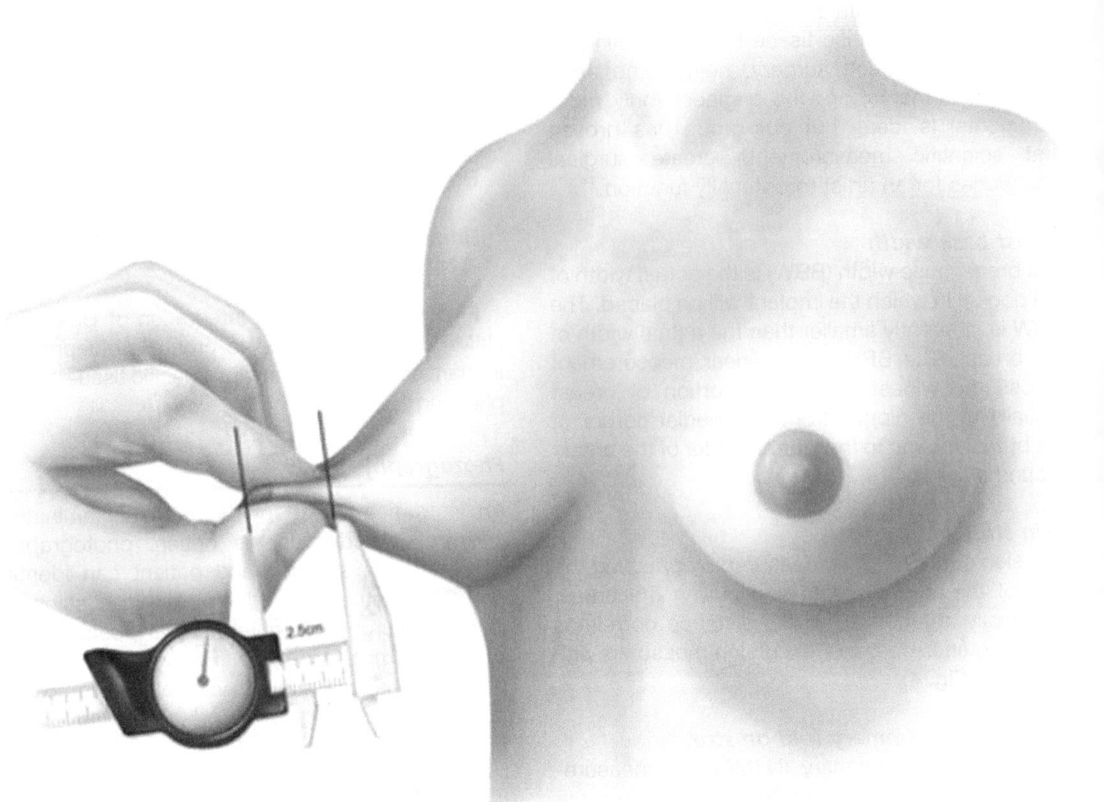

Fig. 4. The SS measurement.

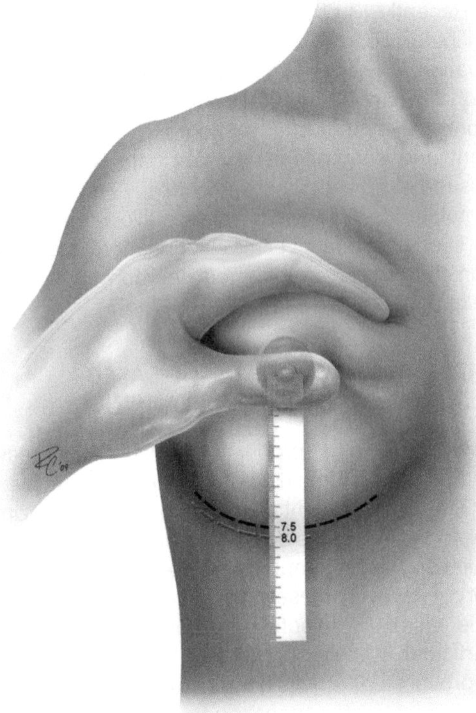

Fig. 5. The N:IMF measurement on stretch.

we now understand tissue-based planning concepts that can help lower reoperation rates for augmentation.[1,9]

Bra/Sizers Limitations

Some surgeons argue that volume is the most important variable in implant selection and suggest using sizers to select an implant. Preoperative sizing consists of placing sample implants in a bra to preview a range of possible results. Typically, the surgeon reviews the height, weight, and body habitus of the patient and then offers a size range of implants. Of note, patients are informed that the sizing bra may add 30 mL to each breast. Also, if a patient desires a saline implant, the selected implant should be 25 mL less than its silicone counterpart to allow for intraoperative overfilling and lower incidence of rippling. Based on this evaluation, a patient then selects 2 implants within 25 mL and the surgeon has the liberty to select the ideal implant based on intraoperative implant sizing and the breast mound. We have found the in-office bra sizer stuffing introduces more unknown variables into implant selection, making it more confusing to patients and actually misleading them in many cases.

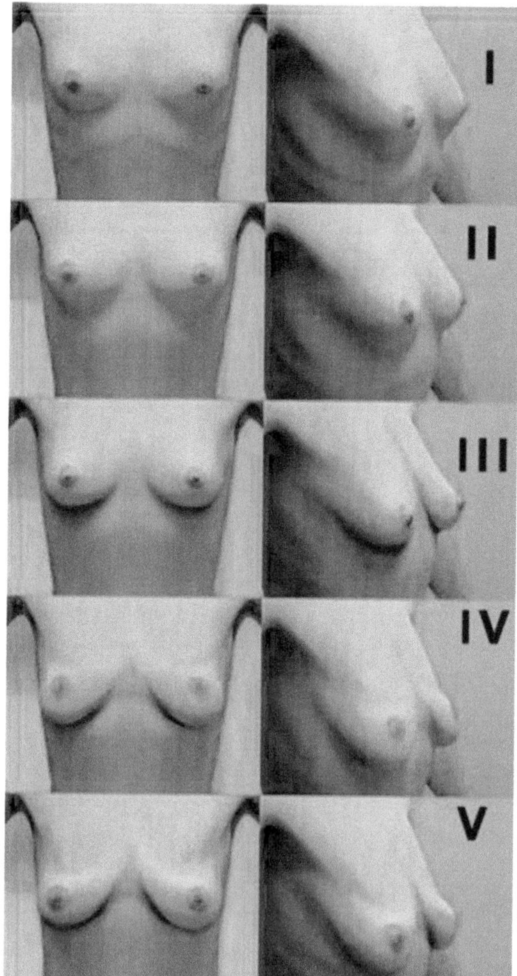

Fig. 6. The 5 breast subtypes based on envelope quality and N:IMF distance on stretch.

Even though this process shares ownership and has been proven to minimize size request changes,[4] this process has some deficiencies. There have been no studies that have compared the accuracy of preoperative breast sizing and postoperative breast volume and shape. This process is not influenced by the objective boundaries of the breast and is a very subjective experience. Furthermore, this process creates preoperative uncertainty and empowers the surgeon instead of the patient to select the final implant. If the surgeon and patient together choose the ideal implant based on the tissue envelope preoperatively, the patient knows the exact implant that will be placed in the operating room and has joint ownership of the implant decision. Furthermore, this process of intraoperative sizers includes increased operative time, which exposes the patient to increased capsular contracture, infection risk, and unwanted effects of general anesthesia (eg, nausea, stiffness). Despite the efforts to include patients in the implant process, the "sizer stuffing methodology" excludes patients from the final implant decision and lacks tissue-based preoperative planning.[4]

High-5 System

Our practice has abandoned the subjective limitations of sizing and uses the tissue-based High-5 system for implant selection and operative planning. By adopting these tenets, our practice has reduced our overall reoperation rate to 2.8% in comparison with the national reoperation rates.[14] The basics of the High-5 process allow the surgeon to make 5 critical decisions for optimal outcomes:

1. Pocket plane
2. Implant size
3. Implant type
4. IMF position
5. Incision

This process is outlined in detail in the 2006 article, "Five critical decisions in breast augmentation using five measurements in 5 minutes: the high five decision support process."[9] However, since its publication, we have made the following advances and simplifications to the 5 steps:

1. As previously discussed, our practice uses a dual-plane pocket for all patients with the exception of true body builders.
2. The measurements of BBW and SS determine optimal fill volume. If the patient is a breast type 1 or 2, the optimal fill volume is reduced further (60 mL and 30 mL, respectively). Any adjustments to the optimal fill based on the patient desires are made. Breast type provides a simpler construct to correlate envelope quality and tissue-based implant selection. Once the final optimal fill is known, 3-dimensional imaging using the desired implant at that optimal fill is performed with the patient.
3. The new inframammary fold incision and ideal postoperative nipple-to-fold distance is extrapolated from the High-5 chart based on the selected implant volume. If the recommended nipple-to-fold distance is greater than the preoperative nipple-to-fold distance, the surgeon should consider altering the fold to the suggested level. A general yet effective formula is a 300-mL implant requires a nipple-to-IMF distance of 8 cm; for every 10-mL volumetric change, the IMF position should adjust by 0.1 cm.

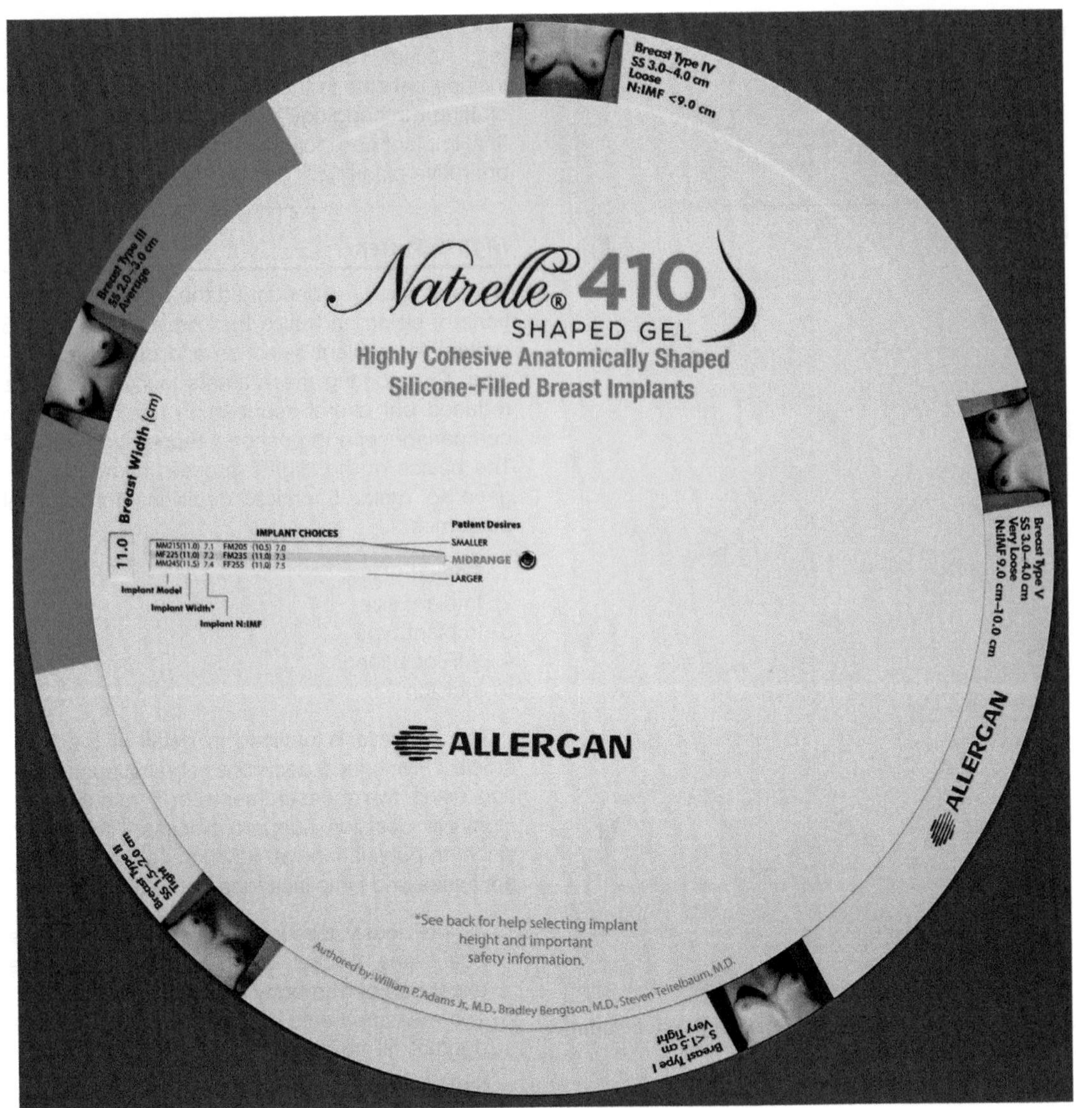

Fig. 7. Integration of BBW, SS, N:IMF distance, and breast type to create a blueprint for implant selection for implant-specific tissue-based planning. (Activas, Inc, Parsippany, NJ.)

4. As previously discussed, our practice uses an IMF approach for all patients. This approach provides optimal control with minimal tissue trauma and reduced exposure to implant contaminants, and passes the "family test"; ie, what incision would we recommend and perform on a family member?

Failure to follow tissue-based planning and natural boundaries of the breast can lead to an unnatural appearance as well as soft tissue distortion with inherent postoperative complications.[5] **Fig. 8** outlines our process for clinical evaluation and patient measurements to execute tissue-based implant selection.

Three-Dimensional Analyses

Even though 3-dimensional imaging has been referenced previously, the concept must be reiterated, as this technology has become an increasingly powerful educational instrument for both the surgeon and patient in the implant decision-making process. Three-dimensional imaging, unlike its historic 2-dimensional counterpart, allows the patient not only to see the breast from various angles but also to simulate postoperative results with the insertion of an implant. Once the surgeon and patient have applied tissue-based preoperative planning to select an implant, the two can visualize the implant in the 3-dimensional model.

Size: Pt. Desires: ☐Natural appearing breast o Unnatural, bulging upper breast
☐Proportionate to protect tissues o Very large
Approximate Desired Cup_______Requests specific cc's:_______
o Pt.Chooses Size o Pt. Leaves Size Choice to Dr. Adams
Implant: o Round o Anatomic o Smooth o Textured
o Saline oSilicone oCohesive o Pt. Leaves Type Choice to Dr. Adams
Pocket Location: ☐PRP oRM oDr. Adams to decide
Incision Location: ☐IM oPA oAX o Incision Choice to Dr. Adams
Pts. Initials_______

Capsular Contracture and Tissue Stretch Factors:
☐Implant choice may affect risk
☐Pt. accepts full responsibility for all costs (hospital and anesthesia) for any surgery necessary to treat capsule, tissue stretch deformities and aging implants. Revision surgery may exceed the costs of the original surgery. Pts. Initials_______

Patient Has Completed, Read and Signed:
☐Pt. Educator Consult ☐Choice Documents
☐Dr Adams website Pt. Ed. Initials: _______

Discussed/Patient Accepts That:
☐The larger the implant , the more risks of sensory loss, tissue damage, and increased risk for re-operations
Pts. Initials_______

Age _____
Height _____ Wt._____lbs
Frame: Sm Med Lrg
Torso: o Nl Wide Nr
Gravida _____
Para _____

Bra **Band** Size: 32, 34, 36
Breast **Cup** Size (Approx.)
Prior to pregnancy____
Largest with preg____
Current Cup Size____
Desired Cup Size____
Previous Breast Disease:
None
Biopsies: o No o Yes
____

Family Hx. Breast Cancer
No Yes
Mother Grandmother Aunt
Maternal Paternal

Previous Mammograms:
☐No ☐Yes
Date: ___________
Interpretation: ☐Normal
☐Other: ___________
Pertinent Medical History:
☐None
____
____
PSH: ___________
____

Smoker:☐No ☐Yes ____
Allergies: ☐NKDA
____
Current Meds, Herbs, Vits:
____

Companion: ___________
Relation: ___________

Specific Limitations Discussed with Patient:

☐Your breasts will never match
☐You may lose some or all sensation
☐You may see or feel edges of your implant due to thin tissues
☐You may require reoperations and additional costs in the future due to implant size requested , your tissue stretch characteristics or capsule you form
☐We give no guarantee of cup size
☐Any reoperation may require an inframammary incision
☐ Other:
____

☐Patient vocalizes under-standing and acceptance of all items checked above. Pt. Initials _________

Breast Masses
☐None
☐Size and Location:
____
____
Larger Breast:
☐Left ☐☐Right
Est. Vol. Diff. _____ cc TBD
Nipple Level
Discrepancy _____ cm N/A
IMF Level
Discrepancy _____ cm N/A
Envelope Compliance
☐Nl ☐Inc ☐☐Dec
☐☐Constricted Lower Env.
☐☐Short, fixed IMF
☐☐Other:
____
☐ **Note Dictated**

Clinical Breast Measurements L/R		**Estimating Desired Breast Implant Volume Based on Breast Measurements and Tissue Characteristics High 5 System**										
Breast BW		**Base Width Parenchyma (cm)**	**10.5**	**11.0**	**11.5**	**12.0**	**12.5**	**13.0**	**13.5**	**14.0**	**14.5**	**15.0**
		Estimated Initial Implant Volume (cc's)	**200**	**250**	**275**	**300**	**300**	**325**	**350**	**375**	**375**	**400**
SS_{MaxStr}		**If SS <2.0, – 30cc**										
		If SS >3.0, + 30cc										
		If SS >4.0, + 60cc										
$N:IMF_{MaxSt}$		**If N:IMF >9.5, + 30cc**										
Breast Type												
Pt. request												
		Total Estimated Implant Volume										
Estimating the Optimal Level of the Inframammary Fold Relative to the Nipple												
		For each volume indicated	**200**	**250**	**275**	**300**		**325**	**350**	**375**		**400**
New IMF		**Set new IMF at N:IMF distance (cm.) (measured under maximal stretch)**	7.0	7.0	7.5	8		8.25	8.5	9.0		9.5

SNN/N:IMF
R /
L /
R / L
BW /
SS /
AD /
SPP
IPP
PP /
PCEF %
C:IMF /
U:IMF /
ChCirc
Dome /
Breast Type:

Notes:

Implant Selected: ________________ **Volume:** _______ **cc** **BaseD**_______**Ht:** _______ **cm.**

1. ST Coverage
SPP >2 SG, DP 1 2 3
SPP <2 RP, DP 1 2 3

4. IMF position _______cm N:IMF
☐Lower fold N:IMFpost____
☐Do not lower fold

5. Incision: ☐IMF ☐RT IMF
☐PA ☐IT IMF
☐TA

Top concerns:

Patient Name: **MRN:**
EDU Date:_______ **Consultation Date:**

Ref:
Resides in Occupation:

Fig. 8. Our intraoperative process for clinical evaluation and patient measurements to execute tissue-based implant selection.

With this postoperative 3-dimensional simulation, the surgeon and patient can confirm expectations based on a scientifically proven technology or make appropriate adjustments in the patient's own picture based on volume and shape to affirm the ideal implant.[15] Previous investigators, including our clinical practice, have verified the accuracy of the preoperative simulation and postoperative images for patient consultation. **Fig. 9** demonstrates an example of a 24-year-old woman who had preoperative breast imaging, preoperative simulation, and postoperative imaging using Allergan (Irvine, CA, USA) Style 15 to 265-mL round implants. Of note, surgeons must caution

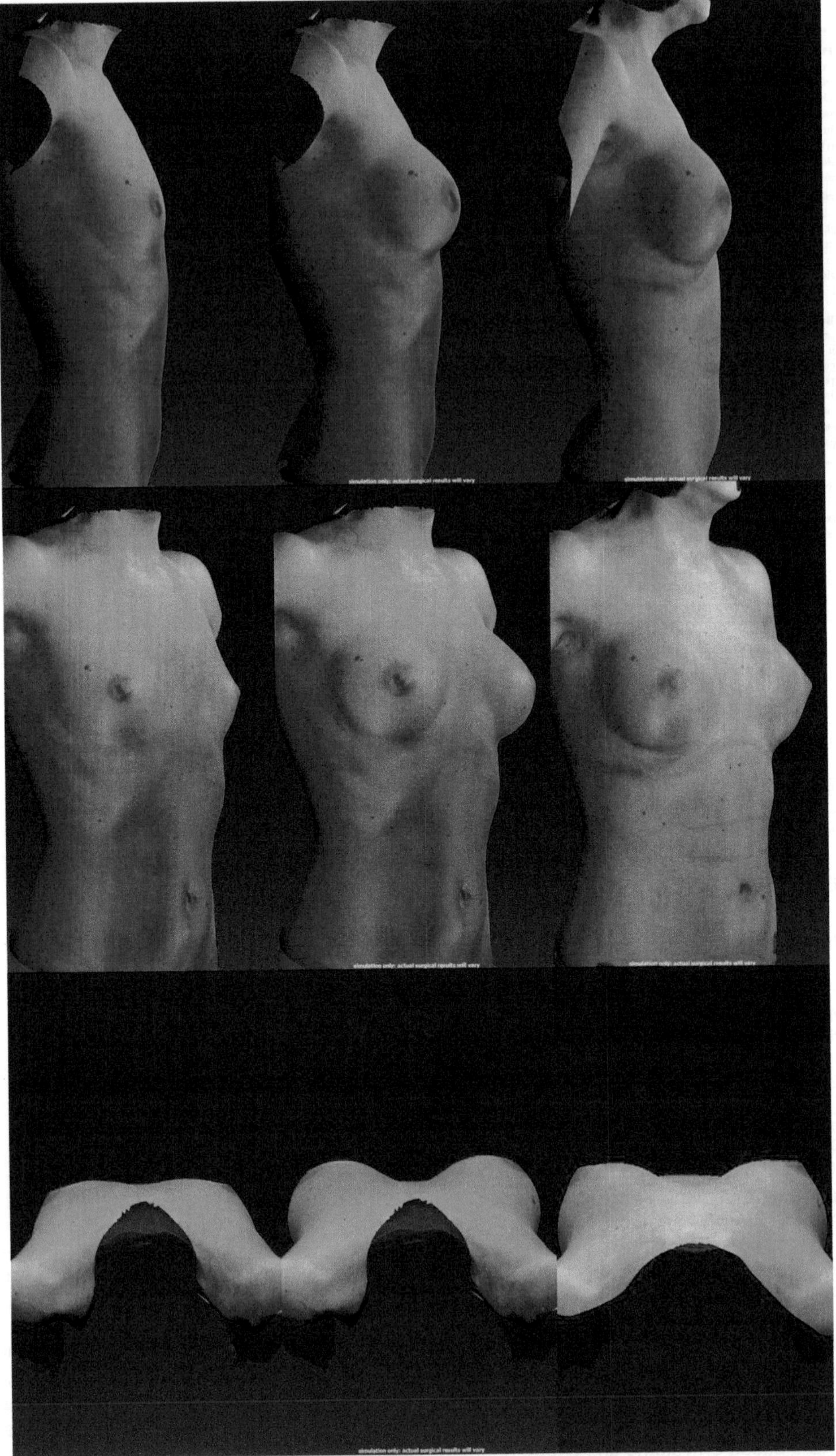

Fig. 9. A 24-year-old woman who had preoperative breast imaging, preoperative simulation, and postoperative imaging using Allergan Style 15 to 265-mL round implants.

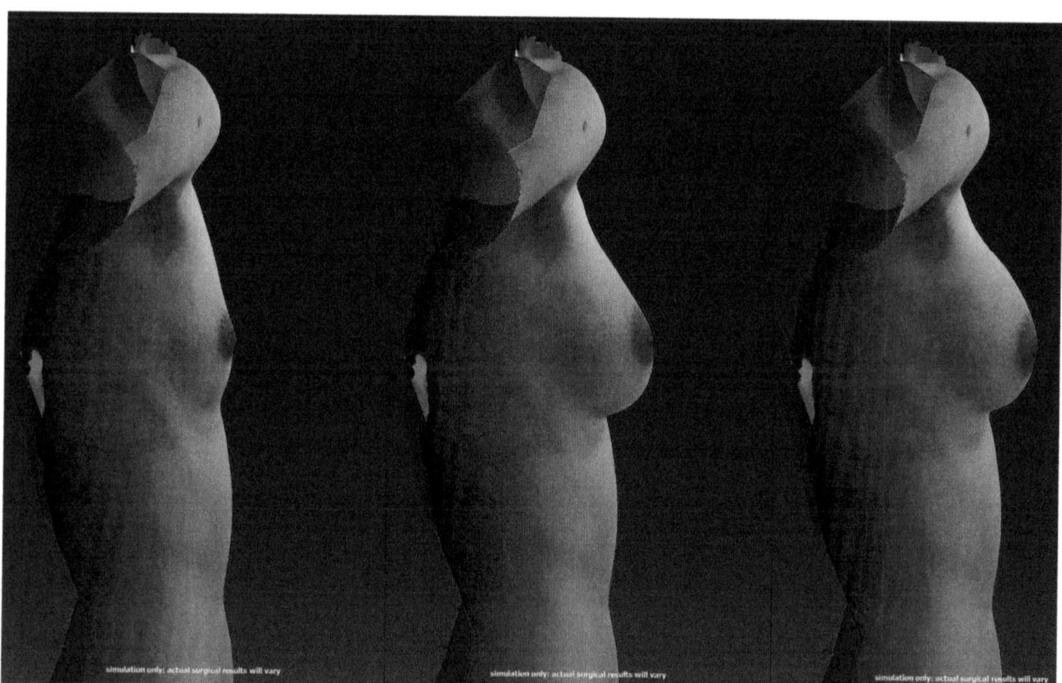

Fig. 10. A preoperative surgical simulation of a 24-year-old woman with an anatomic implant, Allergan FM 410 to 205 mL, and with a round implant, Sientra MP 230 mL.

patients that 3-dimensional imaging is only a simulation and by no means guarantees postoperative results. This is no different from rhinoplasty 3-dimensional imaging, which has been used successfully for many years. Despite this limitation, 3-dimensionalimaging enhances the communication between surgeon and patient and allows the patient to choose an implant based on an actual image of her body. In addition, with the resurgence of anatomic silicone implants in the US market, 3-dimensional imaging may serve as an adjunct to educating patients in different volume and surface characteristics. This technology has been particularly effective in demonstrating differences between a round versus shaped outcome for a given patient. **Fig. 10** represents a preoperative surgical simulation of a 24-year-old woman with an anatomic implant, Allergan FM 410 to 205 mL, and with a round implant, Sientra (Santa Barbara, CA, USA) MP 230 mL.

SUMMARY

Our practice has adopted the philosophy that breast augmentation is not simply a surgical procedure but a process of 4 comprehensive steps. The nonsurgical steps, patient education and tissue-based planning, have been detailed earlier in this article and are essential to optimizing postoperative outcomes and reducing reoperation rates. The surgeon and the patient must assume a mutual responsibility that the implant has been selected based on breast dimensions. Furthermore, they must have a shared understanding of preoperative breast asymmetry and soft tissue limitations. State-of-the-art advances include dedicated education, comprehensive patient/surgeon consultation, surgical forms and analytical sheets, and patient 3-dimensional imaging coupled with tissue-based planning. This breast augmentation process has been transferable to other practices with the same successes, and in the end, with the global adaptation of this approach, the winner is the patient.

Editorial Comments by Bradley P. Bengtson, MD

A great deal is owed to Dr Bill Adams in getting plastic surgeons to think about the surgical procedures that we are performing as a "Process" verses just an event or surgical procedure. The breast augmentation Process may be broken down into four main process categories. Although all are critical, as Dr Adams and colleagues point out, the Patient education, Patient selection and Implant selection are by far and away the most significant. Proper patient evaluation and education using Tissue Base Planning principles and the application of these measurements into the patient assessment is essential in obtaining objective, consistent outcomes and minimizing adverse events, complications and breast revision surgery.

REFERENCES

1. Adams WP Jr. The process of breast augmentation: four sequential steps for optimizing outcomes for patients. Plast Reconstr Surg 2008;122(6): 1892–900.
2. Tebbetts JB. Achieving a zero percent reoperation rate at 3 years in a 50-consecutive-case augmentation mammaplasty premarket approval study. Plast Reconstr Surg 2006;118(6):1453–7.
3. Tebbetts JB, Tebbetts TB. An approach that integrates patient education and informed consent in breast augmentation. Plast Reconstr Surg 2002; 110(3):971–8 [discussion: 979–81].
4. Hidalgo DA, Spector JA. Breast augmentation. Plast Reconstr Surg 2014;133(4):567e–83e.
5. Adams WP Jr, editor. Breast augmentation. 1st edition. New York: McGraw-Hill Professional; 2011.
6. Adams WP Jr, Mallucci P. Breast augmentation. Plast Reconstr Surg 2012;130(4):597e–611e.
7. Tebbetts JB. Dual plane breast augmentation: optimizing implant-soft-tissue relationships in a wide range of breast types. Plast Reconstr Surg 2001; 107(5):1255–72.
8. Tebbetts JB. Dual plane breast augmentation: optimizing implant-soft-tissue relationships in a wide range of breast types. Plast Reconstr Surg 2006; 118(7 Suppl):81S–98S [discussion: 99S–102S].
9. Tebbetts JB, Adams WP. Five critical decisions in breast augmentation using five measurements in 5 minutes: the high five decision support process. Plast Reconstr Surg 2005;116(7):2005–16.
10. Jacobson JM, Gatti ME, Schaffner AD, et al. Effect of incision choice on outcomes in primary breast augmentation. Aesthet Surg J 2012;32(4):456–62.
11. Wiener TC. Relationship of incision choice to capsular contracture. Aesthetic Surg J 2008;32(2):303–6.
12. Wiener TC. The role of betadine irrigation in breast augmentation. Plast Reconstr Surg 2007;119(1):12–5 [discussion: 16–7].
13. Huang GJ, Wichmann JL, Mills DC. Transaxillary subpectoral augmentation mammaplasty: a single surgeon's 20-year experience. Aesthet Surg J 2011; 31(7):781–801.
14. Adams WP. The High Five Process: tissue-based planning for breast augmentation. Plast Surg Nurs 2007;27(4):197–201.
15. Roostaeian J, Adams WP Jr. Three-dimensional imaging for breast augmentation: is this technology providing accurate simulations? Aesthet Surg J 2014;34(6):857–75.

Understanding the Etiology and Prevention of Capsular Contracture

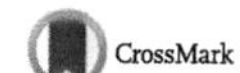

Translating Science into Practice

Simon J. Chong, BHB, MBChB, FRACS,
Anand K. Deva, BSc (Med), MS, FRACS*

KEYWORDS

- Capsular contracture • Biofilm • Breast augmentation • Silicone • *Staphylococcus epidermidis*

KEY POINTS

- Chronic inflammation attributable to the presence of bacterial biofilm is currently the predominant theorem of capsular contracture formation. Conversely, maintenance of implant sterility will prevent capsular contracture.
- The surgical field in breast augmentation is not rendered sterile by standard techniques and perioperative antibiotics.
- Thus, a comprehensive strategy for maintaining implant sterility is critical in preventing bacterial contamination, and is supported by mounting clinical and laboratory evidence.

INTRODUCTION

In an ideal world a medical device, once inserted into the human body, will undergo biological integration with complete tolerance and without any remote-to-implant effects,[1] leading to long-term successful functional and aesthetic outcomes. In the real world, however, medical devices continue to be plagued with a wide spectrum of adverse outcomes, ranging from acute infection to long-term device failure necessitating removal. For breast implants, capsular contracture (CC) represents the most common and most problematic adverse outcome. Following primary augmentation, CC occurs in up to 59% of patients,[2] and is the commonest indication for reoperation.[3,4] Patients undergoing revision surgery for contracture can expect to have recurrence in 18.1% to 39.7% of cases.[5,6] Furthermore, revision surgery is technically more difficult, and satisfaction rates are lower (**Fig. 1**).[6]

Several hypotheses have been forwarded to explain why capsules form and why they progress pathologically around some breast implants, including infection, hematoma, and granulomatous response to free silicone. The most recent, and closest unifying theory is that of septic biofilm formation, elegantly expressed by Adams[7] as an interaction between potentiators and suppressors that come into play when an implant is first inserted into a perimammary space. It is this interplay of factors that leads to either implant

Disclosures: Associate Professor A.K. Deva is a consultant to Allergan, Mentor (J&J), and KCI. He has previously coordinated industry-sponsored research for these companies relating to both biofilms and breast prostheses. Dr S.J. Chong has no affiliations or financial interests to disclose.

Department of Plastic, Reconstructive & Maxillofacial Surgery, Faculty of Medicine and Human Sciences, Macquarie University, Suite 301, Level 3, Macquarie University Clinic Macquarie Park, Sydney NSW 2109, Australia
* Corresponding author.
E-mail address: Anand.deva@mq.edu.au

Clin Plastic Surg 42 (2015) 427–436
http://dx.doi.org/10.1016/j.cps.2015.06.007
0094-1298/15/$ – see front matter

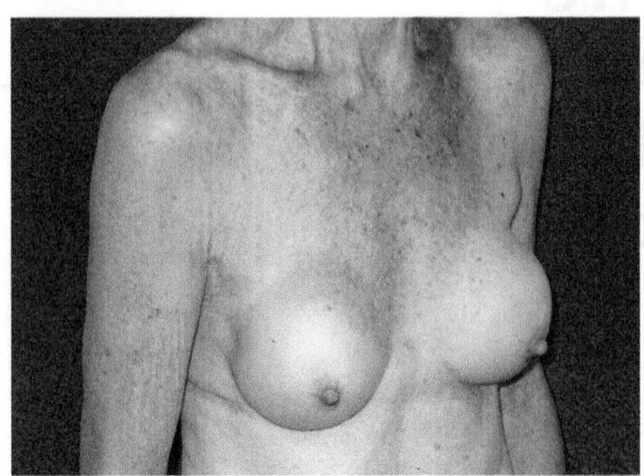

Fig. 1. Patient with bilateral Baker grade IV capsular contracture.

tolerance or progressive peri-implant inflammation and subsequent fibrosis, generating CC (**Fig. 2**).

This review examines the science behind each of these factors, determining their relative importance as either potentiators or suppressors of CC formation. The article also outlines the likely strategies that surgeons can deploy in the operating room to minimize the risk of adverse outcomes in breast augmentation based on the cumulative scientific evidence. In this way, evidence can be used to guide clinicians toward translating the findings of this growing body of research into clinical practice, ultimately for the benefit of patients.

FACTORS INFLUENCING CAPSULAR CONTRACTURE FORMATION

Bacteria and Subclinical Infection (Strong Potentiator)

The deep breast parenchyma is not intrinsically a sterile structure: it contains a penetrating ductal anatomy, populated by flora predominantly consisting of *Staphylococcus epidermidis*.[8–10] The

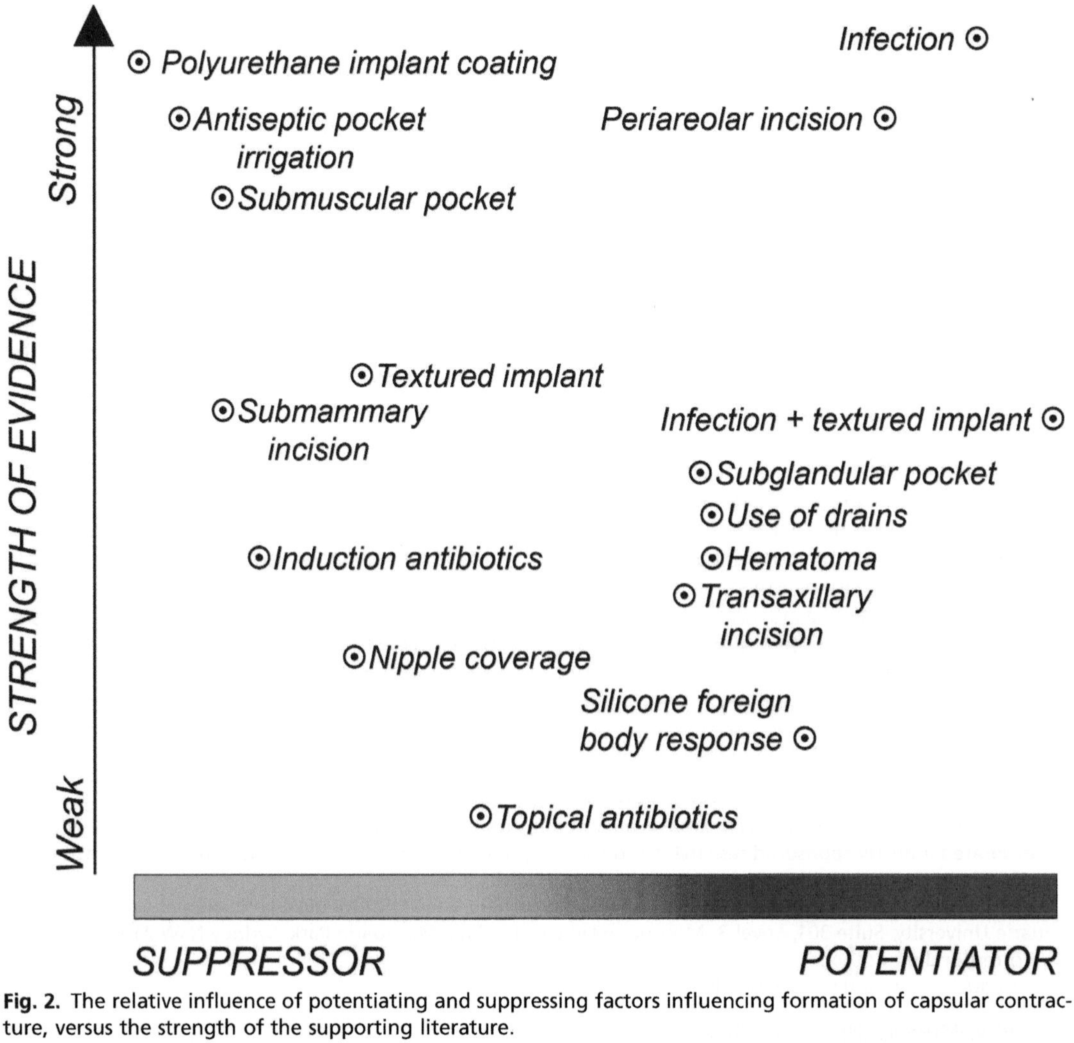

STRENGTH OF EVIDENCE
Strong
Weak
Infection
Polyurethane implant coating
Antiseptic pocket irrigation
Periareolar incision
Submuscular pocket
Textured implant
Submammary incision
Infection + textured implant
Subglandular pocket
Use of drains
Induction antibiotics
Hematoma
Transaxillary incision
Nipple coverage
Silicone foreign body response
Topical antibiotics
SUPPRESSOR
POTENTIATOR

Fig. 2. The relative influence of potentiating and suppressing factors influencing formation of capsular contracture, versus the strength of the supporting literature.

contribution of periprosthetic infection to CC has been recognized for some time, being first proposed by Burkhardt and colleagues[11] in 1981. However, many CCs form without gross clinical infection or positive culture, implying that infection may not be the universal mechanism.

An important step forward was the recognition of periprosthetic bacterial biofilms.[12] Biofilm consists bacteria enclosed within a matrix of their own excreted polysaccharides. This structure allows bacteria to densely adhere to prosthetic and biological surfaces. In this state, bacterial contamination may elude standard microbiological sampling, owing to a paucity of surface bacteria and low metabolic rate. Specialized techniques are required to detect biofilms and identify their contributing microorganisms. The biofilm structure also confers significant resistance against antibiotics, host defenses, and antiseptics.[13–17] There may be other more subtle advantages to the bacteria, such as improved nutrition through promotion of host cell lysis, cooperative metabolism, and horizontal gene transfer (**Fig. 3**).[18]

Through treatment resistance and eliciting a chronic inflammatory response, biofilms may ultimately lead to implant failure in the clinical situation.[19,20] A landmark experiment by Tamboto and colleagues[21] inoculated silicone implants with *S epidermidis* in a porcine model; this was strongly associated with biofilm formation, which itself correlated with a 4-fold increase in CC. It may be that periprosthetic infection has, all along, been a major causative factor in CC formation, and that the ability of biofilms to evade detection by standard sampling methods has confounded our understanding to date. The chronic inflammatory response to *S epidermidis* biofilms is now recognized as a major pathogen in CC.[22,23]

Implant Texturing (Both Suppressor and Strong Potentiator)

Barr and colleagues[8,24] investigated the cytoskeletal reaction of fibroblasts to silicone surfaces. Smooth surfaces predisposed to the planar arrangement of fibroblasts around implants, whereas textured implant surfaces caused fibroblasts to anchor in deep and random patterns. This situation implied an advantage for texturing with respect to CC. The body of conflicting clinical evidence[2,25–34] was unified in 2 meta-analyses in 2006, which concluded a 5-fold superiority of textured over smooth implants, maintained out to 3 years.[35,36]

However, this advantage can be a double-edged sword. When inoculated in vitro, a significantly higher biofilm load is found in textured implants than in smooth implants.[37] This finding suggests that the benefits of texturization may become a liability in infection because of a higher risk of bacterial colonization. With the recent implication of textured implants and biofilms in the causation of anaplastic large cell lymphoma, their use may bear additional scrutiny born of valid concern for oncological safety.[38]

Polyurethane (PU)-coated implants are a notable subset of textured implants. The surface texture is a fibrillar, mesh-like coating, as opposed to having being molded into the silicone or generated through salt removal.[24] This process generates a capsular microarchitecture distinct from textured silicone surfaces, possibly caused by a controlled inflammatory response guided by polyurethane fragment phagocytosis, and lower expression of periprosthetic parallel myofibrils.[39] Previous concerns regarding carcinogenic degradation into 2,4-toluenediamine products have been disproved,[40,41] although the coating does indeed degrade over time, leaving the equivalent of a standard textured silicone surface. PU

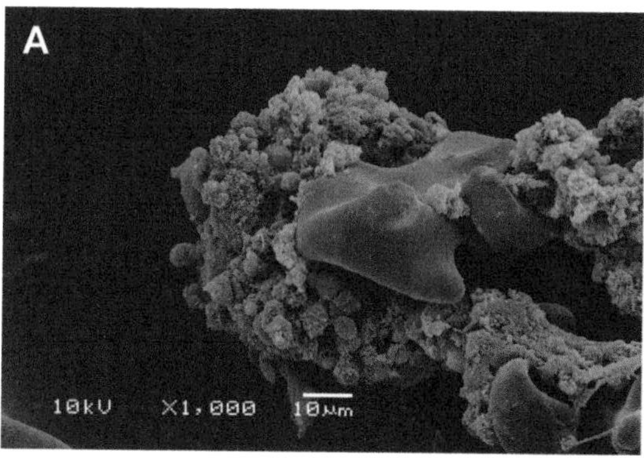

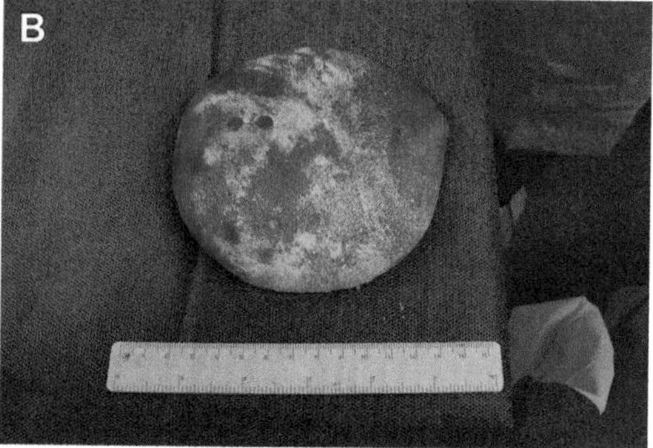

Fig. 3. (*A*) Scanning electron micrograph of biofilm formation on a textured silicone breast implant. (*B*) Intraoperative gross biofilm formation on an explanted textured breast implant.

implants have been shown in numerous studies to have a lower CC rate than other implants.[42–45]

Silicone Foreign Body Reaction (Potentiator)

Despite being chemically stable, silicone is not biologically inert: a universal foreign body reaction is elicited. An issue with older generations of silicone implants was gel bleed through the shell, or mechanical shell rupture, producing free silicone that initiated a granulomatous response.[46] Silicone fillers were hence seen as a potentiating factor in CC formation. However, in modern implants, this is addressed through modified shell characteristics and the use of form-stable cohesive gels.[47] Hence, previous studies implicating implant fillers as a significant potentiator of CC cannot be readily discussed in a contemporary context.[48–50]

Surprisingly, a 2010 literature review by Schaub and colleagues[51] was unable to reliably determine whether a difference existed between silicone and saline with respect to CC rate in cosmetic augmentation. Confounding their meta-analysis was the sheer heterogeneity of implant and technical variables present throughout the literature, in addition to differences in the basic definition of CC.

Incision Choice

Augmentation mammoplasty wounds were previously considered clean,[52] contrary to the now accepted knowledge that the deeply penetrating ductal system is colonized with bacterial flora.[9,10,53] Periareolar bacterial counts have been demonstrated to be 5 times that of the inframammary fold and 4 times that of the axilla.[9] Thus, a periareolar incision may contaminate the sterile field by transecting ductal tissue, and places an implant in contact with bacteria during insertion. In 2008, Wiener[54] demonstrated that a periareolar incision was associated with a 9.5% CC rate, compared with 0.59% for an inframammary incision. The relatively high CC rate in the periareolar group was despite the universal use of povidone-iodine pocket irrigation and perioperative antibiotics. Thus, the evidence clearly supports periareolar incisions as a strong potentiating factor in CC formation; conversely, inframammary incisions are protective. Because of their preference for cohesive gel implants, the authors predominantly use the inframammary incision, as the form-stable implants are difficult to squeeze through a periareolar approach. Should a surgeon elect to use a periareolar incision, the authors would recommend using a plastic insertion sleeve to isolate the implant from the wound tract.

The authors have little experience with transaxillary incisions in their practice. Previous criticisms of hematoma from blind, blunt transaxillary pocket dissection have been addressed through the use of endoscopic direct vision. This technical difference was the basis of a comparison series by Tebbetts,[55] who reported decrease in CC from 4.2% to 1.3% when adopting an endoscopic technique, similar to that reported by Giordano and colleagues.[56] Conversely, a series by Huang and colleagues[57] was largely performed without endoscopic assistance, with a CC rate of 1.9%. Stutman and colleagues[58] did not find any significant difference in infection rates between transaxillary, inframammary, and periareolar incisions, although their retrospective study design was limited by a large number of other variables. Contrary to this, Namnoum and colleagues[59] found a significantly higher rate of CC associated with axillary incisions, but not periareolar, when compared with the inframammary approach.

Submuscular Pocket (Suppressor) Versus Subglandular Pocket (Potentiator)

It has been a consistent finding that the submuscular pocket is protective against CC in comparison with subglandular placement,[59–65] likely because the implant is not exposed to potential colonization by contact with glandular-bearing breast tissue. The subfascial approach may offer a similar advantage.[63] However, the authors are not aware of a trial demonstrating that irrigation of a subglandular pocket with antiseptics reduces the risk of CC relative to that of a submuscular pocket.

Implant Exposure Time (Potentiator)

Through controlled laminar airflow and particular filtration, modern operating theaters are designed to minimize the introduction of particulate contaminants into the sterile surgical field.[66] Despite this, airborne infection is predisposed to by turbulent disruption of settled particles, increased traffic of operating room personnel, talking, and uncovered skin areas.[67,68] It follows that increased open-air exposure time predisposes to infection; increased operative time is associated with increased rates of infection in orthopedic joint replacement procedures.[69] Although there are no data specifically linking increased implant exposure time to CC, the authors recommend that the infection risk be curtailed by only opening implants immediately before insertion.

Induction Intravenous Antibiotics (Suppressor)

Routine use of a single, preincision dose of intravenous antibiotic has been shown to decrease the microbiological load on the intraoperative wound, and the rate of infection in breast implants.[70,71] Extending the duration of antibiotic cover postoperatively does not result in reduced superficial or periprosthetic infections.[71] Once a biofilm is established, a 1000-fold increase in minimum antibiotic concentration may be required to provide bactericidal activity.[72] It would therefore seem reasonable, given that infection can lead to CC let alone gross implant sepsis, to routinely administer prophylactic antibiotics before incision. Yet a recent meta-analysis by Hardwicke and colleagues[73] reported little high-quality contemporary evidence available for analysis: no trials of antibiotics versus controls were found in the preceding 17 years. Only studies comparing antibiotic regimens were available, and no significant difference was found with respect to infection rates. Specifically with respect to CC, the role of systemic antibiotic prophylaxis was concluded as unknown, and overall recommendations could not be made.

Despite these data and in view of the strong evidence favoring subclinical infection as a potentiator of CC, it is the authors' practice to routinely administer a single dose of intravenous antibiotics at anesthetic induction. However, because of known resistance of some *S epidermidis* isolates to methicillin (and thus cephalosporins),[72] antibiotic use does not afford total protection. Wixtrom and colleagues[74] were able to culture *S epidermidis* from 34.9% of nipples and nipple shields at the conclusion of augmentation procedures, despite povidone-iodine surface preparation and preoperative intravenous antibiotics. Other methods of reducing microbial contamination of implants thus remain important adjuncts to reducing the risk of CC.

Pocket Irrigation (Suppressor)

Burkhardt first proposed the subclinical infection model in 1981, and has advocated povidone-iodine pocket irrigation.[11,28,29] Wiener[75] was able to achieve CC rates much lower than those in contemporary publications through routine use of povidone-iodine pocket irrigation. Irrigation with povidone-iodine, cefuroxime, and gentamicin seems to be advantageous over systemic antibiotics alone in significantly reducing CC, even if no difference is observed in infection rates.[51,76] Both Adams and colleagues[77] and Araco and colleagues[78] routinely used pocket irrigation and perioperative antibiotics, and achieved commendably low rates of CC in their respective series. However, infection per se rather than CC formed the focus of their discussions, and there was no comparison between regimens. Pfeiffer and colleagues[79] were forced to withdrawal cephalothin from their routine pocket irrigation because of supply issues, thus creating a trial of antibiotic versus nonantibiotic irrigation. Despite a significant increase in seroma and infection, there was no significant difference in CC rate.

Nipple Coverage (Suppressor)

Collis and colleagues[80] demonstrated that bacterial contamination of the operative field may occur despite adequate skin preparation. These investigators also demonstrated that this may be prevented by placement of an occlusive dressing over the nipple-areola complex, which was subsequently confirmed by Wixtrom and colleagues.[74] Although neither study design was suited to examining the role of nipple shields in preventing CC, Wiener achieved particularly low rates of CC when placing povidone-iodine–soaked gauze over the nipple-areola complex, in addition to pocket irrigation.[75] These studies support the routine use of nipple-areolar dressings to prevent bacterial contamination of the surgical field, a practice that is both inexpensive and easy.

Introduction Sleeves (Suppressor)

As already mentioned, the breast surface and parenchyma may not necessarily be free of bacterial contamination, even in the context of standard sterile technique. Thus, implant contact with the surgical field may cause a breach of sterility. Mladick[81] described the use of introduction sleeves as part of a "no-touch" technique for saline implant insertion. Although a specialized medical device exists expressly for this purpose,[82] the authors have used a cut-off surgical glove as an effective improvisation.[18] Aside from a protective role, sleeves may also ease the inset (and thus decrease handling) of polyurethane implants.[83] Although no comparisons exist to specifically support sleeves as protective against CC, the technique is a simple and inexpensive modification to surgical practice (**Fig. 4**).

Topical Antibiotics (Suppressor)

Use of topical ointments, as opposed to solutions, may increase the dwell time of antibiotic effect on the implant surface. van Heerden and colleagues[84] used punch biopsies of silicone implant shells as substrates for testing commercially available topical antibiotics against *S epidermidis* in broth culture. Biofilm formation did not occur after 7 days when Chloramex®, Fucidin,® or Terramycin® was used. No difference was seen between smooth and textured disks. However, there is little other experience documented in the

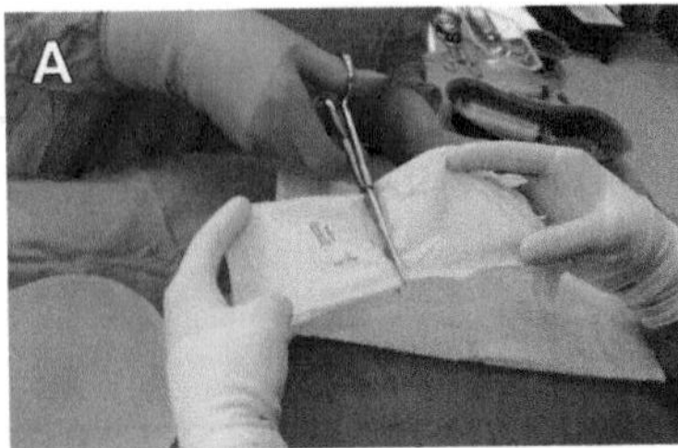
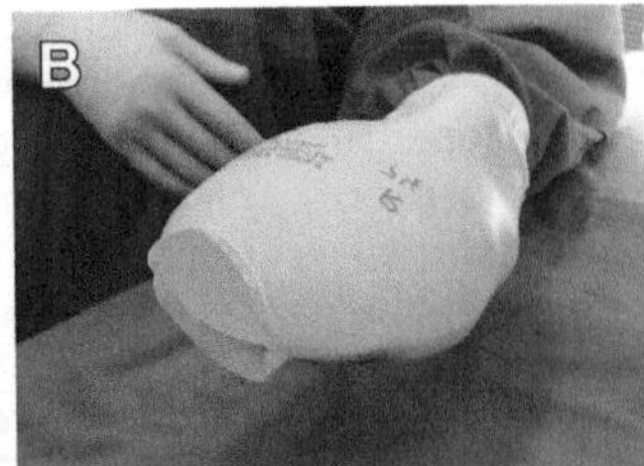
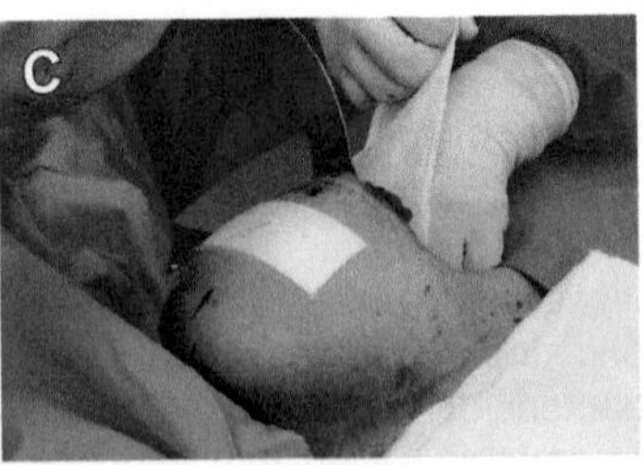

Fig. 4. (*A–C*) Modification of a surgical glove to serve as an improvised introduction sleeve. Minimizing implant contact with skin and divided parenchyma may prevent bacterial contamination.

literature on this topic, making the clinical application unclear.

Hematoma (Potentiator) and Use of Surgical Drains (Potentiator)

An increased CC rate has been demonstrated in the presence of hematoma.[45,50] The cellular and humoral response to hemorrhage products is an intrinsic part of acute wound healing, progressing to inflammation and fibroblastic collagen synthesis. Hematomata may also serve as a culture medium for microorganisms.

This issue raises the possibility that drain use may have a role in reducing CC through hematoma reduction. Conversely, however, drains provide a potential route of implant infection, and biofilm formation has been recognized as little as 2 hours after insertion.[85] Fanous and colleagues[86] reported 319 bilateral augmentations in which drains were routinely used, with the express purpose of hematoma prevention. Rates of infection, hematoma, and CC were all 0%, although there was no control group and other confounders were present. A large series by Araco and colleagues[78] indicated a 5-fold increase in infection associated with drain use; however, their overall CC rate was 0.5%, with no patients having both infection and CC. A prospective study by Henriksen and colleagues[64] associated drainage with a relative risk of 2.3 for CC, although they warn of confounding. A 2013 Cochrane review failed to identify any studies directly assessing drain use in breast augmentation.[87]

Based on the paucity of favorable evidence, the authors do not use drains in augmentation patients, and rely on surgical hemostasis to prevent hematoma formation. A further cautionary tale from Goldberg[88] tells of implants that may be pulled into exposure through the drain opening when the tubing is extracted.

FUTURE DEVELOPMENTS

Isolating the implant from tissue and thereby eliminating the silicone-tissue interaction may be a viable method of preventing CC. Antiadhesion barrier solution has been used to reduce intra-abdominal adhesions. A variety of products are available. Experimental white rat models have demonstrated some efficacy in reducing capsular response to silicone implants,[89–91] although their role in clinical practice is not yet clear.

Acellular human dermis has recently been used for improved lower pole coverage and increased expansion volume in the reconstructive context. Intraoperative samples harvested during expander exchange procedures have demonstrated significantly decreased capsular parameters on histologic analysis.[92] Its role in primary augmentation for preventing CC has not yet been described, although a significant cost issue is anticipated. Similarly, porcine-derived dermis (Strattice®) has been described in revision cases for CC, but not for primary prevention.[93]

Implant coating with surfaces that are either resistant to bacterial adhesion or antimicrobial may be another promising area of research. Jacombs and colleagues[94] demonstrated in a porcine model that polypropylene mesh, coated with minocycline and rifampicin, was able to retard biofilm formation and CC. Microtexturization with metallic nanoparticle technology and carbon nanofilaments are also being explored, but are still experimental at this stage.[95]

SUMMARY

There now exists strong evidence that bacterial contamination of breast implants during insertion is the leading cause of CC. Acknowledging the presence of the additional factors discussed herein, the authors have adopted the following practice points as routine:

1. Administration of intravenous antibiotic prophylaxis at induction
2. Avoidance of periareolar incisions; a dual-plane, subfascial pocket is preferred
3. Use of nipple shields
4. Careful atraumatic dissection to minimize devascularized tissue

5. Avoidance of dissection into the breast parenchyma
6. Thorough and immaculate hemostasis
7. Pocket irrigation with triple antibiotic solution or povidone-iodine
8. Use of new gloves, drapes, and instruments before implant handling
9. Use of an introduction sleeve
10. Minimization of the time of open implant exposure
11. Minimization of manipulation of the implant once in situ
12. Layered closure
13. Avoidance of use of drains
14. Protection of the implant in future procedures with antibiotic prophylaxis

Many of these recommendations are now based on good clinical and laboratory evidence. It is anticipated that ongoing systematic laboratory and clinical research will continue to shed light on both the genesis and prevention of CC. Through such research, clinicians can continue to translate good science into good practice and, ultimately, better outcomes for patients.

Editorial Comments by Bradley P. Bengtson, MD

Capsular Contracture remains the number one complication in nearly every breast implant related study in both reconstruction and aesthetic surgery ever performed. Drs Chong and Deva have among the greatest worldwide experience in both the research of capsular contracture and the Biofilm Theory as a prime factor in its development along with clinical options targeted to decrease its formation. We are slowly progressing from just determining the potential causative factors to employing effective prevention strategies toward the goal of dramatically reducing or eliminating capsular contracture from our practices. Presented are a number of very exciting new findings. It may be that we are on the brink of developing a specific prevention strategy in eliminating the number one implant related complication in our breast implant practices of our time.

REFERENCES

1. Steiert AE, Boyce M, Sorg H. Capsular contracture by silicone breast implants: possible causes, biocompatibility, and prophylactic strategies. Med Devices (Auckl) 2013;6:211–8.
2. Malata CM, Feldberg L, Coleman DJ, et al. Textured or smooth implants for breast augmentation? Three year follow-up of a prospective randomised controlled trial. Br J Plast Surg 1997;50(2):99–105.
3. Cash TF, Duel LA, Perkins LL. Women's psychosocial outcomes of breast augmentation with silicone gel-filled implants: a 2-year prospective study. Plast Reconstr Surg 2002;109(6):2112–21 [discussion: 2122–3].
4. Gabriel SE, Woods JE, O'Fallon WM, et al. Complications leading to surgery after breast implantation. N Engl J Med 1997;336(10):677–82.
5. Cunningham B. The mentor core study on silicone Memorygel breast implants. Plast Reconstr Surg 2007;120(7 Suppl 1):19S–29S [discussion: 30S–2S].
6. Spear SL, Murphy DK, Slicton A, et al. Inamed silicone breast implant core study results at 6 years. Plast Reconstr Surg 2007;120(7 Suppl 1):8S–16S [discussion: 17S–8S].
7. Adams WPJ. Capsular contracture: what is it? What causes it? How can it be prevented and managed? Clin Plast Surg 2009;36(1):119–26.
8. Barr S, Hill E, Bayat A. Current implant surface technology: an examination of their nanostructure and their influence on fibroblast alignment and biocompatibility. Eplasty 2009;9:e22.
9. Bartsich S, Ascherman JA, Whittier S, et al. The breast: a clean-contaminated surgical site. Aesthet Surg J 2011;31(7):802–6.
10. Thornton JW, Argenta LC, McClatchey KD, et al. Studies on the endogenous flora of the human breast. Ann Plast Surg 1988;20(1):39–42.
11. Burkhardt BR, Fried M, Schnur PL, et al. Capsules, infection, and intraluminal antibiotics. Plast Reconstr Surg 1981;68(1):43–9.
12. Deva AK, Chang IC. Bacterial biofilms: a cause for accelerated capsular contracture? Aesthet Surg J 1999;19(2):130–3.
13. Mah TF, O'Toole GA. Mechanisms of biofilm resistance to antimicrobial agents. Trends Microbiol 2001;9(1):34–9.
14. Mah TF, Pitts B, Pellock B, et al. A genetic basis for *Pseudomonas aeruginosa* biofilm antibiotic resistance. Nature 2003;426(6964):306–10.
15. Borriello G, Werner E, Roe F, et al. Oxygen limitation contributes to antibiotic tolerance of Pseudomonas aeruginosa in biofilms. Antimicrob Agents Chemother 2004;48(7):2659–64.
16. Fux CA, Wilson S, Stoodley P. Detachment characteristics and oxacillin resistance of *Staphyloccocus aureus* biofilm emboli in an in vitro catheter infection model. J Bacteriol 2004;186(14):4486–91.
17. Fux CA, Costerton JW, Stewart PS, et al. Survival strategies of infectious biofilms. Trends Microbiol 2005;13(1):34–40.
18. Deva AK, Adams WP Jr, Vickery K. The role of bacterial biofilms in device-associated infection. Plast Reconstr Surg 2013;132(5):1319–28.
19. Leid JG, Shirtliff ME, Costerton JW, et al. Human leukocytes adhere to, penetrate, and respond to *Staphylococcus aureus* biofilms. Infect Immun 2002;70(11):6339–45.

20. Jesaitis AJ, Franklin MJ, Berglund D, et al. Compromised host defense on *Pseudomonas aeruginosa* biofilms: characterization of neutrophil and biofilm interactions. J Immunol 2003;171(8):4329–39.
21. Tamboto H, Vickery K, Deva AK. Subclinical (biofilm) infection causes capsular contracture in a porcine model following augmentation mammaplasty. Plast Reconstr Surg 2010;126(3):835–42.
22. Pajkos A, Deva AK, Vickery K, et al. Detection of subclinical infection in significant breast implant capsules. Plast Reconstr Surg 2003;111(5):1605–11.
23. Netscher DT. Subclinical infection as a possible cause of significant breast capsules. Plast Reconstr Surg 2004;113(7):2229–30.
24. Barr S, Hill E, Bayat A. Patterning of novel breast implant surfaces by enhancing silicone biocompatibility, using biomimetic topographies. Eplasty 2010; 10:e31.
25. Shapiro MA. Smooth vs rough: an 8-year survey of mammary prostheses. Plast Reconstr Surg 1989; 84(3):449–57.
26. Coleman DJ, Foo IT, Sharpe DT. Textured or smooth implants for breast augmentation? A prospective controlled trial. Br J Plast Surg 1991;44(6):444–8.
27. Copeland M, Choi M, Bleiweiss IJ. Silicone breakdown and capsular synovial metaplasia in textured-wall saline breast prostheses. Plast Reconstr Surg 1994;94(5):628–33 [discussion: 634–6].
28. Burkhardt BR, Demas CP. The effect of Siltex texturing and povidone-iodine irrigation on capsular contracture around saline inflatable breast implants. Plast Reconstr Surg 1994;93(1):123–8 [discussion: 129–30].
29. Burkhardt BR, Eades E. The effect of Biocell texturing and povidone-iodine irrigation on capsular contracture around saline-inflatable breast implants. Plast Reconstr Surg 1995;96(6):1317–25.
30. Tarpila E, Ghassemifar R, Fagrell D, et al. Capsular contracture with textured versus smooth saline-filled implants for breast augmentation: a prospective clinical study. Plast Reconstr Surg 1997;99(7): 1934–9.
31. Hakelius L, Ohlsen L. Tendency to capsular contracture around smooth and textured gel-filled silicone mammary implants: a five-year follow-up. Plast Reconstr Surg 1997;100(6):1566–9.
32. Collis N, Coleman D, Foo IT, et al. Ten-year review of a prospective randomized controlled trial of textured versus smooth subglandular silicone gel breast implants. Plast Reconstr Surg 2000;106(4):786–91.
33. Fagrell D, Berggren A, Tarpila E. Capsular contracture around saline-filled fine textured and smooth mammary implants: a prospective 7.5-year follow-up. Plast Reconstr Surg 2001;108(7):2108–12 [discussion: 2113].
34. Poeppl N, Schreml S, Lichtenegger F, et al. Does the surface structure of implants have an impact on the formation of a capsular contracture? Aesthetic Plast Surg 2007;31(2):133–9.
35. Wong CH, Samuel M, Tan BK, et al. Capsular contracture in subglandular breast augmentation with textured versus smooth breast implants: a systematic review. Plast Reconstr Surg 2006;118(5): 1224–36.
36. Barnsley GP, Sigurdson LJ, Barnsley SE. Textured surface breast implants in the prevention of capsular contracture among breast augmentation patients: a meta-analysis of randomized controlled trials. Plast Reconstr Surg 2006;117(7):2182–90.
37. Jacombs A, Tahir S, Hu H, et al. In vitro and in vivo investigation of the influence of implant surface on the formation of bacterial biofilm in mammary implants. Plast Reconstr Surg 2014;133(4):471e–80e.
38. Hu H, Jacombs A, Vickery K, et al. Chronic biofilm infection in breast implants is associated with an increased T cell lymphocytic infiltrate—implications for breast implant associated lymphoma. Plast Reconstr Surg 2015;135:319–29.
39. Vazquez G, Pellon A. Polyurethane-coated silicone gel breast implants used for 18 years. Aesthetic Plast Surg 2007;31(4):330–6.
40. Hester TR Jr, Ford NF, Gale PJ, et al. Measurement of 2,4-toluenediamine in urine and serum samples from women with Meme or Replicon breast implants. Plast Reconstr Surg 1997;100(5):1291–8.
41. Hester TR Jr, Tebbetts JB, Maxwell GP. The polyurethane-covered mammary prosthesis: facts and fiction (II): a look back and a "peek" ahead. Clin Plast Surg 2001;28(3):579–86.
42. Melmed EP. Polyurethane implants: a 6-year review of 416 patients. Plast Reconstr Surg 1988;82(2): 285–90.
43. Hester TR Jr, Nahai F, Bostwick J, et al. A 5-year experience with polyurethane-covered mammary prostheses for treatment of capsular contracture, primary augmentation mammoplasty, and breast reconstruction. Clin Plast Surg 1988;15(4):569–85.
44. Handel N, Silverstein MJ, Jensen JA, et al. Comparative experience with smooth and polyurethane breast implants using the Kaplan-Meier method of survival analysis. Plast Reconstr Surg 1991;88(3): 475–81.
45. Handel N, Cordray T, Gutierrez J, et al. A long-term study of outcomes, complications, and patient satisfaction with breast implants. Plast Reconstr Surg 2006;117(3):757–67 [discussion: 768–72].
46. Barker DE, Retsky MI, Schultz S. "Bleeding" of silicone from bag-gel breast implants, and its clinical relation to fibrous capsule reaction. Plast Reconstr Surg 1978;61(6):836–41.
47. Bondurant S, Ernster V, Herdman R. Safety of silicone breast implants. Institute of Medicine (US) Committee on the safety of silicone breast implants. Washington, DC: National Academies Press (US); 1999.

48. Asplund O. Capsular contracture in silicone gel and saline-filled breast implants after reconstruction. Plast Reconstr Surg 1984;73(2):270–5.
49. Gylbert L, Asplund O, Jurell G. Capsular contracture after breast reconstruction with silicone-gel and saline-filled implants: a 6-year follow-up. Plast Reconstr Surg 1990;85(3):373–7.
50. Handel N, Jensen JA, Black Q, et al. The fate of breast implants: a critical analysis of complications and outcomes. Plast Reconstr Surg 1995;96(7):1521–33.
51. Schaub TA, Ahmad J, Rohrich RJ. Capsular contracture with breast implants in the cosmetic patient: saline versus silicone—a systematic review of the literature. Plast Reconstr Surg 2010;126(6):2140–9.
52. Perrotti JA, Castor SA, Perez PC, et al. Antibiotic use in aesthetic surgery: a national survey and literature review. Plast Reconstr Surg 2001;109(5):1685–93.
53. Courtiss EH, Goldwyn RM, Anastasi GW. The fate of breast implants with infections around them. Plast Reconstr Surg 1979;63(6):812–6.
54. Wiener TC. Relationship of incision choice to capsular contracture. Aesthetic Plast Surg 2008;32(2):303–6.
55. Tebbetts JB. Axillary endoscopic breast augmentation: processes derived from a 28-year experience to optimize outcomes. Plast Reconstr Surg 2006;118(7 Suppl):53S–80S.
56. Giordano PA, Rouif M, Laurent B, et al. Endoscopic transaxillary breast augmentation: clinical evaluation of a series of 306 patients over a 9-year period. Aesthet Surg J 2007;27(1):47–54.
57. Huang GJ, Wichmann JL, Mills DC. Transaxillary subpectoral augmentation mammaplasty: a single surgeon's 20-year experience. Aesthet Surg J 2011;31(7):781–801.
58. Stutman RL, Codner M, Mahoney A, et al. Comparison of breast augmentation incisions and common complications. Aesthetic Plast Surg 2012;36(5):1096–104.
59. Namnoum JD, Largent J, Kaplan HM, et al. Primary breast augmentation clinical trial outcomes stratified by surgical incision, anatomical placement and implant device type. J Plast Reconstr Aesthet Surg 2013;66(9):1165–72.
60. Biggs TM, Yarish RS. Augmentation mammaplasty: a comparative analysis. Plast Reconstr Surg 1990;85(3):368–72.
61. Puckett CL, Croll GH, Reichel CA, et al. A critical look at capsule contracture in subglandular versus subpectoral mammary augmentation. Aesthetic Plast Surg 1987;11(1):23–8.
62. Gutowski KA, Mesna GT, Cunningham BL. Saline-filled breast implants: a Plastic Surgery Educational Foundation multicenter outcomes study. Plast Reconstr Surg 1997;100(4):1019–27.
63. Stoff-Khalili MA, Scholze R, Morgan WR, et al. Subfascial periareolar augmentation mammaplasty. Plast Reconstr Surg 2004;114(5):1280–8 [discussion: 1289–91].
64. Henriksen TF, Fryzek JP, Holmich LR, et al. Surgical intervention and capsular contracture after breast augmentation: a prospective study of risk factors. Ann Plast Surg 2005;54(4):343–51.
65. Stevens WG, Nahabedian MY, Calobrace MB, et al. Risk factor analysis for capsular contracture: a 5-year Sientra study analysis using round, smooth, and textured implants for breast augmentation. Plast Reconstr Surg 2013;132(5):1115–23.
66. Lidwell OM, Lowbury EJ, Whyte W, et al. Effect of ultraclean air in operating rooms on deep sepsis in the joint after total hip or knee replacement: a randomised study. Br Med J (Clin Res Ed) 1982;285(6334):10–4.
67. Mangram AJ, Horan TC, Pearson ML, et al. Guideline for prevention of surgical site infection, 1999. Centers for Disease Control and Prevention (CDC) Hospital Infection Control Practices Advisory Committee. Am J Infect Control 1999;27(2):97–132 [quiz: 133–4; discussion: 96].
68. AORN. Recommended practices for traffic patterns in the perioperative practice setting. Perioperative standards and recommended practices. Denver (CO): AORN, Inc; 2013. p. 121–4.
69. Willis-Owen CA, Konyves A, Martin DK. Factors affecting the incidence of infection in hip and knee replacement: an analysis of 5277 cases. J Bone Joint Surg Br 2010;92(8):1128–33.
70. Gylbert L, Asplund O, Berggren A, et al. Preoperative antibiotics and capsular contracture in augmentation mammaplasty. Plast Reconstr Surg 1990;86(2):260–7 [discussion: 268–9].
71. Khan UD. Breast augmentation, antibiotic prophylaxis, and infection: comparative analysis of 1,628 primary augmentation mammoplasties assessing the role and efficacy of antibiotics prophylaxis duration. Aesthetic Plast Surg 2010;34(1):42–7.
72. Uckay I, Pittet D, Vaudaux P, et al. Foreign body infections due to *Staphylococcus epidermidis*. Ann Med 2009;41(2):109–19.
73. Hardwicke JT, Bechar J, Skillman JM. Are systemic antibiotics indicated in aesthetic breast surgery? A systematic review of the literature. Plast Reconstr Surg 2013;131(6):1395–403.
74. Wixtrom RN, Stutman RL, Burke RM, et al. Risk of breast implant bacterial contamination from endogenous breast flora, prevention with nipple shields, and implications for biofilm formation. Aesthet Surg J 2012;32(8):956–63.
75. Wiener TC. The role of betadine irrigation in breast augmentation. Plast Reconstr Surg 2007;119(1):12–5 [discussion: 16–7].

76. Giordano S, Peltoniemi H, Lilius P, et al. Povidone-iodine combined with antibiotic topical irrigation to reduce capsular contracture in cosmetic breast augmentation: a comparative study. Aesthet Surg J 2013;33(5):675–80.
77. Adams WPJ, Rios JL, Smith SJ. Enhancing patient outcomes in aesthetic and reconstructive breast surgery using triple antibiotic breast irrigation: six-year prospective clinical study. Plast Reconstr Surg 2006;117(1):30–6.
78. Araco A, Gravante G, Araco F, et al. Infections of breast implants in aesthetic breast augmentations: a single-center review of 3,002 patients. Aesthetic Plast Surg 2007;31(4):325–9.
79. Pfeiffer P, Jorgensen S, Kristiansen TB, et al. Protective effect of topical antibiotics in breast augmentation. Plast Reconstr Surg 2009;124(2):629–34.
80. Collis N, Mirza S, Stanley PR, et al. Reduction of potential contamination of breast implants by the use of 'nipple shields'. Br J Plast Surg 1999;52(6):445–7.
81. Mladick RA. "No-touch" submuscular saline breast augmentation technique. Aesthetic Plast Surg 1993;17(3):183–92.
82. Moyer HR, Ghazi B, Saunders N, et al. Contamination in smooth gel breast implant placement: testing a funnel versus digital insertion technique in a cadaver model. Aesthet Surg J 2012;32(2):194–9.
83. Castello MF, Han S, Silvestri A, et al. A simple method to inset and position polyurethane-covered breast implants. Aesthetic Plast Surg 2014;38(2): 365–8.
84. van Heerden J, Turner M, Hoffmann D, et al. Antimicrobial coating agents: can biofilm formation on a breast implant be prevented? J Plast Reconstr Aesthet Surg 2009;62(5):610–7.
85. Dower R, Turner ML. Pilot study of timing of biofilm formation on closed suction wound drains. Plast Reconstr Surg 2012;130(5):1141–6.
86. Fanous N, Salem I, Tawile C, et al. Absence of capsular contracture in 319 consecutive augmentation mammaplasties: dependent drains as a possible factor. Can J Plast Surg 2004;12(4):193–7.
87. Stojkovic CA, Smeulders MJ, Van der Horst CM, et al. Wound drainage after plastic and reconstructive surgery of the breast. Cochrane Database Syst Rev 2013;(3):CD007258.
88. Goldberg HM. Drains and breast implants. Plast Reconstr Surg 1988;81(6):990.
89. Lew DH, Yoon JH, Hong JW, et al. Efficacy of antiadhesion barrier solution on periimplant capsule formation in a white rat model. Ann Plast Surg 2010; 65(2):254–8.
90. Park SO, Han J, Minn KW, et al. Prevention of capsular contracture with Guardix-SG((R)) after silicone implant insertion. Aesthetic Plast Surg 2013; 37(3):543–8.
91. Yang JD, Kwon OH, Lee JW, et al. The effect of montelukast and antiadhesion barrier solution on the capsule formation after insertion of silicone implants in a white rat model. Eur Surg Res 2013;51(3–4): 146–55.
92. Basu CB, Leong M, Hicks MJ. Acellular cadaveric dermis decreases the inflammatory response in capsule formation in reconstructive breast surgery. Plast Reconstr Surg 2010;126(6):1842–7.
93. Hester TR Jr, Ghazi BH, Moyer HR, et al. Use of dermal matrix to prevent capsular contracture in aesthetic breast surgery. Plast Reconstr Surg 2012;130(5 Suppl 2):126S–36S.
94. Jacombs A, Allan J, Hu H, et al. Prevention of biofilm-induced capsular contracture with antibiotic-impregnated mesh in a porcine model. Aesthet Surg J 2012;32(7):886–91.
95. Taylor E, Webster TJ. Reducing infections through nanotechnology and nanoparticles. Int J Nanomedicine 2011;6:1463–73.

Three-dimensional Imaging and Simulation in Breast Augmentation

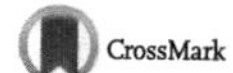

What Is the Current State of the Art?

Mark D. Epstein, MD[a,*], Michael Scheflan, MD[b]

KEYWORDS

- Vectra • Breast augmentation • 3D computer simulation • Breast implants
- Computerized stereoscopic imaging • Photogrammetry

KEY POINTS

- Computerized capture of three-dimensional objects with the ability to create three-dimensional representations (surfaces) is now possible.
- These surfaces can be rotated freely in space
- This technology has been applied to the capture of the female breast.
- Calculations of volume and measurement parameters can be obtained with accuracy.
- Simulations of breast augmentation are possible by treating the breast model as an elastic solid and inserting an implant of known dimensions and volume under the breast.
- Software programmed algorithms are implemented to deform the breast by the implant while maintaining breast tissue volume constant, thereby producing a simulation of the augmented breast.
- This technology has been applied to the consultation process of the breast augmentation procedure, improving patient understanding and facilitating communication between patient and surgeon.

INTRODUCTION

Because the focus of this article is on the current state of the art in three-dimensional (3D) computer simulations in breast augmentation, the historical aspects of the development of this technology are not addressed here. A basic explanation of the method by which 3D images are obtained and processed is presented, followed by a discussion of how this technology is used in the authors' clinical practices. This technology is continually evolving, with major advances not only in the quality and accuracy of image capture but also in the postproduction processing and simulation of potential surgical results.

Classic examples of two-dimensional images are drawings and photographs. Depth perception is the ability to perceive the environment in 3 dimensions, as well as to naturally understand

Disclosures: Advisory board of Vectra imaging system for Canfield Scientific; consultant for Allergan, Inc; developer of Epstein Breast Implant Retractor, Black and Black, Inc; developer of Epstein Breast Retractors, ASSI, Inc; speaker for Pacira pharmaceuticals (M.D. Epstein). Consultant, investigator, and advisory board member for Allergan; consultant for TEI Bioscience, Boston MA; Vectra steering committee member for Canfield Scientific; consultant for Stem Cell Medicine, Jerusalem, Israel (M. Scheflan).

[a] Center for Aesthetic Surgery, 2500 Route 347, Building 22A, Stony Brook, NY 11790, USA; [b] Scheflan Plastic Surgery, 10 Habarzel Street, Tel Aviv 69710, Israel
* Corresponding author.
E-mail address: mepstein@epsteinplasticsurgery.com

Clin Plastic Surg 42 (2015) 437–450
http://dx.doi.org/10.1016/j.cps.2015.06.013
0094-1298/15/$ – see front matter

the relative distance of objects (ie, what is in the foreground vs what is in the background). Two-dimensional images by definition lack true depth and require the intervention of the brain to provide depth by means of a database of monocular visual cues that are created through visual learning over time. Visual cues can be either binocular (based on slightly differing images present by each eye) or monocular (based on cues for which only 1 eye is needed, such as perspective, object size, texture, and grain). Perceptions of depth and 3 dimensions are based on both monocular and binocular cues. In contrast, stereoscopy is the creation or enhancement of the illusion of depth in an otherwise flat, two-dimensional image by creating binocular vision, and is the basis of the technology behind 3D imaging in breast augmentation.

Stereopsis is the perception of 3D structure and depth based on visual information presented to the brain from 2 eyes (binocular vision). Humans, like most other creatures, have 2 eyes that are at the same vertical level on the head, but are at different positions horizontally. When focused on a subject, the images projected on the retinas of each of the two eyes vary very slightly. This horizontal (binocular) disparity is caused by the horizontal separation of the two eyes, also known as parallax. This information is then transmitted to the visual cortex, where the resultant perception is of 3D structure with depth.

A stereoscopic camera has 2 lenses and 2 sensors or film frames positioned at the same vertical level but separated (usually horizontally), producing 2 slightly dissimilar images that, when viewed with a stereoscope (each eye sees only 1 of the 2 different images), the brain perceives as a 3D image. The brain is able to receive these 2 dissimilar images and convert them into a perception of a 3D structure.

Take a photograph and scan it into a computer and look at that photograph on a flat computer screen. Both images are two-dimensional. Any perception of three dimensionality is caused by monocular cues seen on either the original photograph or its scanned-in version. If a photograph of a subject is taken with a stereoscopic digital camera, there are 2 slightly different photographic files and a computer to process them. It now becomes possible to create stereopsis: the perception of 3D realism based on binocular vision as obtained from 2 different digital cameras. This ability is the basis of the current, state-of-the-art 3D imaging.

COMPUTERIZED STEREOSCOPIC IMAGING

When processing binocular images, the brain is trying to reconcile identical visual content shown from 2 slightly different perspectives. A computer does this as well, but in a slightly different way. The surface of an image sensor is divided into a matrix of tiny units called pixels. Pixels are analogous to the rods and cones in the retina. They see color and intensity. In order to reconcile slightly dissimilar images on 2 sensors, pixels that are recording light information on exactly the same tiny portion of the subject need to be matched. To do this, the computer needs an algorithm. For instance, select one pixel from camera A and find the corresponding pixel on camera B, which is recording the same part of the subject. This selection can be accomplished by looking at groups of pixels and concentrating on either defining features or a specific area on the subject. Skin does not have many strong defining features, although skin contains texture, including pores, fine lines, and pigmentation differences, thus providing a pattern to match one camera image against another. An area on one camera's sensor is selected and the computer tries to find a corresponding area on the other camera's sensor by pattern recognition[1,2] (**Fig. 1**).

CAMERA CALIBRATION

The only way to determine where in space a subject lies is to have a method of calibration such that the location of the 2 cameras relative to each other in space is known. One commonly used method is the Tsai algorithm, originally described in 1987. A white card with a series of dots of known distance apart is used, and an L is used as a calibration standard. An image of this card is taken and subsequently the cameras can be calibrated[3] (**Fig. 2**).

Following the Tsai calibration, which calibrates each camera separately, there is a global optimization to refine the accuracy. Photogrammetrists call this bundle adjustment: see Ref.[4] for an example. Once the cameras are calibrated, when an image is taken of a subject, any corresponding point on the subject can be taken and, based on where that point appears on each image sensor, the location of that point in space can be determined. This process is repeated until the entire image is processed and all pixels on the 2 sensors that share a corresponding point on the subject are accounted for. For any image, the clinician can now associated an individual ray in space for each pixel. Where the 2 rays for a given corresponding pair of related pixels intersect in space is a point on the surface of a given subject (**Fig. 3**).

Each image sensor captures a portion of the subject not visualized on the other sensor. These areas that lie in the periphery of the stereoscopic view of the camera are discarded.

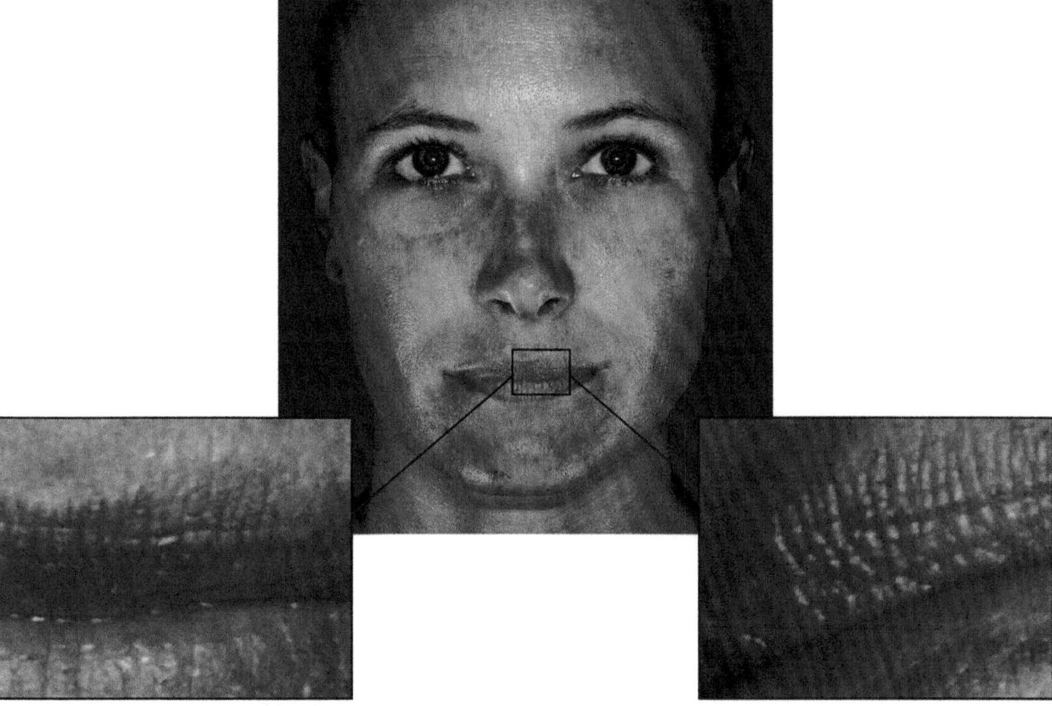

Fig. 1. Two slightly differing images of a woman's lips, with defining features (rhytides) within the lips that make it possible to reconcile the 2 images by pattern recognition. When this process is complete, each pixel on one camera sensor can be made to correspond with another pixel on the other camera's sensor.

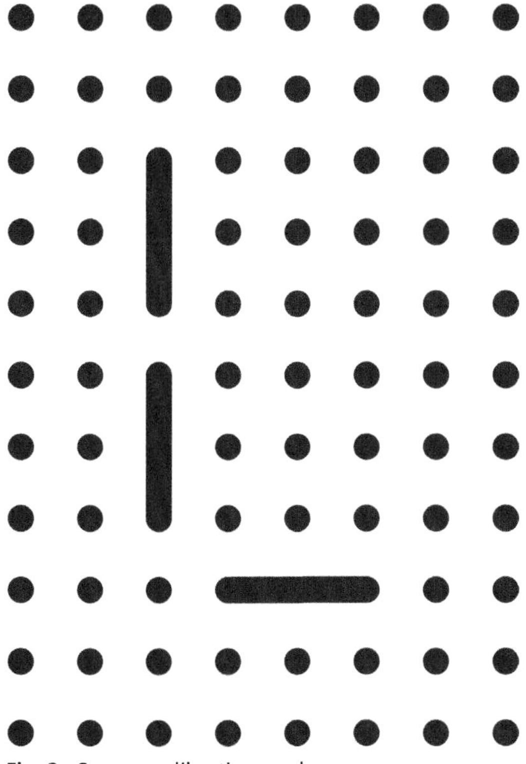

Fig. 2. Camera calibration card.

THE THREE-DIMENSIONAL SURFACE

When all the patches of the subject are assembled, a 3D surface is created. This surface can be rotated in space or manipulated as desired, and is the beginning of a 3D representation of a subject. There are limitations in the quantity of the surface of the subject that can be captured in this manner. A stereoscopic camera set up in this manner cannot capture enough usable surface to permit computerized simulation. To rectify this problem, multiple stereoscopic cameras can be set up and all calibrated together. For instance, if there are 3 pairs of stereoscopic cameras set up to the right, left, and front of the subject; 3 separate, overlapping surfaces can be created. Because all 3 pairs of cameras are calibrated together at the same time, every point in space of each of the 3 surfaces is known. By viewing all 3 surfaces together, the surfaces overlap to produce a seamless, larger 3D surface encompassing approximately 220° around the subject. For every point in space, only 1 pair of cameras is responsible for identifying where a given patch is by deciding which set of cameras is recording the greatest amount of pixels. This process of joining the surfaces together is called stitching (**Fig. 4**).

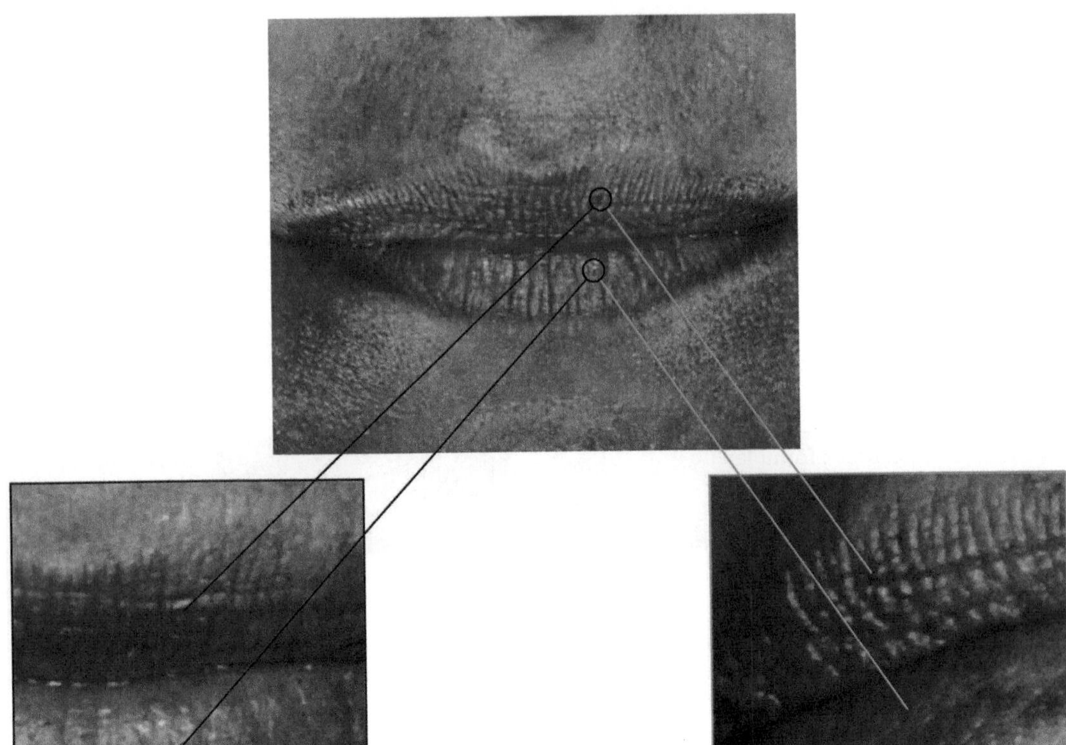

Fig. 3. Two representative points on a woman's lips are shown, along with where they appear on each of the 2 image sensors. Because the relative positions of the cameras are known, the positions of the 2 points on the upper lip in space are determined.

Photogrammetry is the process of obtaining measurements from photographs and determining the exact position of a subject's surface points. Photogrammetry is complex and beyond the scope of this article, but it involves computational geometry, algebra, trigonometry, numerical analysis, calculus, partial differential equations, and statistics!

CREATING A USABLE THREE-DIMENSIONAL SURFACE

At this point, a 3D surface of a woman's anterior chest wall and breasts can be created. A wire-frame model is created by tiling the surface with very small triangles. Color is then projected onto the surface to represent the skin surface.

COMPUTER SIMULATION

In order to perform simulations, the computer algorithms have to be able to interpret the contours of a 3D surface. This interpretation is accomplished through the process of land marking. Earlier versions of software required manual placement of landmarks; however, the process is now automated and fairly accurate. The ability to manually adjust the landmarks improves precision with simulation. The surface may also be cropped as desired. Cropping does not affect the simulations; it only serves to clean the images up from an aesthetic point of view.

The next step is to consider each breast in isolation of the chest wall. A finite element model is used to treat the isolated breast as an elastic solid. Much like the way the surface of a subject is tiled with adjoining triangles, the interior of the breast is filled with adjoining tetrahedrons. A tetrahedron is a polyhedron composed of 4 triangular faces, or sides, and 4 vertices, or corners, where the 3 faces meet. Knowing the volume and quantity of the tetrahedrons permits calculations of volume. The accuracy of these calculations depends on accurate placement of the landmarks that are used to determine the locations of the borders of the breast with respect to the chest wall. After tetrahedralization is completed, the surface of the breast is tiled with triangles and the skin is painted (ie, added) on top (**Fig. 5**).

SIMULATION OF BREAST AUGMENTATION

Once the surface of the breast is defined and its volume is known, simulation of breast

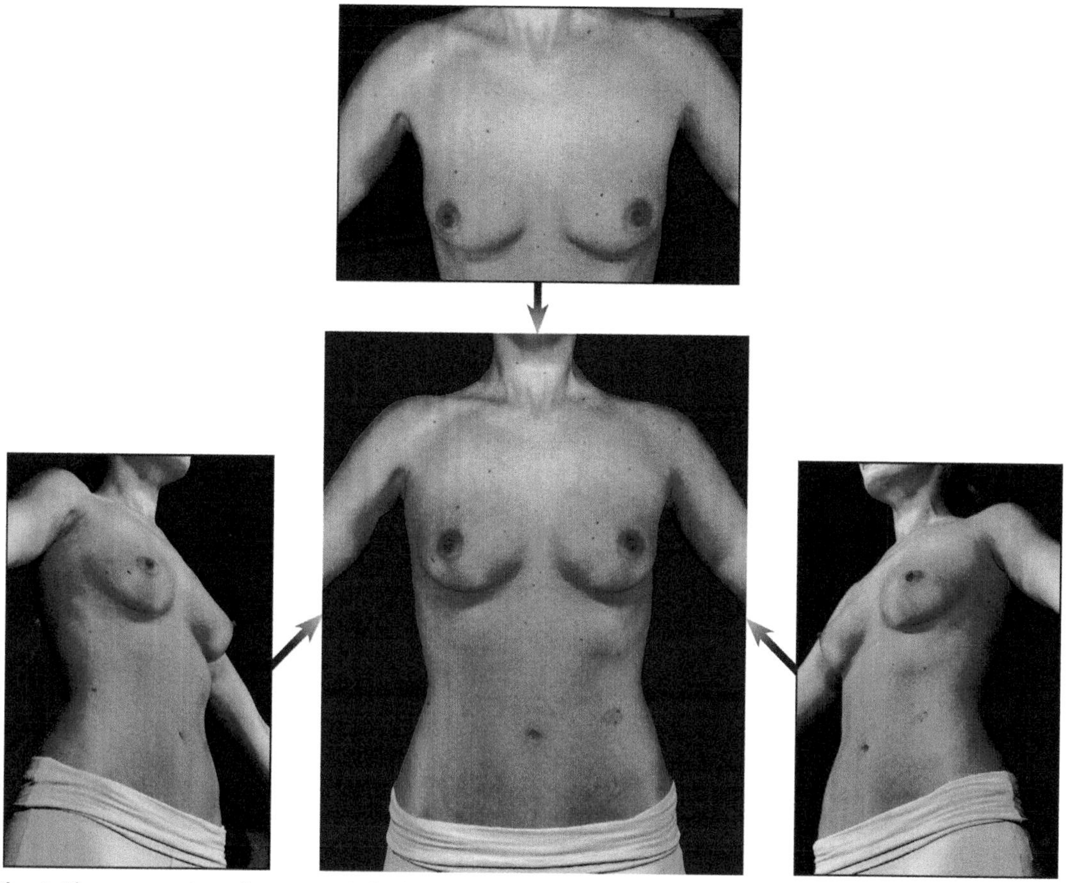

Fig. 4. Three separate surfaces are stitched together to produce a 220° surface.

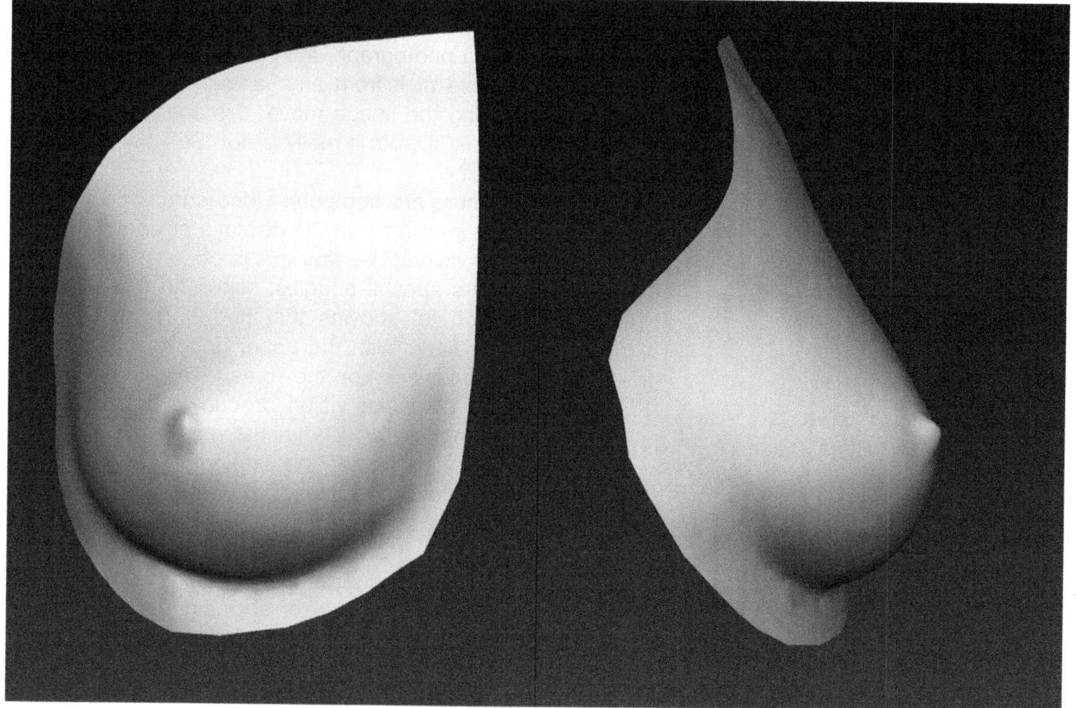

Fig. 5. Isolation of the breast from the chest wall.

augmentation with placement of an implant can be accomplished. A library of different implant shapes (round vs anatomic) can be created with the exact dimensions and volumes of breast implants from several manufacturers. Just as in surgery, in which the breast is detached from the chest wall, this can also be done using computer modeling of the breast. The breast can be treated as an elastic solid and deformed by an underlying implant based on the way the computerized algorithm is constructed. These parameters can be altered to simulate the stiffness of the implant filler. The implant volume is defined, and its shape and dimensions are known and can therefore be represented by tetrahedrons (**Fig. 6**), just as the breasts are. The underlying implant can now deform the overlying breast to simulate augmentation. Because the volume of the breast is known and does not change (not accounting for postsurgical atrophy), the overlying breast can change shape with its volume held constant by the software, thus providing greater accuracy to the simulation process (**Fig. 7**). The final contours of the surface of the torso can be produced, initially as a gray surface (**Fig. 8**). A gray surface is devoid of the distraction of skin texture and color, thus better revealing the surface contours. The skin can then be painted onto the gray surface (see **Fig. 8**).

MASTOPEXY: AUGMENTATION

Once there is a wireframe model of the breast, the surgeon has numerous options. With the right algorithm, the breast contours can be modified as desired. One of the most challenging tasks has been to simulate a mastopexy. This process involves modification of the size and movement of the nipple areolar complex, removal of skin, and reshaping and redistribution of parenchyma. Creating an algorithm to do this is a difficult task, but this has been done for periareolar, circumvertical, and Wise-pattern mastopexies. Once the mastopexy has been simulated and any adjustments in contour made, then an implant can be added to the simulation as described earlier. Again, having control of the total isolated breast volume and keeping it constant allows the clinician to obtain a more realistic result during simulation (**Fig. 9**).

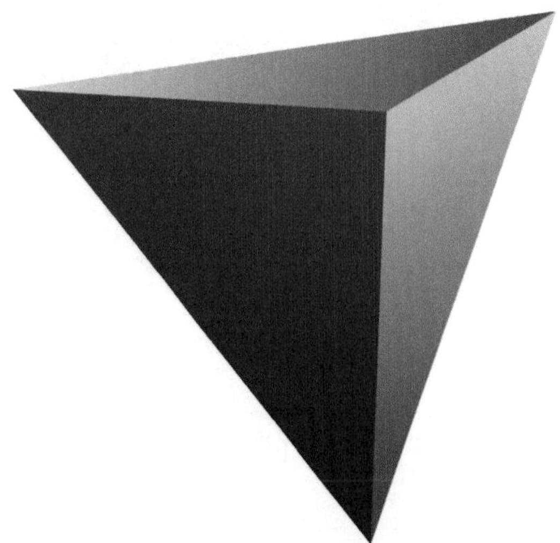

Fig. 6. A single tetrahedron, the basic element of volume in a three-dimensional surface.

IS THIS THREE-DIMENSIONAL?

The computer screen shows a two-dimensional image of a 3D surface. The difference between this 3D surface and a regular jpeg image is that this 3D surface can be freely rotated in space and viewed from any perspective, or manipulated (ie, augmentation) as discussed earlier. The resultant image is still two-dimensional when viewed on the computer screen. However, the act of rotating the image (motion) is a monocular visual cue of 3 dimensionality.

CREATING A TRUE THREE-DIMENSIONAL IMAGE

With a two-dimensional image on the screen that, for all intents and purposes, looks 3D because, unlike a photograph, it can be rotated in space and looked at it from any vantage point. Along with seeing the image move, this cues the brain that this is 3D, but it really is not. So what is the next step?

There are computer video cards and monitors that support true 3D displays of data via binocular vision. The way this is done is that the user wears special goggles, similar to those used to watch 3D movies that had 1 red filter and 1 blue filter. With the paper goggles off, a double image is seen on the screen. That is the technology: binocular vision producing stereopsis; the perception of 3 dimensions. To achieve this with a computer the technology makes a few substitutions. Instead of using a stereoscopic camera, the computer takes the 3D surface and presents it as 2 slightly different images based on a differing perspective. The 3D computer display is capable of showing these 2 images. The paper goggles are replaced by a sophisticated 3D goggle that has 2 shutters in place of the red and blue plastic lenses. These shutters are essentially an LCD screen that can go from

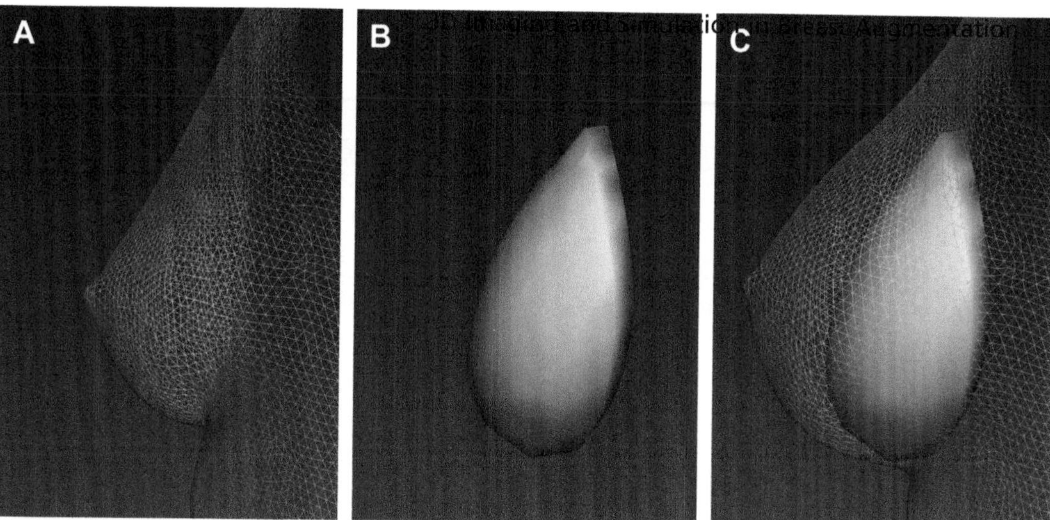

Fig. 7. Tetrahedralization of the breast alone (*A*), implant alone (*B*), and augmented breast (*C*).

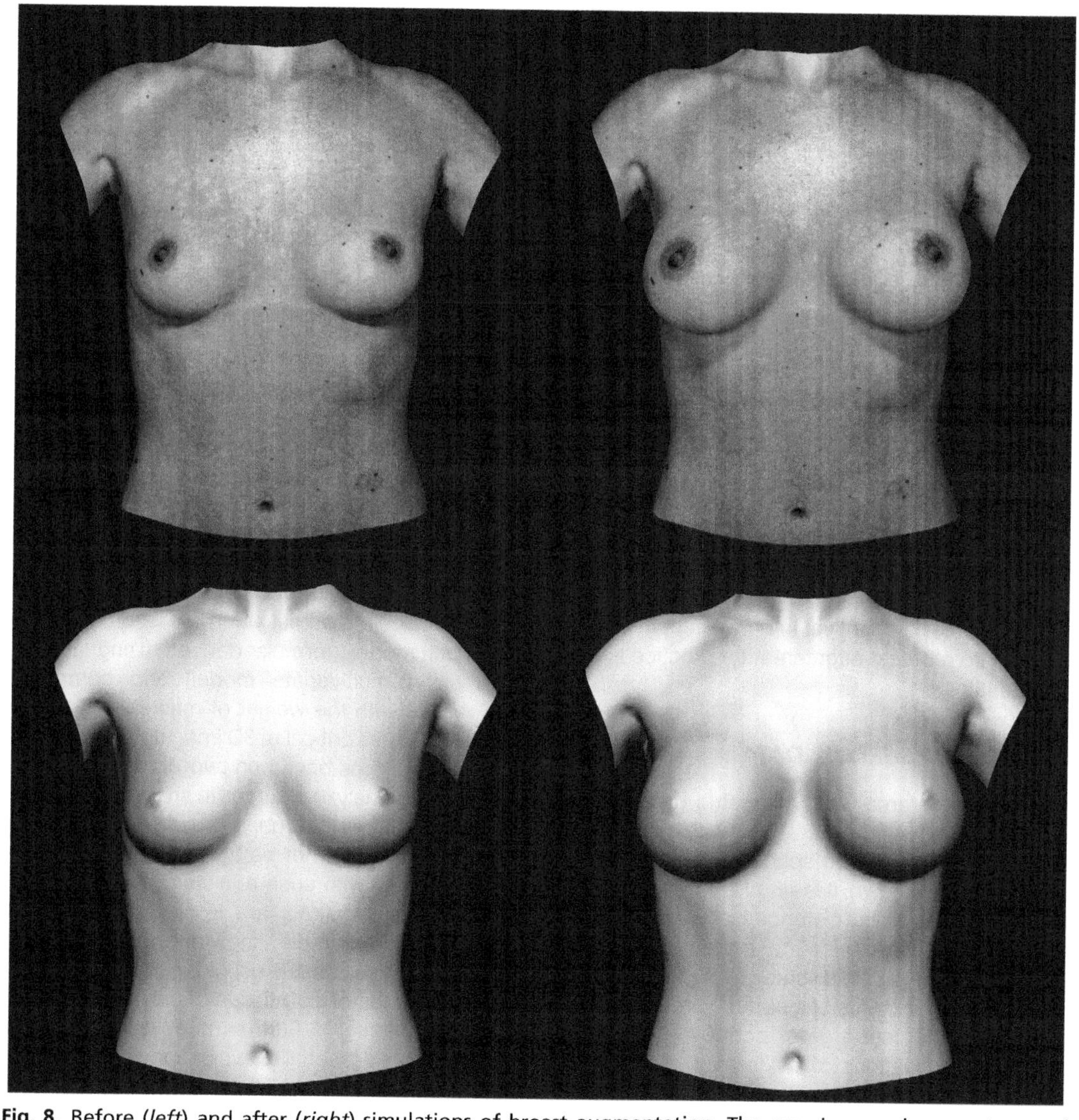

Fig. 8. Before (*left*) and after (*right*) simulations of breast augmentation. The gray images show contour and depth. Next, the skin is then painted onto the gray surface as a final step.

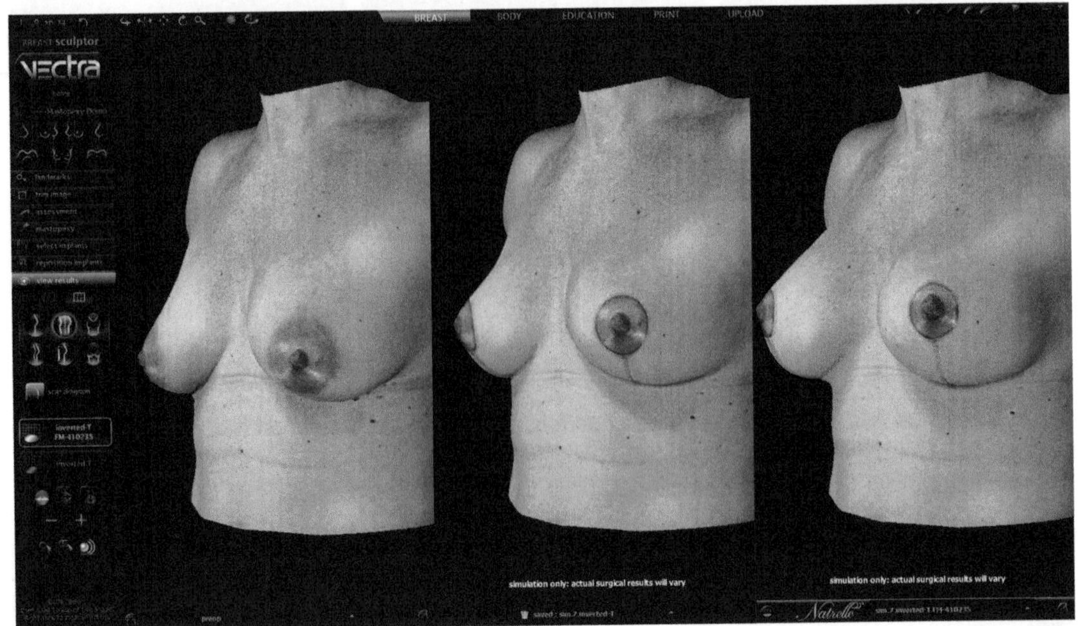

Fig. 9. Before surgery (*left*), simulation of mastopexy only (*middle*), and simulation of augmentation with implant plus mastopexy (*right*).

clear to opaque and back again very quickly. A small infrared transmitter connected to the computer located in the same room sends a synchronization signal to the goggles to tell the goggles which lens is to be opaque and which is to be transparent. This process is in synchronization with the computer display. Now the eyes are receiving a true binocular image of what is displayed on the computer screen.

At this point there is a 3D surface that can be rotated with any degree of freedom, can be morphed to simulate surgery, and can be viewed with a true 3D perspective. Integration of this technology into a breast augmentation practice is discussed later.

ANALYSIS OF SURFACE DATA

Linear, surface area, and volumetric data can be obtained from 3D surfaces with accuracy. Because the location in space of every point on a 3D surface is known, it is simple to make a determination of the linear distance between 2 points, or even to measure the surface area of a section of the surface (eg, keloid scars).[5] Volumetric determinations of segments of a surface are also easily made. The greatest area of controversy is volumetric determinations of the breast as a whole. The breast needs to be isolated from the chest wall and its borders properly defined, which requires 2 processes: accurate placement of landmarks on the breast, especially the medial and lateral breast landmarks; and accurate estimation of the chest wall surface so that the breast can be separated from it.[6,7] Studies have shown high correlation between MRI and 3D imaging techniques with regard to both estimation of breast volume and position of the chest wall.[8,9] One criticism regarding the use of 3D imaging is that this technology is not available to all plastic surgeons. To this end, there are published articles attempting to obtain such data using other means. In one study, anthropometric landmarks were used to calculate breast volume based on a mathematical model (formula derived using a linear regression multivariate model) and comparing the results with the weight of mastectomy specimens.[10] Others critical of 3D imaging have created analysis systems based on two-dimensional photographs to analyze changes in shape and proportion after breast surgery; however, volumetric calculations could not be obtained. This failure is a critical flaw with such a system, because volumetric determinations are important in surgical planning. For example, knowing the difference in breast volume can be used for setting a target for fill volumes of soft tissue expanders in breast reconstruction.[11,12] Furthermore, volumetric calculations are essential to evaluations of fat transfer to the breast,[11] and to analysis after various techniques of breast reduction.[13–15] 3D imaging technology has also been use in planning differential amounts of tissue resection and assessment of postoperative results in breast reduction surgery.[16,17]

THREE-DIMENSIONAL IMAGE CAPTURE, COMPUTER SIMULATION, AND BREAST AUGMENTATION

There are several approaches to using this technology in a clinical breast augmentation practice. The first question to address is whether or not this technology is useful to the surgeon and the patient. One study of patients who underwent breast augmentation using 3D imaging concluded that patients prefer having 3D imaging available; they think that the preoperative computer simulations yielded accurate portrayals of their surgical result, assisted them in choosing an implant; and they would choose the same implant again. An independent panel of surgeons compared the computer simulations with the surgical results and noted the greatest accuracy with regard to breast projection, width and height, with the least accuracy in predicting intermammary distance. Eighty-six percent of patients rated the simulations as very accurate in predicting their surgical result.[18] Another study concluded that 3D computerized imaging is very helpful in implant selection when correcting breast asymmetry during augmentation.[19]

HOW THE AUTHOR INTEGRATES THIS TECHNOLOGY INTO HIS PATIENT WORK FLOW (EPSTEIN)

In speaking with my colleagues who offer this technology to their patients, there are 2 different ways to use this during a patient consultation. The first thing that you must ask yourself when contemplating adding this equipment to your office is the following: do I let the patient guide me in selecting implant size or do I guide the patient? To ask the question another way: do you give the patient sample implants, socks filled with rice, bags of water, and so forth to place into their bras to select implant size or do you follow the principles of soft tissue–based planning[20,21] in selecting an implant size, telling the patient that this is the implant size that they should consider? A discussion of the merits and criticisms of each methodology is beyond the scope of this article so those issues are not addressed here. However, how the data are used and the capabilities of the imaging system are determined by your practice philosophy with regard to implant size selection. My personal bias is toward soft tissue–based planning; however, you can adjust your consultation toward patient selection of implant size if you choose to do so.

IMPLEMENTING THE TECHNOLOGY INTO YOUR CONSULTATION WORKFLOW

First decide who is going to take the images of the patient, and at what point in the consultation this will be done. Some surgeons have a nurse or patient coordinator in charge of the imaging, and even have a dedicated room set up for this purpose. I am going to inject some personal bias into this article because I have had a 3D imaging system (Vectra X3, Canfield Scientific, Fairfield, NJ) since 2009 and have imaged more than 1000 patients with this system.

My preference is to have the imaging system in the same room in which the consultation is conducted. If the patient is imaged in one room and moved to another, there is the inconvenience to consider because the patient is disrobing, getting dressed to move to the examination room, and then disrobing again. This decision is a personal matter for the surgeon. If the imaging system is not in the consultation room, then a computer should be available to the surgeon to display the 3D images. I strongly recommend against doing all imaging activities in one room and the examination in another. The surgeon needs to review the images, as well as the simulations, with the patient during the consultation process.

I have my imaging system in one of my examination rooms and this room is used for all primary breast augmentation consultations. The room is not large, only 2.4 × 3 m (8 × 10 feet), but is just large enough to have the imaging system against a side wall, because I also have a photo studio in the same room, with strobe lighting with soft boxes up on the ceiling in the corners of the room. To save space, I have the computer monitor mounted to the wall to the right of the capture system, with a keyboard and mouse on a keyboard shelf also mounted to the wall just below the monitor (**Fig. 10**). The computer is inside a cabinet in an adjoining room just on the other side of the wall, behind the capture system. This arrangement avoids having a large computer cart in my examination room for which no additional space exists. It is a very clean installation and does not physically get in my way. There is ample room for the patient (and her guests) to stand around the monitor and view the images. Printing hard copy images is essential for the patient to take home and this is done via a network color laser printer (Xerox Phaser 8560, Xerox Corporation, Norwalk, CT) in the surgical coordinator's office. The surgical coordinator sees which images are printed, so

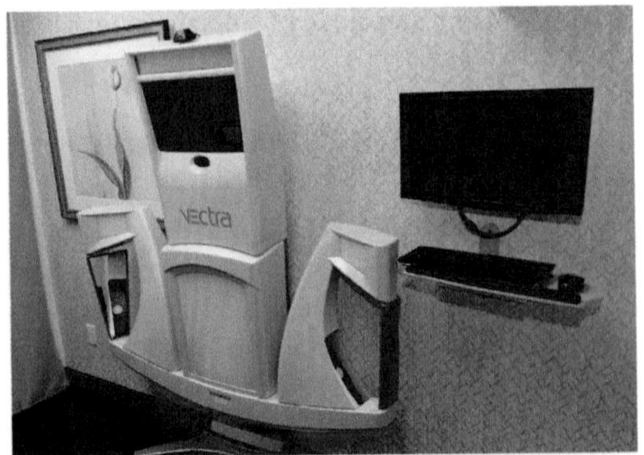

Fig. 10. Installation of Vectra imaging system at the practice of the author MDE. (*Courtesy of* Canfield Scientific, Inc, Fairfield, NJ; with permission.)

she can look at the implant type and create all the relevant quotes before I finish the consultation. Images can also be uploaded during the consultation for the patient to view at home via a secure portal hosted by the imaging system manufacturer. This process also provides metrics that I can analyze to see whether or not my patients are logging in from home, thus allowing me to obtain a cursory gauge of their interest.

After I hold my introductory discussion about breast augmentation, I then proceed with capturing a 3D image of the patient's breasts. While the image is processing, which takes about 1 to 2 minutes, I perform a breast examination and take appropriate measurements of the breasts. Once the image is on the screen, I then adjust the landmarks and save the preoperative image to the chart. Next, I review the measurements obtained and, based on my examination of the breasts and these measurements, I determine what I consider to be the best implant size for the patient. I usually produce a simulation using a round as well as a shaped implant.

Sometimes the patient is totally amenable to soft tissue–based planning as described by Tebbetts[20] and Tebbetts and Adams,[21] but sometimes they want some input in the size based on the images they see. I think that it is very important to caution the patient that the simulations are just that; a computerized estimation of how they will look after breast augmentation. It is important that they understand that they cannot heavily scrutinize the images because the simulation is not an exact representation of how they will look after surgery. It is common for the simulation to make the breasts appear farther apart than they will be, and this seems to be the most common concern that the patients have after surgery, even more than the size. The next issue is size. I try to show how proportionality and aesthetic balance are more important than the numerical size of the implant and the cup size letter. If the surgeon does not get this across to the patient, then the patient will continue pushing for a larger implant than is desired. I explain to the patient how the computer can increase their breast size almost without limits but, in reality, the tissues have limits of elasticity and this must be respected. Sometimes it is helpful to discuss (and show) the consequences of using an implant larger than recommended. The software that my imaging system uses has an array of useful tools that allow me to incrementally increase or decrease the implant size by 1 size at a time, show the simulation in either 1 window by itself or in 2 or 3 windows to show preoperative versus 1-implant or 2-implant scenarios, add a bikini top or tank top, move the images into several different positions for comparison, superimpose preoperative and simulation images, add a mastopexy when indicated, as well as several other useful things.

If you prefer a more patient-directed discussion regarding implant size, you can take a different approach: instead of showing the patient how she would look with the implant that you think is best for her, you may allow her to select implants and then show how she may look with those sizes. I caution against this practice because I think that it may lead to women selecting implants that are too large for their breasts, much like the practice of allowing them to place sizer implants or bags of rice or water inside their bras, but that is a different matter. As much as some patients like using sizers, I never use them during the consultation practice because it can lead to the patient requesting implants that are too large for their breasts, which is against the concept of soft tissue–based planning, and, furthermore, it potentially loses all the benefits gained by using this process for implant selection.

After the surgery is completed, the imaging system is still useful as a means of postoperative documentation of surgical results. I usually take images every 4 months or so for the first year, because the results are generally fairly stable by then, although age-associated changes still occur as time goes on. On the 4-month visit, I obtain a capture of the patient's breasts and then do a side-by-side comparison, preoperative and postoperative, and I conservatively estimate that about 90% of women have forgotten what they looked like before breast augmentation surgery. I then print comparison photos and for them to take home.

If you are following and analyzing your surgical results, even if only subjectively, subsequent 3D image capture is essential. For inframammary incisions, you it provides an excellent view of the scars, which are otherwise often difficult to photograph well with a standard camera, even under the studio lighting conditions that I use. The patients have to lean back, the lighting hits the breasts tangentially rather than straight on, and autofocus based on contrast changes is difficult for faded scars.

For patients who require a mastopexy, 3D imaging can show the results following periareolar, circumvertical, as well as Wise-pattern mastopexies. The resultant image can then be adjusted for placement of an implant as desired.

HOW THE AUTHOR INTEGRATES THIS TECHNOLOGY INTO HIS PATIENT WORK FLOW (SCHEFLAN)

In the last decade, I have been using the process of education, assessment, selection of implants, surgical technique, and postoperative management as described by Tebbetts and Adams[21] for patients having breast augmentation.

In 2008, I added the 3D capturing technology to my practice armamentarium and have captured images of 2451 patients since then.

The 3D imaging technology of Vectra has become an integral part of my everyday practice. It is the cornerstone of my breast and facial documentation, consultation, communication, planning, and assessment of results.

In breast augmentation consults, the system contributes to strengthen, validate, and bring alive my manual measurements and provide a 3D analysis of breast and chest wall shape and symmetry. Often minor asymmetries that were previously unnoticed become apparent and quantifiable.

At this point the surgeon may use the education checklist in the system, pointing out the patient's soft tissues and skeletal particularities and asymmetries and stating that these cannot be completely corrected with surgery. It is used to augment the current informed consent process.

Three-dimensional imaging assists in the choice of implant selection and the formulation of a treatment plan. It is pivotal in simulating outcomes and capturing follow-ups (short and long term), accurately comparing the preoperative with postoperative conditions in 1 click.

Before having the Vectra technology, I used the Bio dimensional system developed by Allergan and Constantin Stan, MD, to help the consultation process. Since then I have used the Allergan Natrelle sizer (**Fig. 11**) kit to add an additional breast on, personal dimension to the patient. I have found that there is good correlation between the 3D Vectra images in clothing and the Bio dimensional shaped sizers in an appropriate bra and tank top. For a while after adopting the Vectra technology, I have thought that patients do not need the sizer step, but have reverted back to doing it following popular demand.

Except for the picture taking, I do it all myself. In most practices, the surgeon does not take the images; instead they are taken by a nurse, a patient coordinator, or a photographer. In other practices the nurse does the measurements and creates simulations ahead of the final discussion with the surgeon, who presents these simulations to the patient and alters them if they do not suit her tastes.

Following are the 10 steps I pursue with patients seeking aesthetic breast enhancement surgery with implants. All are done in 1 room (**Fig. 12**).

1. Relevant medical history.
2. Physical examination and breast measurements.
3. Three-dimensional and two-dimensional picture taking.
4. Put the patient in an appropriate circumference-fitting bra with shaped (back side concave) sizers, selected according to her tissue-based measurements. Add T-shirt top.
5. Sit with patient in front of Vectra screen and select 2 implant scenario options (according to manual and computer-generated measurements) within the suggested range offered by the software, along with the patient's feedback on your proposed in-bra enhancement.
6. Show the patient the before and after options on 1 screen, put her in a bikini top, show the after option (transparent) on top of the before option (solid), and present from all angles.
7. Choose the implants. The decision is made by the patient guided by the surgeon, in front of the screen with the patient still wearing the bra and respective sizers (**Fig. 11**) and tank top in front of the mirror.
8. The last step is a description of the surgery, postoperative management/recovery, and potential adverse events.
9. Questions and answers.
10. The patient now moves to the next room to visit the patient coordinator, receives a quote along with written information, and schedules surgery. All patients return for another, shorter consultation visit before surgery.

Following the introduction and integration of this revolutionary 3D photography system into my structured process of breast augmentation, patient acceptance rates for surgery has significantly increased and the process of the consultation has become more educational, predictable, precise, and enjoyable for patients and surgeon alike.

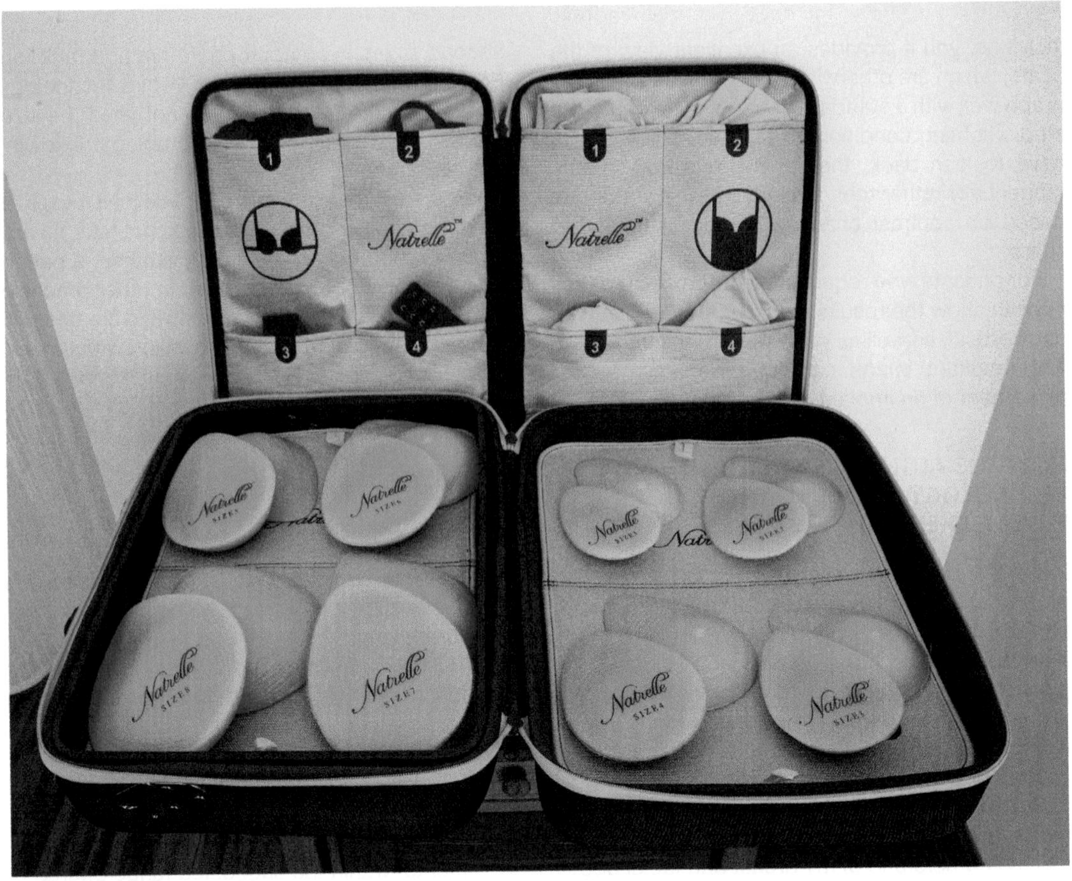

Fig. 11. Sizers used by MS.

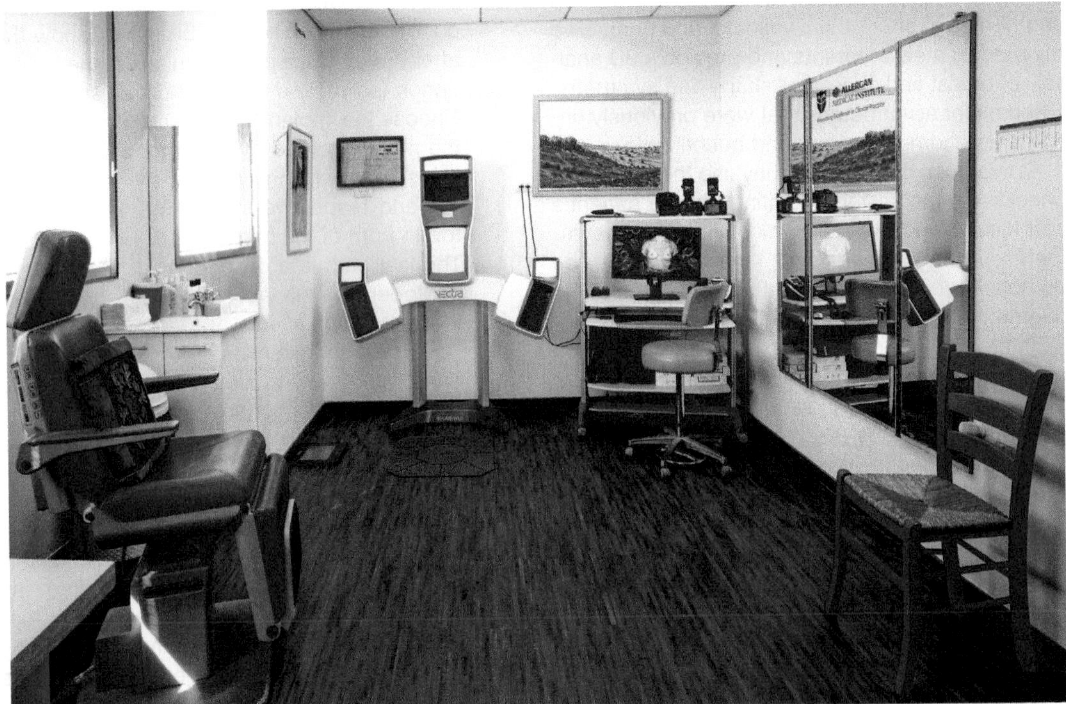

Fig. 12. Installation of Vectra imaging system and examination room at the practice of the author MS.

SUMMARY

Three-dimensional image capture and computer simulation has come a long way since the early days of stereoscopic cameras. The principles of photogrammetry were first described several decades ago, before the existence of the earliest computers. Modern computers permit real-time image processing and analysis as well as prediction of surgical results following breast augmentation. This technology has now been applied in the surgical consult room and has enabled patients to benefit by being offered an enhanced visual understanding of their potential surgical results and by being more involved in the process of implant selection, even if this is directed by the surgeon.

ACKNOWLEDGMENTS

The authors thank the following members of the Vectra team at Canfield Scientific Inc: Dennis O'Neal for his assistance with the illustrations, patient case studies, and video production; Paul Otto and Gideon Amos for their assistance in understanding and describing photogrammetry; and Saija Autrand for her illustrations. Without their assistance, this article would not have been possible.

Editorial Comments by Bradley P. Bengtson, MD

3-D imaging and simulation has absolutely transformed my practice. Although this technology may be used for the face and body, where this technology is the most accurate by far is in the breast. Current systems are so accurate they can predictably simulate outcomes with only a few percent variance from the actual final outcome. I utilize this technology mainly as an educational tool. It allows the surgeon and the patient to align their expectations and for the surgeon to show and highlight asymmetries in ways and positions patients are completely unaware. It is the best way for patients to visualize their range of outcomes, has completely replaced any before and after images to try and compare, and allows the surgeon to show significant asymmetries and walk through the procedure. It also is a great marketing tool: "See your Afters...Before". New modules now also allow for mastopexy simulation, mastopexy with fat transfer and augmentation mastopexy outcomes for comparison. The future is exciting with modules for breast reduction, reconstruction and revision in progress which will allow for removal of devices of known volume or removal of specific volumes to be worked into the simulation.

REFERENCES

1. Otto GP, Chau TKW. 'Region-growing' for matching of terrain images. Image Vis Comput 1989;7(2):83–93.
2. Gruen A. Least squares matching: a fundamental measurement algorithm. In: Atkinson KB, editor. Close range photogrammetry and machine vision. Dunbeath, Caithness (United Kingdom): Whittles Publishing; 1996. p. 217–55.
3. Tsai AR. A versatile camera calibration technique for high-accuracy 3D machine vision metrology using off-the-shelf TV cameras and lenses. IEEE J Robot Autom 1987;3(4):323–44.
4. Triggs B, McLauchlan P, Hartley R, et al. Bundle adjustment – a modern synthesis. In: Zisserman A, Szeliski R, editors. Vision algorithms: theory and practice. New York: Springer-Verlag; 2000. p. 298–372.
5. Stekelenburg CM, van der Wal Martijn BA, Knol DL. More three-dimensional digital stereophotogrammetry: a reliable and valid technique for measuring scar surface area. Plast Reconstr Surg 2013;132(1):204–11.
6. Eder M, Papadopulos NA, Kovacs L. Breast volume determination in breast hypertrophy. Plast Reconstr Surg 2007;120(1):356–7.
7. Swanson EA. Measurement system for evaluation of shape changes and proportions after cosmetic breast surgery. Plast Reconstr Surg 2012;129(4):982–92.
8. Kovacs L, Eder M, Hollweck R, et al. New aspects of breast volume measurement using 3-dimensional surface imaging. Ann Plast Surg 2006;57:602–10.
9. Kovacs L, Eder M, Hollweck R. Comparison between breast volume measurement using 3D surface imaging and classical techniques. Breast 2006;6(2):137–45.
10. Longo B, Farcomeni A, Ferri G. The BREAST-V: a unifying predictive formula for volume assessment in small, medium, and large breasts. Plast Reconstr Surg 2013;132(1):1e–7e.
11. Lewis PG, Mattison GL, Kim HY, et al. Abstract 29: evaluation of 3D photographic imaging as a method to measure differential volumes in reconstructed breast tissue. Plast Reconstr Surg 2014;133(3S):39.
12. Fadl A, Kumar N, Quan M, et al. 121C: using 3-dimensional analysis to quantify volumetric changes in the breast. Plast Reconstr Surg 2010;125(6):83.
13. Choi M, Quan M, Fadl A, et al. Defining pseudoptosis (bottoming out) 3 years following short-scar medial pedicle reduction mammaplasty. Plast Reconstr Surg 2010;126:64.
14. Quan M, Fadl A, Tepper O, et al. 191C: one-year outcome study comparing the bottoming-out process in inferior pedicle versus medial pedicle breast reduction techniques. Plast Reconstr Surg 2010;125(6):125.

15. Quan M, Fadl A, Tepper O, et al. 157C: defining pseudoptosis (bottoming out) 3 years following short-scar medial pedicle reduction mammoplasty. Plast Reconstr Surg 2010;125(6):105.
16. Tepper O. 3D imaging for planning and analysis in aesthetic breast surgery. Plast Reconstr Surg 2009;124(4S):108–9.
17. Tepper OM, Choi M, Small K, et al. An innovative three-dimensional approach to defining the anatomical changes occurring after short scar-medial pedicle reduction mammaplasty. Plast Reconstr Surg 2008;121(6):1875–85.
18. Donfrancesco A, Montemurro P, Hedén P. Three-dimensional simulated images in breast augmentation surgery: an investigation of patients' satisfaction and the correlation between prediction and actual outcome. Plast Reconstr Surg 2013;132(4):810–22.
19. Liu C, Luan J, Mu L, et al. The role of three-dimensional scanning technique in evaluation of breast asymmetry in breast augmentation: a 100-case study. Plast Reconstr Surg 2010;126(6):2125–32.
20. Tebbetts JB. A system for breast implant selection based on patient tissue characteristics and implant-soft tissue dynamics. Plast Reconstr Surg 2002;109: 1396–409 [discussion:1410–5].
21. Tebbetts JB, Adams WP. Five critical decisions in breast augmentation using five measurements in 5 minutes: the high five decision support process. Plast Reconstr Surg 2005;116:2005–16.

Shapes, Proportions, and Variations in Breast Aesthetic Ideals

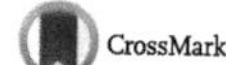

The Definition of Breast Beauty, Analysis, and Surgical Practice

Patrick Mallucci, MBChB, MD, FRCS, FRCS (Plast)[a,b,*],
Olivier Alexandre Branford, MA, MBBS, PhD, MRCS, FRCS (Plast)[a,c]

KEYWORDS

• Aesthetic • Augmentation • Beauty • Breast • Ideal • Natural • Perfect • Proportion

KEY POINTS

- Few studies in the plastic surgical literature are useful in planning an ideal breast.
- Simplicity is key to obtaining consistently beautiful and natural results.
- There are 4 key features that define an attractive breast geometrically.
- The lower pole is critical in determining breast beauty.
- The ICE principle can be used as a template to reliably achieve beautiful breasts.

INTRODUCTION

Many sculpted, painted, and photographed women with beautiful natural breasts have adorned the history of art. However, until recently there have been few objective data in the plastic surgical literature to define an aesthetically pleasing template for breast shape and proportion. An essential part of aesthetic surgery is an understanding of the aesthetic ideals of the body. Such guidelines allow for interpretation, manipulation, and modification to create or recreate a determined aesthetic outcome. The Greeks and the Romans first set out to define ideals of beauty and proportion. Plato compared human proportions with the ideal columns of a Greek temple, while Vitruvius, a Roman author and architect, also spoke of ideal human and facial proportion, and his writings formed the basis of Leonardo da Vinci's Vitruvian Man in the late fifteenth century. In the latter, the division of the face into thirds and fifths form part of the iconic da Vinci images correlating ideal human shape with geometry.

More recently much has been written about such norms, particularly in the face,[1–3] and with regards to orthognathic angles and proportions,[4] which act as guides in facial reconstruction and craniofacial surgery. Similarly, in the nose the precise establishment of nasal proportion by Gunter and colleagues[5] has led to a template for basic nasal ideals: a "map" for aesthetic rhinoplasty. In addition, Burget and Menick[6,7] have described aesthetic units of the nose to serve as a guide for nasal reconstruction.

Financial disclosure: No external sources of support, funding, or benefits were received for this project by any of the authors, who have no commercial interest to disclose.

[a] Department of Plastic Surgery, The Cadogan Clinic, 120 Sloane Street, London SW1X 9BW, UK; [b] Department of Plastic Surgery, Royal Free Hampstead NHS Trust, Pond Street, London NW3 2QG, UK; [c] Department of Plastic Surgery, The Royal Marsden, Fulham Road, London SW3 6JJ, UK
* Corresponding author. The Cadogan Clinic, 120 Sloane Street, London SW1X 9BW, UK.
E-mail address: pat.mallucci@googlemail.com

Clin Plastic Surg 42 (2015) 451–464
http://dx.doi.org/10.1016/j.cps.2015.06.012
0094-1298/15/$ – see front matter

Although much has been written on breast form, it has not been subject to such precise definitions of beauty. Vague terms have often been used to describe desirable characteristics such as proportion, harmony, shape, and flow.[8,9] However, these are not objective or measurable parameters. Others have applied measurements to certain criteria but not as identifiers of beauty or aesthetic ideal. The often referred to "Penn triangle" described an equilateral triangle based on nipple distance from the suprasternal notch observed in a selected group of women with attractive breasts.[10] It does not, however, define shape or form, or any other key components that might be responsible for the attractiveness of those breasts. Indeed, it is perfectly possible to have the Penn dimensions and still have an unattractive breast.

Hauben and colleagues[11] examined breast-nipple-areola proportion in 50 randomly selected female volunteers. Their group included women aged between 24 and 64 years in addition to women with body mass indices ranging from 20.4 to 30.8 kg/m^2. This observational study on a random population showed no correlation of the findings with breast attractiveness.

Fabié and colleagues[12] examined breast proportions in photographs of 70 volunteer women and 1 mannequin, and selected the 10 women who obtained the best scores given by a panel of 20 people including plastic surgeons and lay people. The findings highlighted that nipple position was significant in determining aesthetic proportion in the breast as determined by sternal notch to nipple distance, relative to trunk height. However, the initial population of women included in their study was not selected for the attractiveness of their breasts.

A small study by Hsia and Thomson[13] examined breast profile through hand-drawn line drawings analyzing differences in preference between surgeons and patients, suggesting that the latter prefer a less natural look than the former. Although the numbers are too small to draw any real conclusions, the importance of breast profile was highlighted as a parameter for assessment.

ANALYSIS OF BREAST BEAUTY

The authors previously identified key objective parameters defining the aesthetic ideal of the breast in 2 studies: an observational analysis of 100 models with natural breasts,[14] and a population analysis with 1315 respondents.[15]

In the first of these articles, 100 consecutive topless models with natural breasts were studied. These models were chosen from the Sun newspaper Web site (published in the United Kingdom by News International Ltd). This publication has the tenth greatest circulation in any language in the world, and exclusively photographs topless models who have not had aesthetic breast procedures. The models' breasts were analyzed to establish whether a pattern of identifiable features was common to all of them as clear indices of their attractiveness. Four key features were identified and are shown in **Box 1** and **Fig. 1**.

Perhaps the most significant observation was of the upper pole to lower pole (U:L) distribution, the so-called 45:55 ratio, defining the lower pole as consistently slightly fuller than the upper pole. This observation is a fundamental one, and contravenes conventional notions of upper pole fullness as being a desirable end goal of breast augmentation.

Fig. 2 demonstrates a good result whereby the attractive 4 key features of the breast have been maintained after augmentation. Clinical examples of poor results in aesthetic breast surgery are shown in **Figs. 3** and **4**, illustrating that deviation from these norms yields a less attractive breast: the greater the deviation, the less attractive the breast (**Figs. 3** and **4**).

The importance of these findings lies in the ability to define an "aesthetic template" that might ultimately serve as a guide for surgical planning and implant selection through a better understanding of aesthetic goals.

POPULATION ANALYSIS

As a verification of their previous findings, the authors designed and conducted a population analysis to test the hypothesis that the observations made in the first study[14] were more widely recognized as markers of breast beauty.[15]

A total of 1315 respondents of all ages, sexes, social class, and ethnic backgrounds were asked to rank the attractiveness of images of 4 women with varying breast sizes. Each of the women's breasts were morphed into 4 different proportions: one of the key features was the U:L percentage proportion, corresponding to ratios of 35:65,

Box 1
Critical ideals of breast beauty

- Upper pole to lower pole ratio (U:L) of 45%:55% (ie, slightly fuller lower pole than upper pole): the "45:55 breast"
- Skyward-pointing nipple (20° mean angle)
- Straight/mildly concave upper pole slope
- Tight lower pole convexity

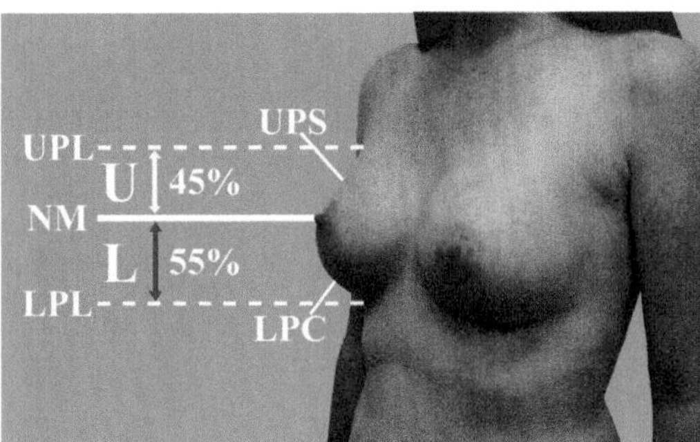

Fig. 1. Representative three-quarter profile view with standard breast parameters as used in the survey: upper pole to lower pole ratio (U:L), nipple angulation, and contour of upper and lower poles. The breast shown has an upper to lower pole ratio of 45:55, straight upper pole, skyward-pointing nipple, and convex lower pole. L, lower pole; LPC, lower pole convexity; LPL, lower pole line; NM, nipple meridian; U, upper pole; UPL, upper pole line; UPS, upper pole slope. (*From* Mallucci P, Branford OA. Population analysis of the perfect breast: a morphometric analysis. Plast Reconstr Surg 2014;134:437; with permission.)

45:55, 50:50, and 55:45. **Fig. 5** shows an example image panel for the patient with a larger breast size. Rankings were analyzed according to population demographics: Effects of age, sex, nationality, and ethnicity were evaluated. The responses of 53 plastic surgeons were also included.

The overwhelming finding from the population study was that all subgroups found the 45:55 proportion across the 4 image panels the most attractive of the breast forms presented. Key findings are shown in **Box 2**.

Comparisons of different demographic groups revealed the most interesting findings of the study, shown in **Figs. 6** and **7**. Perhaps most strikingly, 85% of women younger than 40 years (n = 467) ranked the 45:55 as the most attractive breast type, statistically significantly more ($P < .05$) than the 76% of women older than 40 years (n = 193) (see **Fig. 7**). This observation reflects preference in the prime captive age group for breast augmentation: 7 out of 8 women younger than 40 years had a greater preference for the more natural breast shape as opposed to 1 out of 8 who chose the 50:50 ratio. This finding is clearly an important consideration in planning for breast augmentation for either preference in this cohort. The change in profile selection with age is interesting, with the more mature group choosing more upper pole fullness, perhaps as a reflection of their own loss of projection over time.

Perhaps the most striking observation was that overall, 90% of men (n = 655) ranked the 45:55 as the most attractive breast compared with 82% of women (n = 660) (see **Fig. 7**). This difference was statistically significant ($P<.001$), and is in stark contrast to previously misplaced assumptions that men prefer oversized or "fake" breasts, a view that has long been held as a clichéd interpretation of male preference.

Another commonly held assumption is that cultural/ethnic background has a significant influence on perception of beauty. This population study suggests otherwise and does not support this view: All continents ranked the 45:55 as the preferred breast type, as shown in **Fig. 8**, and even individuals from cultures with the lowest

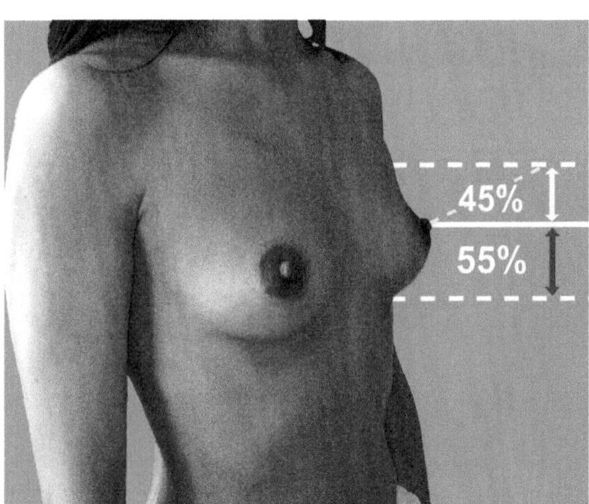

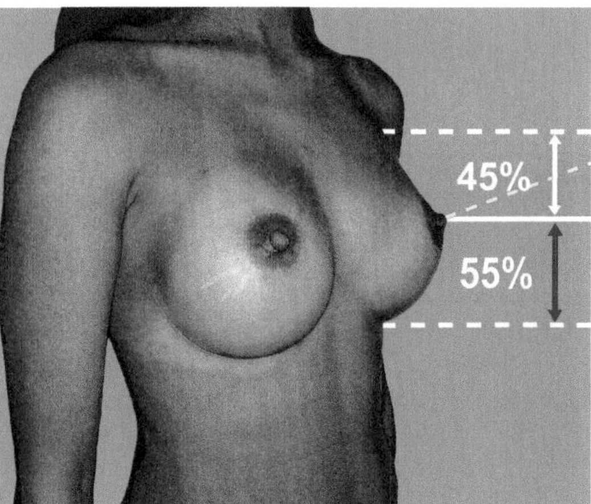

Fig. 2. Breast augmentation patient. (*Left*) Preoperative view. (*Right*) Postoperative view. Three-quarter profile view of a patient with a good result following breast augmentation whereby the 45:55 ratio, upper pole contour, upward-pointing nipple, and lower pole convexity have been maintained. (*From* Mallucci P, Branford OA. Concepts in aesthetic breast dimensions: analysis of the ideal breast. J Plast Reconstr Aesthet Surg 2012;65:10; with permission.)

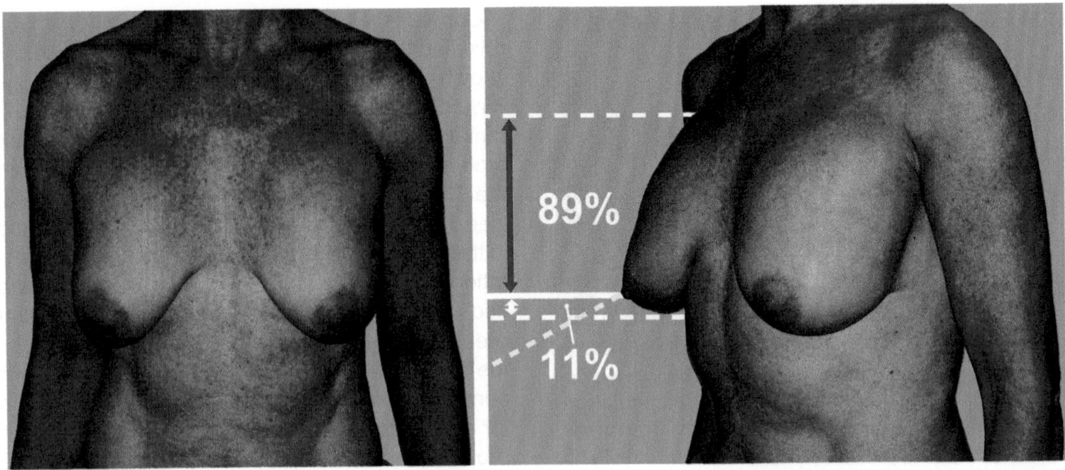

Fig. 3. Analysis of poor postoperative result following breast augmentation. (*Left*) Anteroposterior view. (*Right*) Three-quarter view. The U:L ratio is grossly disproportionate, at 89:11. There is upper pole convexity and downward-pointing nipples. (*From* Mallucci P, Branford OA. Concepts in aesthetic breast dimensions: analysis of the ideal breast. J Plast Reconstr Aesthet Surg 2012;65:12; with permission.)

degree of preference preferred the 45:55 ratio in approximately 75% of cases.

It is also significant that of the 53 plastic surgeons questioned, 94% selected the 45:55 as the preferred "look" even though the majority will not seek to replicate this proportion in patients asking for breast augmentation.

The population study reaffirmed the previous findings that the 45:55 ratio has universal appeal in defining the ideal breast.[14] The observation that in the naked breast a slightly fuller lower pole is more desirable than upper pole fullness is fundamental and is the basis of the 45:55 ratio. The combination of this ratio and the other previously identified parameters visually resonates with all subgroups. Although there is some variation throughout, the overwhelming selection of the 45:55 distribution suggests that breast beauty has universal appeal that largely transcends cultural, sex, and age differences, probably a truism for all things "beautiful" whereby there is a generality of recognition. Past assumptions that a full upper pole is deemed as attractive are not supported by these findings, and as such this study challenges conventional thought about breast attractiveness whereby historically, emphasis has

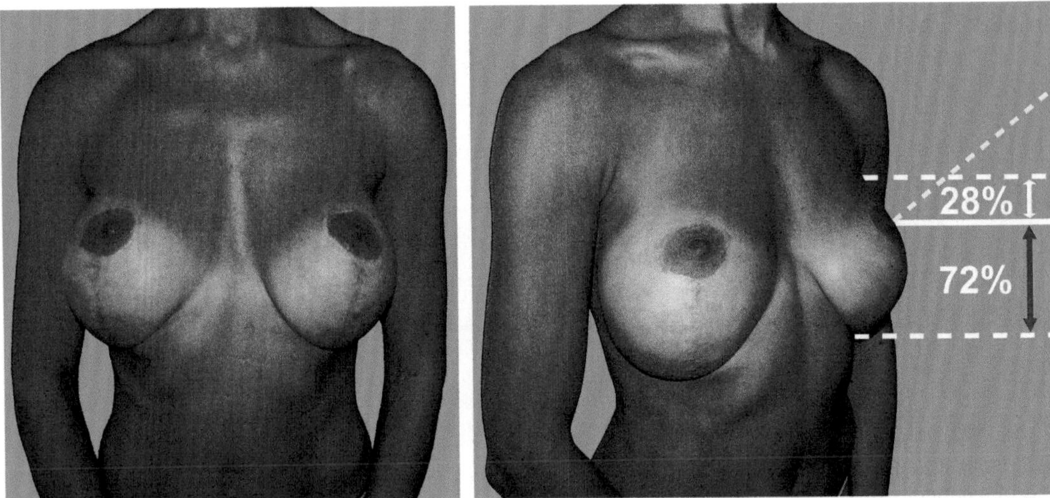

Fig. 4. Vertical scar mastopexy. (*Left*) Anteroposterior view. (*Right*) Three-quarter view. In this case the bottoming out of the breast is associated with a U:L ratio of 28:72. (*From* Mallucci P, Branford OA. Concepts in aesthetic breast dimensions: analysis of the ideal breast. J Plast Reconstr Aesthet Surg 2012;65:12; with permission.)

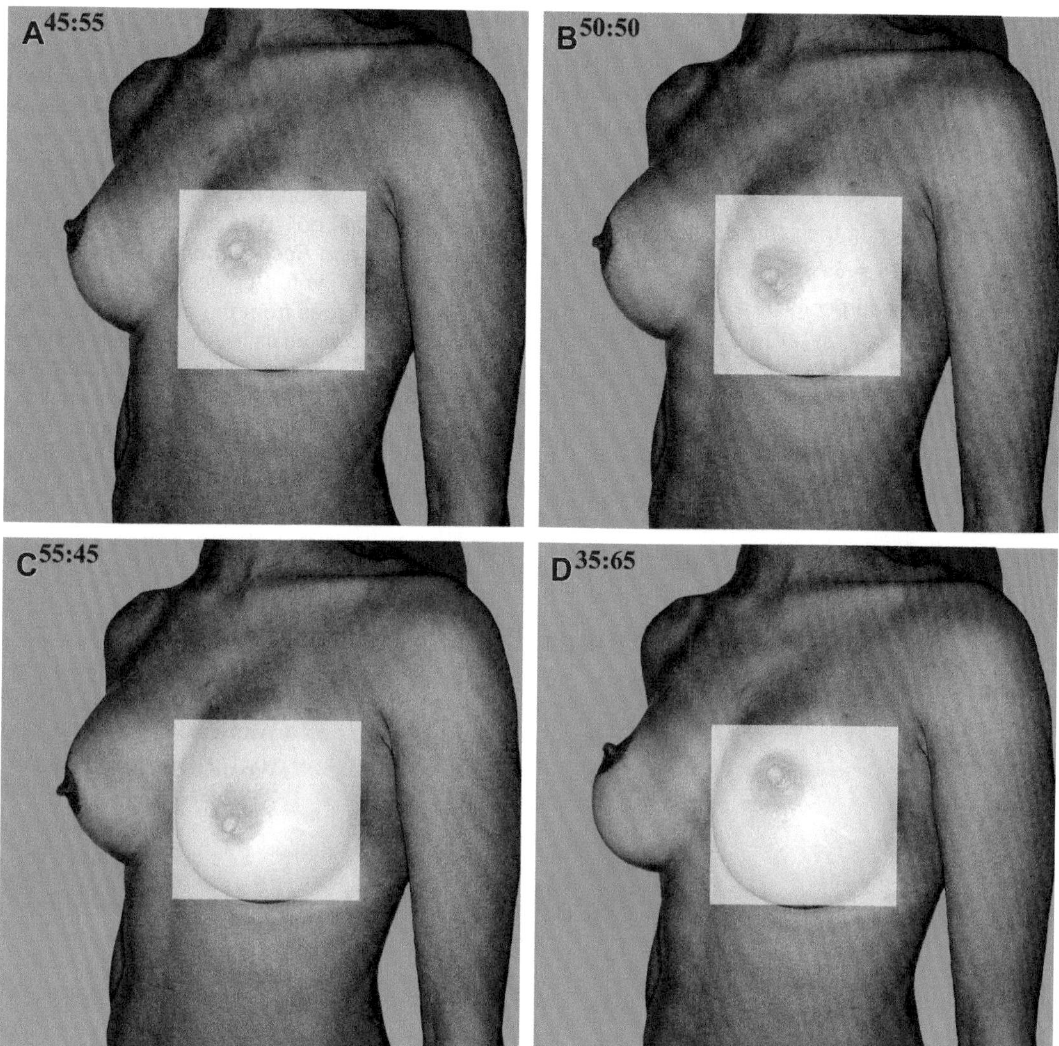

Fig. 5. (*A–D*) Randomized image panel of patient with large breast size. The U:L percentage ratios are shown for each image; these were not shown in the study questionnaire but are shown here for clarity. (*From* Mallucci P, Branford OA. Population analysis of the perfect breast: a morphometric analysis. Plast Reconstr Surg 2014;134:440; with permission.)

been placed on upper pole fullness as a desirable end goal in breast augmentation.

The pressure to fill the upper pole has infiltrated the mind set of both patient and physician, even though there appears to be no evidence that this is a desirable feature to either parties in most cases.[15] The authors postulate that fullness of the upper pole is a desired look in clothing and that women tend to picture themselves clothed rather than thinking of the naked breast. Paradoxically the desired clothed look does not equate to attractiveness in the naked breast; that is, exaggerated upper pole fullness is not attractive out of clothing. This observation is critical for both patient and physician in understanding aesthetic goals. It is a subtle concept that becomes visually obvious when images are shown to patients as part of their discussion.

AESTHETIC TEMPLATE

These 2 studies have together provided the basis for defining an aesthetic template around which to plan and aim for in all forms of aesthetic breast surgery, from reduction/mastopexy to breast augmentation and also in reconstruction.[14,15] The template based on the 45:55 ratio essentially defines the beauty of a natural youthful breast. These

Box 2
Key findings of population analysis of the ideal breast

Breasts with a U:L ratio of 45:55 were universally scored highest, notably by:

- 82% of women overall (n = 660)
- 87% of women in their thirties (n = 190)
- 90% of men (n = 655)
- 94% of plastic surgeons (n = 53)
- 92% of North Americans (n = 89)
- 95% of South Americans (n = 23)
- 86% of Europeans (n = 982)
- 87% of Caucasians (n = 1016)
- 87% of Asians (n = 209)

studies recognize that most women (and men) seek natural beauty in their breasts, and that the desire for an overfilled and oversized look seems to have infiltrated practice without challenge over the past decades. The negative consequences of oversizing are well established and among the most common reasons for reoperation.[16]

A recent online poll (Rohrich, Chief Editor of the journal *Plastic and Reconstructive Surgery*) asked respondents to vote for their favored breast shape using images from the authors' population analysis (http://journals.lww.com/plasreconsurg/Pages/videogallery.aspx?videoId=538&autoPlay=true). Of the 1201 votes cast, the overwhelming majority selected the 45:55 ratio, acting as an independent international validation of the results of the study (**Table 1**).

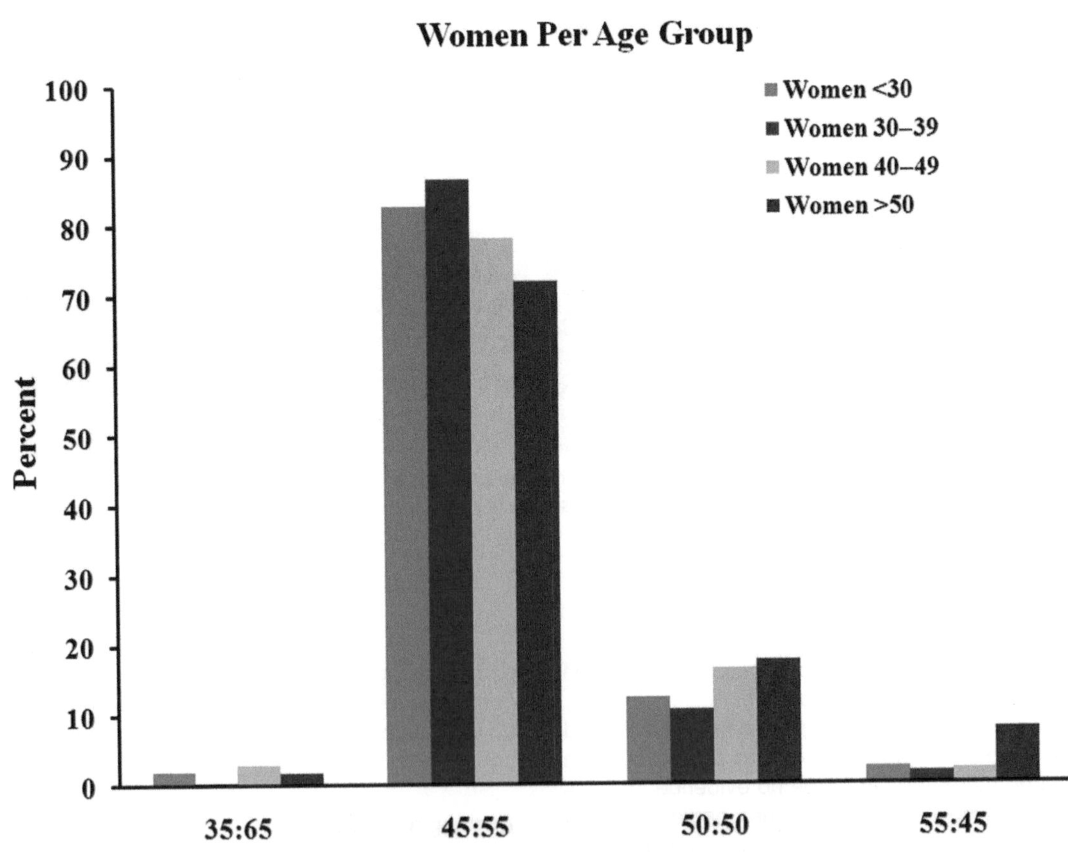

Fig. 6. Mean percentage of women in different age groups choosing each breast proportion as their first choice. There was a statistically significant difference in the percentage of women in their thirties and women in their forties choosing the 45:55 breast type ($P<.05$), with the younger women preferring the more natural 45:55 breast type. (*From* Mallucci P, Branford OA. Population analysis of the perfect breast: a morphometric analysis. Plast Reconstr Surg 2014;134:443; with permission.)

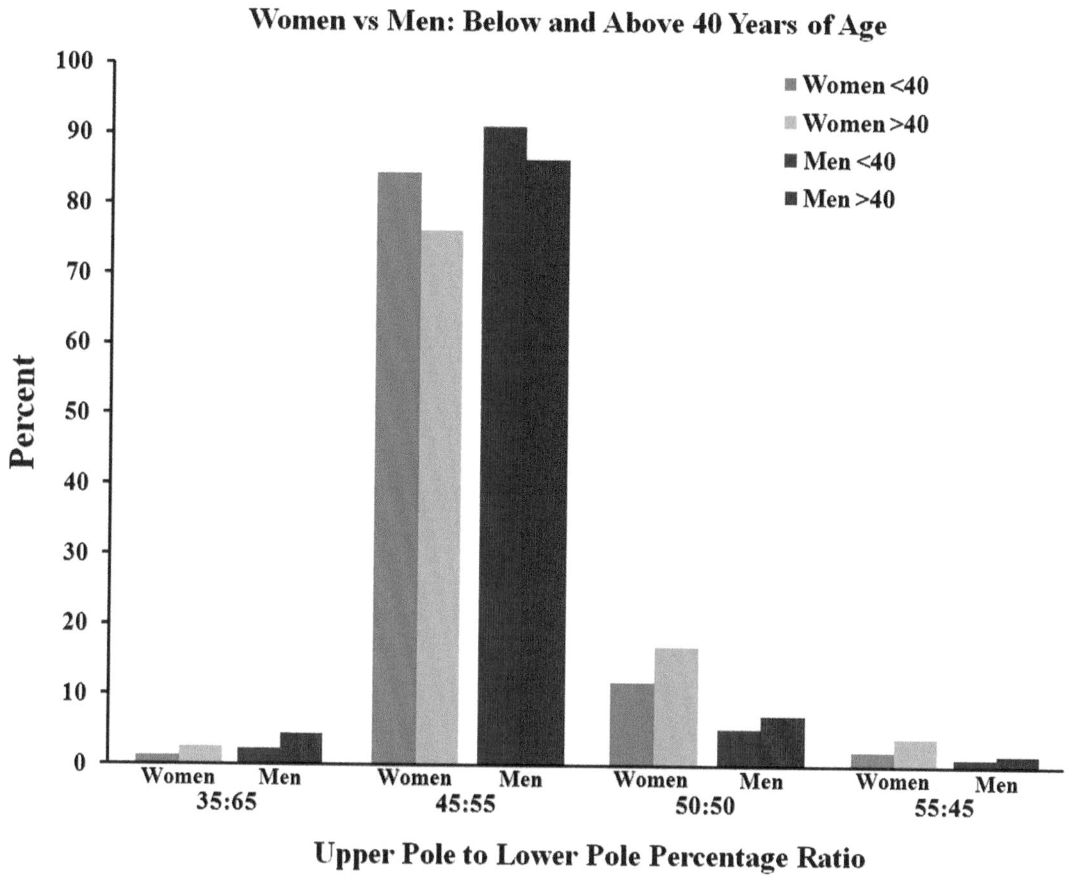

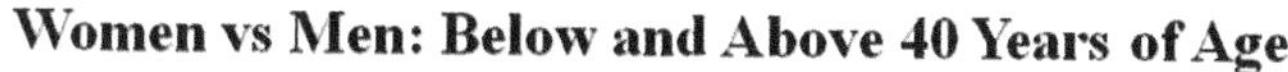

Fig. 7. Mean percentage of women and men choosing each breast proportion as their first choice, subdivided into those younger than 40 years and those older than 40 years for each sex. (*From* Mallucci P, Branford OA. Population analysis of the perfect breast: a morphometric analysis. Plast Reconstr Surg 2014;134:443; with permission.)

There are several examples, from Ancient Greece to the present day, of the 45:55 ratio. The Venus de Milo, long held as a classical and ephemeral icon of nude beauty, has the 4 key features[14] (**Fig. 9**). Manet's Olympia (**Fig. 10**), first exhibited in the 1865 Paris Salon, depicts a woman with these 4 key features and is modeled on Titian's Venus of Urbino (1538). Helmut Newton, a prolific, widely imitated art fashion photographer whose photographs regularly appeared in Vogue and other publications, photographed several women with breasts with the 4 key features.

TREATMENT GOALS AND SURGICAL PLANNING

The breast template described has formed the basis for surgical planning to recreate the 45:55 proportion in breast augmentation. The authors have developed a simple formula to help achieve consistent results: the ICE formula (Mallucci P, Branford OA: Design for natural breast augmentation: the 'ICE' principle. Plast Reconstr Surg. Submitted for publication.) (see later discussion).

Tebbetts and others have advocated the concept of tissue-based implant selection using the template of the breast, the tissue distribution, and quality to guide implant selection rather than to be led solely by patient choice.[17–19] This approach has greatly contributed to a "healthier" selection of implants with the long-term interests of the patient in mind. The combination of this philosophy with aesthetic goals in place leads to an optimal outcome. The quantitative interplay between skin envelope, implant dimensions, and implant placement determines the postoperative proportions, and therefore beauty, of that breast.

In addition, many other systems have been implemented to guide implant selection: biodynamic

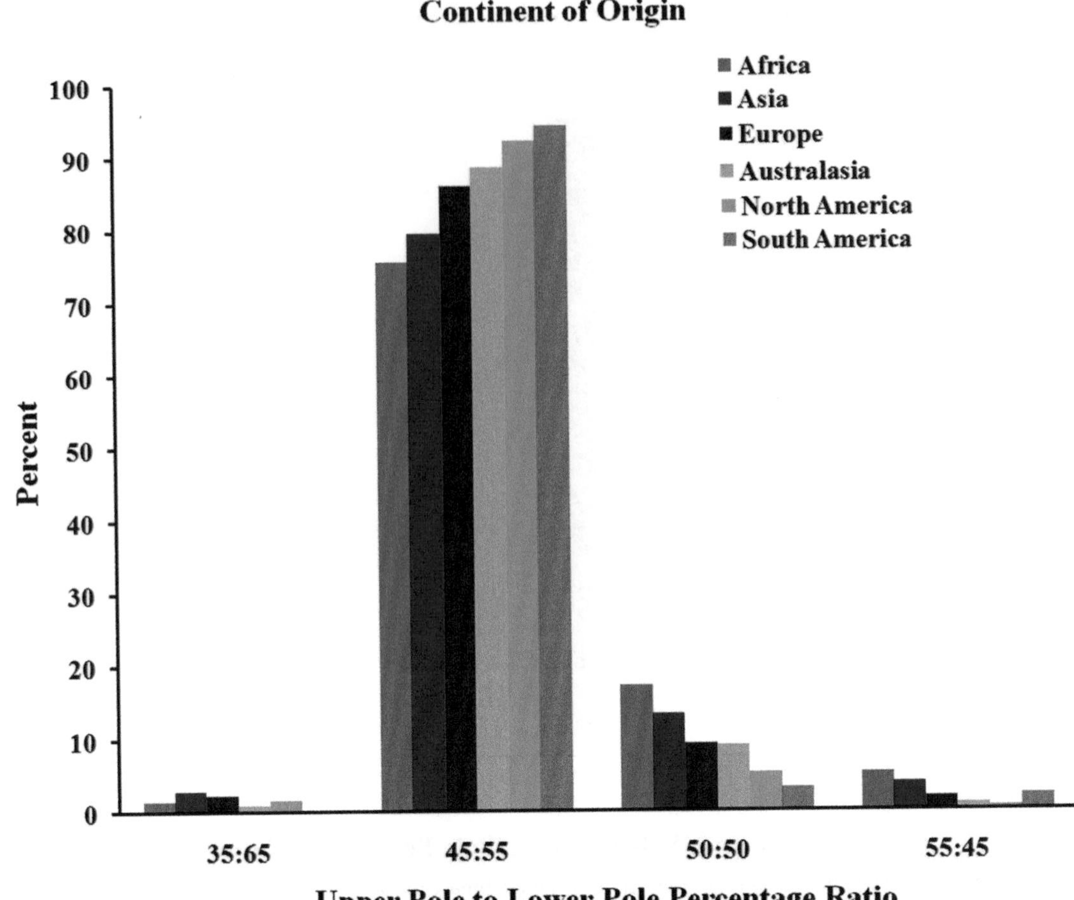

Fig. 8. Mean percentage of respondents from different continents of origin choosing each breast proportion as their first choice. (*From* Mallucci P, Branford OA. Population analysis of the perfect breast: a morphometric analysis. Plast Reconstr Surg 2014;134:445; with permission.)

(Allergan), BodyLogic (Mentor), and Vectra 3D imaging, to name but a few. Although they are useful adjuncts to implant selection for both patient and physician, they fall short of defining the end goal in terms of aesthetic definition of the breast.

Table 1
Votes in online poll for different breast proportions

Upper Pole to Lower Pole Ratio (U:L)	Response (N = 1201)
45:55	70% (n = 839)
50:50	27% (n = 322)
55:45	2% (n = 29)
35:65	1% (n = 11)

The ICE formula (Mallucci P, Branford OA: Design for natural breast augmentation: the 'ICE' principle. Plast Reconstr Surg. Submitted for publication.) is a simplification of previous methods which, though accurate, have often been deemed as complex and difficult for many to put into practice (eg, Heden the Akademikliniken (AK) method). The ICE formula is based around the vertical positioning of the implant relative to the nipple-areolar complex (NAC) and takes into account that a projecting object will recruit skin from the chest wall onto the breast. If that object exceeds the natural capacity of the lower pole of the breast, the inframammary fold (IMF) is lowered as chest wall skin is recruited upward. One of the key calculations is to try to predict this movement and to what extent the fold is lowered, so that the inframammary incision lies in the new fold, or neo-IMF. The authors' preferred incision is via an

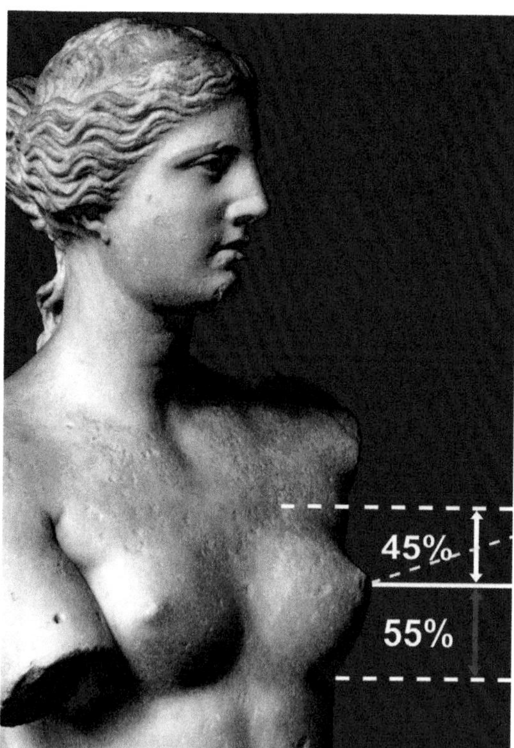

Fig. 9. The Venus de Milo statue at the Louvre, created sometime between 130 and 100 BC, possesses the 45:55 ratio. (*From* Mallucci P, Branford OA. Reply: Population analysis of the perfect breast: a morphometric analysis. Plast Reconstr Surg 2015;135:644e; and *Courtesy of* Plastic and Reconstructive Surgery © 2014, with permission.)

inframammary approach, as its placement is crucial in defining the lower pole of the breast and determines precisely the position of the implant.

MEASUREMENT PRINCIPLES

The authors use breast-base width to act as a guide for initial implant selection, as previously described by many investigators.[17,19]

For a given implant the next most important questions are;

1. What are the demands of the implant on the lower pole of the breast?
2. What is the capacity of the lower pole of the breast?

The capacity of the lower pole of the breast, in simplistic terms, is measured as the distance of from the nipple to the IMF on maximum stretch. The effect of the implant on the capacity will be a function of the height of the implant and how much of that vertical height lies below the level of the NAC, in addition to the projection of the implant away from the horizontal plane. If the latter 2 measurements exceed the natural capacity, the excess will be the extra skin needed to be recruited into the lower pole, namely, the amount the fold needs to be lowered.

To recreate the 45:55 proportion for an anatomic implant, it is positioned at its midpoint relative to the NAC, because the lower half of an anatomic implant is more loaded in volume than the upper half corresponding with the desired look (**Fig. 11**). For a round implant, slightly more of the implant is placed bellow the NAC (ie, 55% and 45% above the NAC) to recreate the differential in volume distribution (see **Fig. 11**).

The 3 key determinants of IMF position are summarized in **Box 3**.

THE ICE FORMULA

In summary, based on previous discussion, the calculation of the new fold position for a given anatomical implant is as follows.

(Implant height/2 + projection) − (Existing capacity (nipple-IMF on maximal stretch)) = Excess skin required *or* distance by which IMF needs to be lowered

or: I − C = E,

where I is implant dimensions (height + projection); C is capacity of lower pole (nipple-IMF on stretch); and E is excess skin required in the lower pole (ie, lowering of IMF).

For example, for an anatomic implant with a height of 10 cm and a projection of 5 cm, if it is placed at the midpoint of the NAC, the vertical height below the NAC is 5 cm + projection of 5 cm, so a total of 10 cm of skin will be required below the NAC.

If the nipple to IMF distance on stretch is 8.5 cm, the degree to which the fold needs to be lowered is:

I = 5 + 5

C = 8.5

I − C = E;

therefore, E = 10 − 8.5 = 1.5: this is the excess skin required or degree to which the IMF needs to be lowered.

If I and C are the same, E = 0; in other words, the IMF does not have to be moved, as the capacity of the breast matches that required for the selected implant.

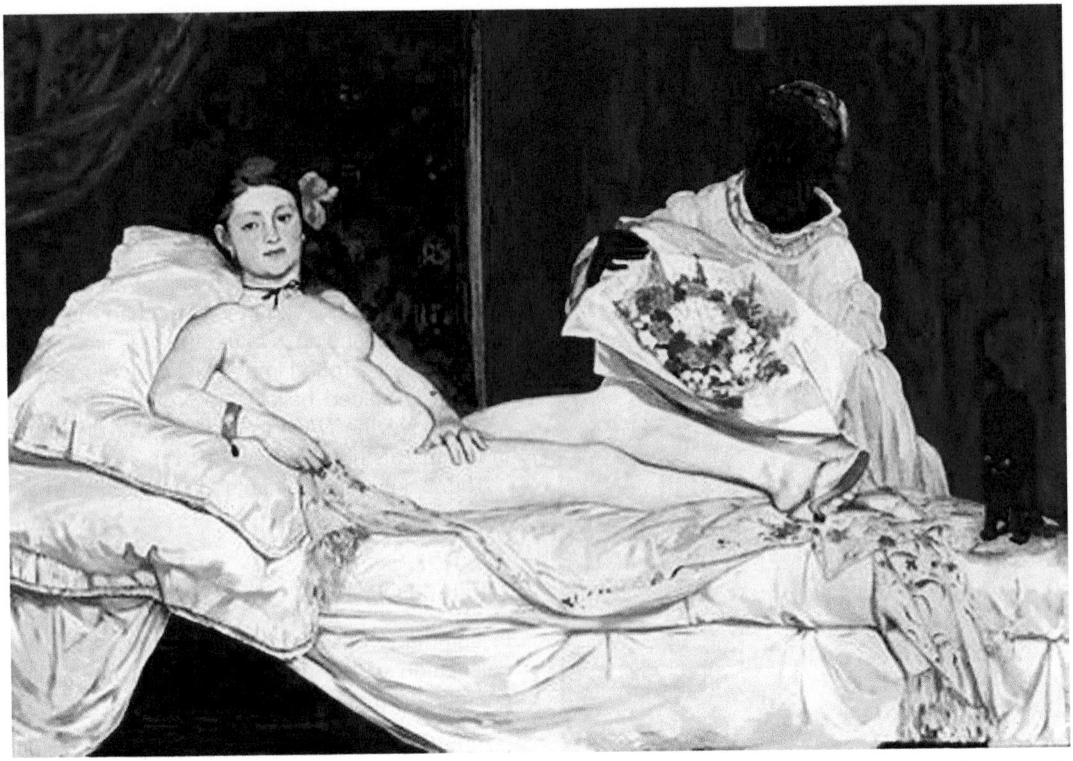

Fig. 10. Manet's Olympia (1860s), also showing the beauty of the 45:55 ratio with a straight upper pole and tight lower pole convexity.

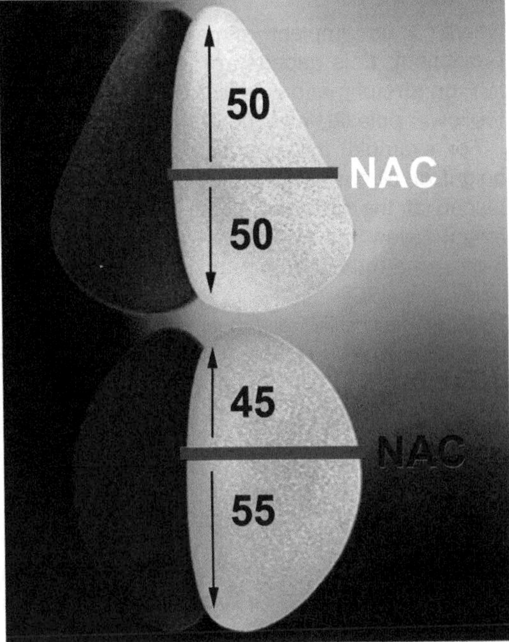

Fig. 11. Diagram showing position of implant meridian relative to the NAC in the ICE formula for an anatomic implant at 50:50 position (above) and a round implant at 45:55 position (below).

If I − C = 2, the fold needs to be lowered by 2 cm. It is then a matter of judgment whether such lowering of the IMF will be suitable for that particular fold or breast to avoid a double-bubble deformity. If this is deemed too big a distance, the wrong implant has been selected and a smaller implant with lesser height and projection needs to be selected such that I − C = 1 or less.

ANALYSIS OF THE ICE PRINCIPLE

To test the accuracy of the ICE formula for producing consistent results, the authors conducted a

Box 3
Key determinants of inframammary fold position

- The vertical position of the implant relative to the nipple-areola complex (note that if this is low, it drives the implant lower)
- Implant projection (as this recruits skin onto the chest wall)
- Capacity of lower pole (ie, nipple–inframammary fold on stretch)

prospective study in 50 consecutive patients undergoing primary breast augmentation via an inframammary incision with anatomic or round implants. The ICE formula was applied to all cases to calculate the position of the IMF.

Patients were photographed preoperatively and postoperatively in standardized three-quarter profile views using high-resolution digital photography. Photographs were uploaded into Adobe Photoshop CS4 (Adobe Systems, Inc, San Jose, CA, USA), and the preoperative and postoperative measurements were made using the ruler function according to the 4 key parameters previously identified.[15] In addition, the position of the IMF scar, as a marker of the overall precision of surgical planning, was measured as a percentage of the distance from the center of the nipple to the new IMF.

A clinical example is shown in **Figs. 12–14**. The ICE formula calculations are shown in **Fig. 12**. In this patient an anatomic implant was used with a height of 10.6 cm and a projection of 4.6 cm, thus giving an implant meridian to lowest aspect of implant height of 5.3 cm (as already described, anatomic implants are loaded in the lower pole, so these are placed at 50:50). The nipple to IMF distance under stretch was 8.5 cm, so in this case:

I. What you need = 9.9 cm = Implant meridian to lowest aspect of implant (5.3 cm) + Implant projection (4.6 cm)
C. What you have = Nipple to IMF distance under stretch (8.5 cm)
E. Extra skin required = What you need (9.9 cm) – What you have (8.5 cm) = 1.4 cm

I = 9.9 (ie, 1/2 of implant height – 5.3 cm + 4.6 cm of implant projection)

C = 8.5 cm (nipple-IMF on stretch)

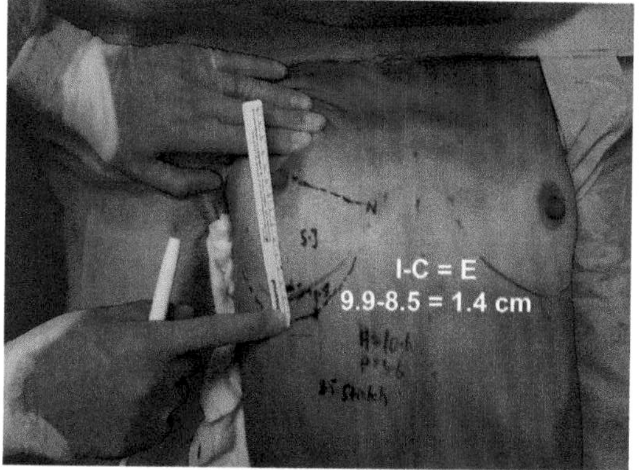

Fig. 12. Intraoperative planning using the ICE formula. Here the I – C = E calculation is shown corresponding to the ICE formula calculation shown in the main text.

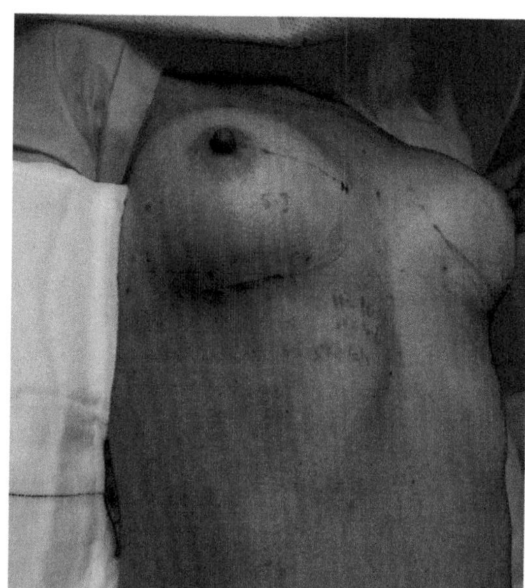

Fig. 13. Intraoperative result using the ICE formula on the patient shown in **Fig. 12**. This photograph shows that the incision ends up precisely in the inframammary fold.

$$I - C = E$$

$$9.9 - 8.5 = 1.4$$

Therefore, the IMF was lowered by 1.4 cm. It is clear from the intraoperative and postoperative photographs that the scar lay precisely in the IMF.

RESULTS

In this study the authors created a system whereby the creation of the look previously defined could be put into practice; that is, to try and replicate as closely as possible the 4 key parameters described earlier.[14,15] The ICE formula has been used to put concept into surgical planning. The 50 patients observed conformed much more closely to the 4 key parameters postoperatively than preoperatively (**Figs. 15** and **16**, **Tables 2** and **3**). If one compares the change in U:L ratios for both left and right sides combined, patients went from a mean preoperative U:L ratio of 52:48 to a mean postoperative U:L ratio of 45:55, an improvement of 7% without mastopexy. Nipple angulation changed from 11° skyward to 19° skyward. The box-and-whisker charts show not only that the medians approximated closely to the 4 key parameters previously described but also that the spread of data was greatly narrowed postoperatively. This result indicates that using the

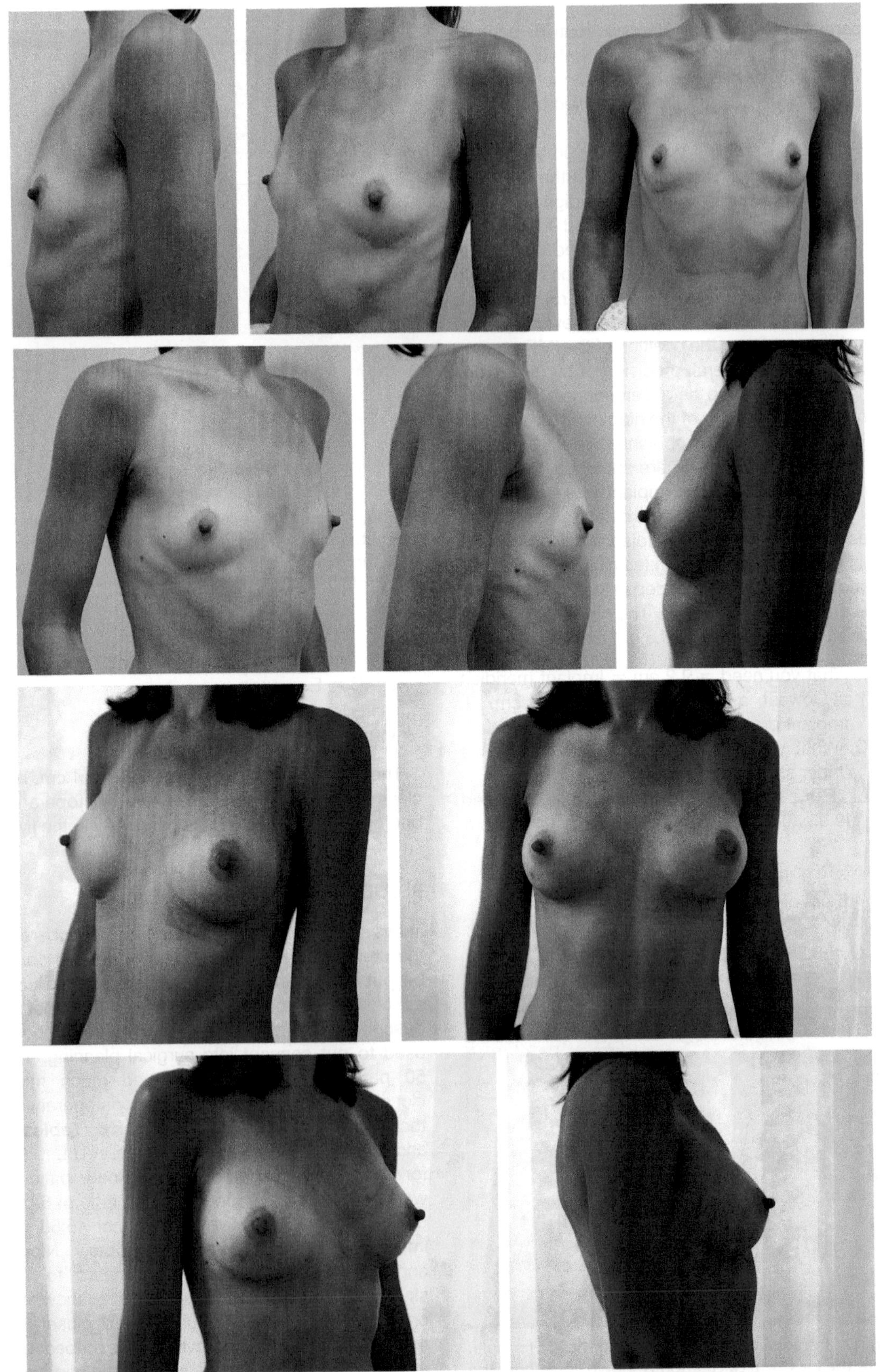

Fig. 14. Preoperative and postoperative pictures of breast augmentation patient shown in **Figs. 12** and **13**.

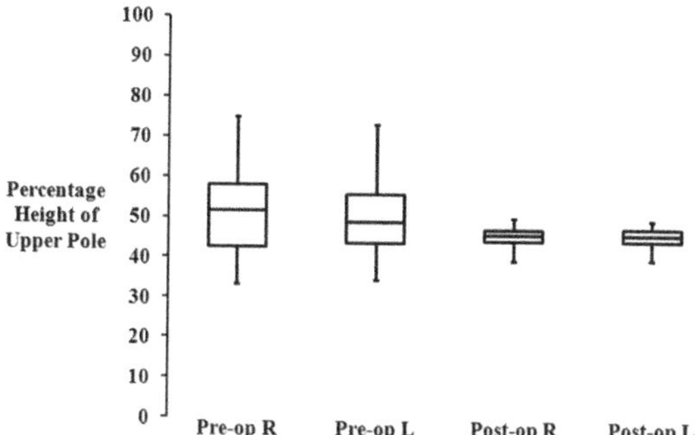

Fig. 15. Box-and-whisker plots of change in percentage of breast attributed to the upper pole for left and right sides, showing close approximation to the 45:55 ratio and reduced spread of data postoperatively. Minimum, maximum, median, and quartiles are shown.

ICE formula reduces variability in outcomes. The accuracy of incision placement relative to the IMF was 99.7% on the right and 99.6% on the left, with a standard error of only 0.2% on both sides. The authors have thus shown, using a simple formula for surgical planning in breast augmentation, that an ideal breast may be achieved consistently and with precision.

DISCUSSION

Tebbetts and Adams[17] have determined the position of the IMF based on implant volume and have also shown, using 5 measurements, that a biodimensional approach to implant selection is crucial in reducing reoperation rates.[17] Hedén has detailed the Akademikliniken method in surgical planning, although this has not yet been published. He uses a large number of parameters, including soft-tissue and implant characteristics, including "lower ventral curvature" of implant, implant height, implant projection, base diameter, breast height, skin elasticity, and glandular thickness, to compute IMF incision placement. There is a difficulty in techniques that take into account too many variables: the complexity may outweigh the usefulness of the techniques, the importance of some variables may be overestimated, and some parameters are in reality difficult to quantify and are therefore open to error.

The ICE formula is a simplification of this, taking into consideration 2 implant parameters (height and projection), and the soft-tissue, base-width, and nipple to IMF-on-stretch values. The results show that despite this simplification, implant position and IMF incision placement are very accurate and crucial to the aesthetic outcome.

Precise location of the incision in the IMF is critical, as it is the defining marker of the lower pole of the breast. Poor incision placement affects implant position and the entire aesthetic of the lower pole of the breast. Although the principle can be applied equally to round or anatomic implants, creation of the "natural look" with a 45:55 outcome undoubtedly lends itself more to anatomic implants. The increasing availability of anatomic implants in the United States following Food and Drug Administration approval may signal a tidal change in approaches to breast augmentation.

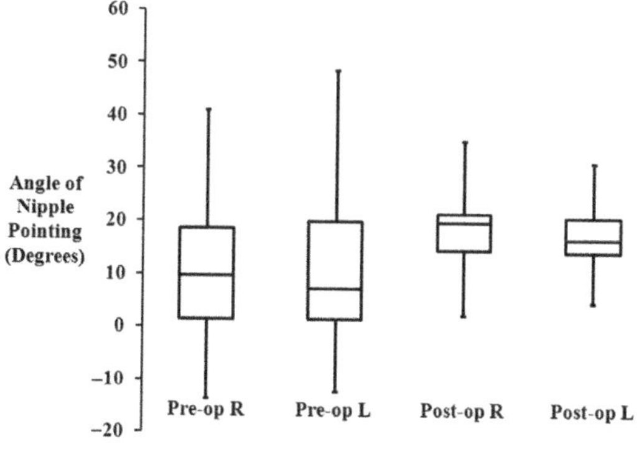

Fig. 16. Box-and-whisker plots of angle of nipple pointing for left and right sides, showing approximation to the 20° skyward nipple angulation and reduced spread of results postoperatively. Minimum, maximum, median, and quartiles are shown.

Table 2
Mean preoperative and postoperative U:L ratio for right (R) and left (L) sides for 50 consecutive breast augmentation patients

Preoperative R	51.5:48.5
Preoperative L	52.6:47.4
Postoperative R	45.3:54.7
Postoperative L	45.5:54.5

Table 3
Mean preoperative and postoperative nipple angulation (°) for right (R) and left (L) sides for 50 consecutive breast augmentation patients

Preoperative R	11.7
Preoperative L	11.2
Postoperative R	18.7
Postoperative L	18.3

SUMMARY

Understanding what constitutes breast beauty is essential for those carrying out aesthetic breast surgery. The authors' published work challenges some preconceived ideas about breast attractiveness. The notion that upper pole fullness is desirable in the naked breast is not upheld by these studies; in fact, the opposite is suggested. A beautiful breast is beautiful in its lower pole; this is the look of a perfectly formed youthful but natural breast, and is the basis of the 45:55 principle. Upper pole fullness is more often a desired look in clothing, and it is important to make this distinction in being able to guide and best advise patients about desired outcomes. The template set out here is intended as an "aesthetic guide" for both patients and surgeons alike. The development of the ICE formula is the practical extension and application of these aesthetic principles. It can be used as a basis for design in breast augmentation surgery to achieve more predictable and consistent outcomes.

The aesthetic ideal presented herein goes very much hand in hand with safe practice, and is an extension of tissue-based implant planning previously described. The end goal is to produce more acceptable, longer lasting results and, ultimately, more beautiful breasts.

Editorial Comments by Bradley P. Bengtson, MD

Few plastic surgeons would argue that the best outcomes and results are a blend of both Art and Science. Leonardo da Vinci was probably the most well-known proponent of attributing mathematical measurements and proportions to the concepts of beauty. Although "beauty is in the eye of the beholder" and there are certainly differences in what plastic surgeons and patients are looking for in breast shapes and volumes, Dr Mallucci has identified four key components that are important in determining aesthetic outcomes. He also points out the opposite being true as well when these key principles are violated or not present preoperatively, the aesthetics of the breast are clearly not ideal. Regardless of your belief or use of measurements, there is no question that plastic surgeons are looking at their breast outcomes in much more objective ways both pre- and post-operatively and the trend is certainly for more objective data to support out aesthetic eye and confirm our concepts of beauty in addition to use tissue based planning to lower our revision rates by respecting breast measurements and tissue tolerances of the soft tissues.

REFERENCES

1. Ricketts RM. Divine proportion in facial esthetics. Clin Plast Surg 1982;9:401–22.
2. Farkas LG, Kolar JC. Anthropometrics and art in the aesthetics of women's faces. Clin Plast Surg 1987; 14:599–616.
3. Powell N, Humphries B. Proportions of the aesthetic face. New York: Thieme-Stratton; 1984.
4. Elsalanty ME, Genecov DG, Genecov JS. Functional and aesthetic endpoints in orthognathic surgery. J Craniofac Surg 2007;18:725–33.
5. Gunter JP, Rohrich RJ, Adams WP Jr. Dallas rhinoplasty: nasal surgery by the masters. St Louis (MO): Quality Medical Publishing; 2007.
6. Burget GC, Menick FJ. The subunit principle in nasal reconstruction. Plast Reconstr Surg 1985;76: 239–47.
7. Burget GC. Aesthetic restoration of the nose. Clin Plast Surg 1985;12:463–80.
8. Brody GS. The perfect breast: is it attainable? Does it exist? Plast Reconstr Surg 2004;113:1500–3.
9. Blondeel PN, Hijjawi J, Depypere H, et al. Shaping the breast in aesthetic and reconstructive breast surgery: an easy three-step principle. Part IV—aesthetic breast surgery. Plast Reconstr Surg 2009;124:372–82.
10. Penn J. Breast reduction. Br J Plast Surg 1955;7: 357–71.
11. Hauben DJ, Adler N, Silfen R, et al. Breast-areola-nipple proportion. Ann Plast Surg 2003;50:510–3.
12. Fabié A, Delay E, Chavoin JP, et al. Plastic surgery application in artistic studies of breast cosmetic. Ann Chir Plast Esthet 2006;51:142–50 [in French].
13. Hsia HC, Thomson JG. Differences in breast shape preferences between plastic surgeons and patients seeking breast augmentation. Plast Reconstr Surg 2003;112:312–20 [discussion: 321–2].
14. Mallucci P, Branford OA. Concepts in aesthetic breast dimensions: analysis of the ideal breast. J Plast Reconstr Aesthet Surg 2012;65:8–16.
15. Mallucci P, Branford OA. Population analysis of the perfect breast: a morphometric analysis. Plast Reconstr Surg 2014;134:436–47.
16. Tebbetts JB, Teitelbaum S. High- and extra-high-projection breast implants: potential consequences for patients. Plast Reconstr Surg 2010;126:2150–9.
17. Tebbetts JB, Adams WP. Five critical decisions in breast augmentation using five measurements in 5 minutes: the high five decision support process. Plast Reconstr Surg 2006;118:35S–45S.
18. Heden P. Mastopexy augmentation with form stable breast implants. Clin Plast Surg 2009;36: 91–104, vii.
19. Adams WP Jr. The process of breast augmentation: four sequential steps for optimizing outcomes for patients. Plast Reconstr Surg 2008;122:1892–900.

The Laminated Nature of the Pectoralis Major Muscle and the Redefinition of the Inframammary Fold

Clinical Implications in Aesthetic and Reconstructive Breast Surgery

Melvin M. Maclin II, MD[a,*], Olivier A. Deigni, MD, MPH[b], Bradley P. Bengtson, MD[c]

KEYWORDS

• Pectoralis major muscle • Inframammary fold • Subpectoral augmentation • Breast augmentation • Breast reconstruction • Acellular dermal matrix • Breast inflection points • Chest wall anatomy

KEY POINTS

- The inframammary fold (IMF) is a critical landmark and aesthetic structure in breast surgery, yet it is poorly understood.
- The skin envelope is considered a separate entity from the chest wall; however, its surgical manipulation is not independent of chest wall anatomy.
- The pectoralis major muscle is a key structure in both cosmetic and reconstructive surgery, and its structure and performance are related to its inferior costal origins.
- A better understanding of the relationship of the IMF, pectoralis, and chest wall anatomy can offer improved outcomes in breast surgery.

INTRODUCTION

The breast is appreciated aesthetically and clinically for its shape, projection, and volume. Multiple techniques have evolved over the years to modify, enhance, or recreate the breast mound. To this end surgical techniques have evolved to manipulate the breast skin envelope, soft tissues, and chest wall anatomy, with and without prosthetic devices. The pectoralis major specifically is altered for pocket dissection and implant coverage. Both the aesthetic and reconstructive surgeons are intimately aware of its relationship to the chest wall and the breast soft tissues. Both are able to achieve outstanding outcomes; however, the authors present an alternative appreciation of the pectoralis and its relationship to the breast. The authors liken the comparison to the tale retold by John Saxe of the 6 blind wise men and the elephant (**Fig. 1**). Although Saxe claims the learned men were wrong, the authors propose to illustrate a broader perspective on the nature of the pectoralis.

[a] Parkcrest Plastic Surgery, 845 North New Ballas Court, Suite 300, St Louis, MO 63141, USA; [b] St Louis University, St Louis, MO, USA; [c] Bengtson Center for Aesthetics & Plastic Surgery, Michigan State University, East Lansing, MI, USA

* Corresponding author.

E-mail address: drmaclin@earthlink.net

Clin Plastic Surg 42 (2015) 465–479
http://dx.doi.org/10.1016/j.cps.2015.06.011

The Blind Men and the Elephant, John Godfrey Saxe (1816–87)

It was six men of Indostan
To learning much inclined,
Who went to see the Elephant
(Though all of them were blind),
That each by observation
Might satisfy his mind.

The First approached the Elephant,
And happening to fall
Against his broad and sturdy side,
At once began to bawl:
"God bless me! but the Elephant
Is very like a WALL!"

The Second, feeling of the tusk,
Cried, "Ho, what have we here,
So very round and smooth and sharp?
To me 'tis mighty clear
This wonder of an Elephant
Is very like a SPEAR!"

The Third approached the animal,
And happening to take
The squirming trunk within his hands,
Thus boldly up and spake:
"I see," quoth he, "the Elephant
Is very like a SNAKE!"

The Fourth reached out an eager hand,
And felt about the knee
"What most this wondrous beast is like
Is mighty plain," quoth he:
"'Tis clear enough the Elephant
Is very like a TREE!"

The Fifth, who chanced to touch the ear,
Said: "E'en the blindest man
Can tell what this resembles most;
Deny the fact who can,
This marvel of an Elephant
Is very like a FAN!"

The Sixth no sooner had begun
About the beast to grope,
Than seizing on the swinging tail
That fell within his scope,
"I see," quoth he, "the Elephant Is very like
a ROPE!"

And so these men of Indostan
Disputed loud and long,
Each in his own opinion
Exceeding stiff and strong,
Though each was partly in the right,
And all were in the wrong!

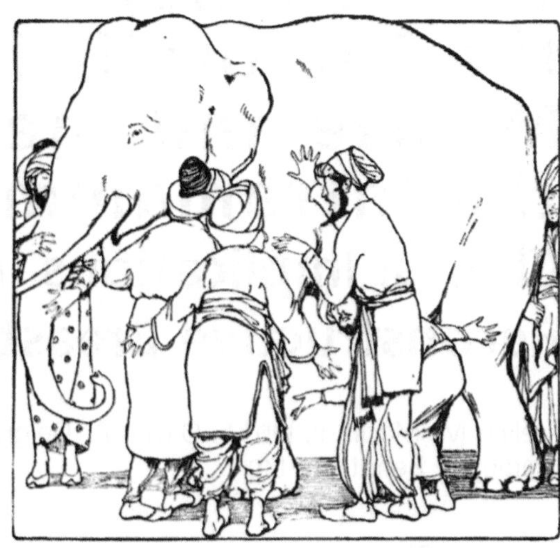

Fig. 1. The blind men and the elephant. (*From* Holton MA, Curry CM. Holton-Curry readers, volume 4. Chicago: Rand McNally & Company; 1914.)

REVIEW OF THE LITERATURE

The IMF is a critical visual marker for the breast, and its importance in both aesthetic and breast reconstruction surgery is the foundation of achieving acceptable results as emphasized by Carlson, the first of the wise men describing the IMF as an aesthetic structure.[1] Yet its structure and definition have been difficult to understand.[2,3] To compound this, the relationship of the IMF with chest wall anatomy is only casually understood. A broader appreciation of the IMF as it relates to the skin, muscle, and chest wall aids in obtaining improved outcomes. Observations from clinical and cadaveric dissection are described to broaden this appreciation.

In a cadaveric study by Maillard and Garey,[4] the IMF was approached from a subglandular approach with the breast soft tissues bluntly dissected off the chest wall until resistance was encountered. A crescent-shaped ligamentous band was identified stretching between the superficial surface of the pectoralis major muscle and the overlying skin. Bayati and Seckel[5] later identified the IMF as a ligamentous structure arising from the periosteum of the fifth rib medially and extending to the interspace between the fifth and sixth ribs laterally. The ligament inserts onto the deep dermis in the region of the inframammary skin fold. In this study, the IMF was approached from a subpectoral approach with the pectoralis bluntly dissected off the chest wall. After avulsion of the insertions of the pectoralis muscle off the fifth rib, the ligament they identified at the inframammary crease resisted further blunt dissection inferiorly. From this resistance the IMF serves a suspensory role. Further dissection beyond this area of resistance risks loss of support structure for an implant and with future bottoming out and double-bubble phenomenon. The second of the wise men describing the IMF as a physical support structure for the implant.

Whether the IMF exists as a ligamentous structure or a dense collagen network, the IMF functions as a zone of adherence between the dermis and the underlying pectoralis fascia.[3] How this zone exists is poorly understood. In a study of 20 fresh cadavers, Matousek and Corlett[6] identified a network of fascial condensations around the breast (**Fig. 2**). This fascial ring around the breast provides fixation between the deep muscle fascia and the anterior breast capsule. Inferiorly from the level of the fifth rib and inserting on the inferior pole of the breast they have named the triangular fascial condensation (**Fig. 3**). Furthermore, they identified short horizontal ligaments arising from the deep fascia of the rectus abdominis to Scarpa fascia and inserting into the inferior limit of the fold. Thus, the third wise man appreciating the IMF as part of the fascial framework of the breast.

The pectoralis and the IMF are considered separate structures that are related only by proximity. As mentioned previously, the relationship with the pectoralis muscle is only vaguely understood. A study by Nanigian and Wong[7] examined the IMF as it relates to the inferior origin of the pectoralis major muscle. In a study of 20 female cadavers and 10 patients with planned mastectomy, the inframammary crease was marked transcutaneously with methylene blue and then approached internally along the superficial surface of the pectoralis muscle. The inferior origin of the pectoralis was identified visually, and the distance to the blue markings was measured. The average distance of the IMF below the visually identified inferior pectoralis origin was approximately 2 cm in both groups. The rib origin of the pectoralis was not identified, and the pectoralis muscle was not dissected from its inferior origin in this study. Madsen and Chim[8] later evaluated the anatomic variance of the pectoralis muscle in the context of breast reconstruction. Fifty patients who underwent mastectomy were evaluated preoperatively and intraoperatively, and the relationship of the pectoralis origin with the IMF was assessed. The

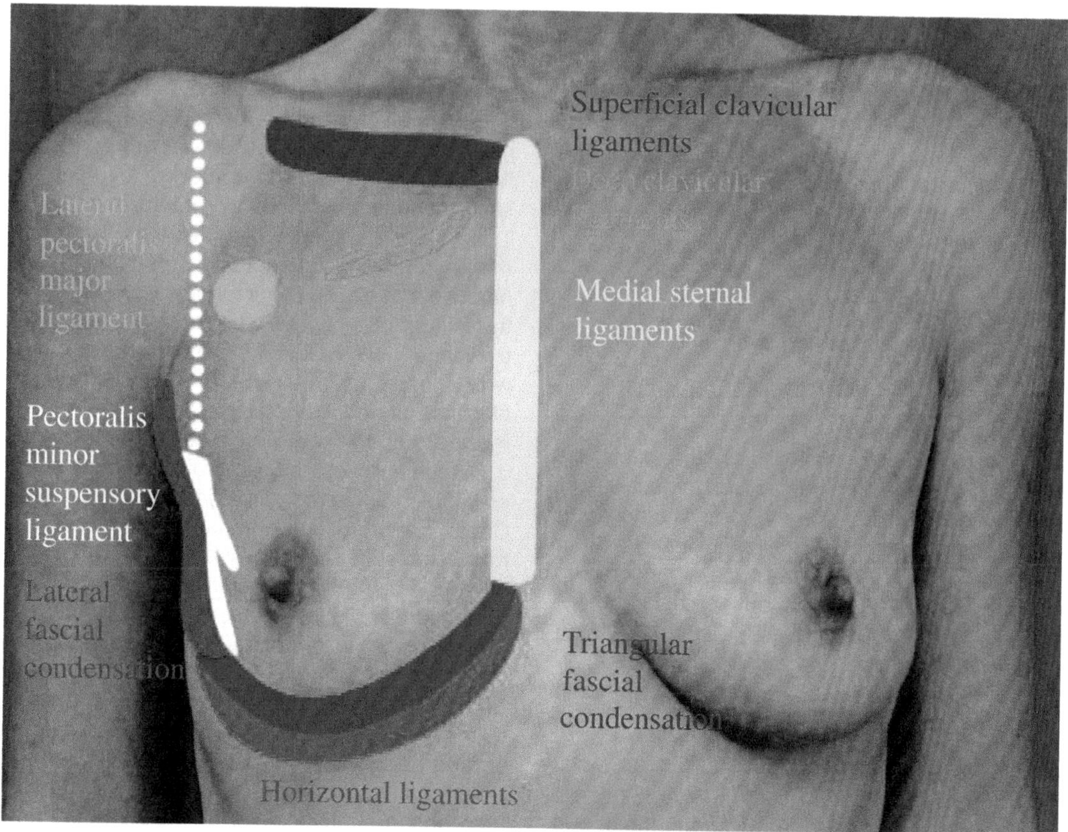

Fig. 2. The surface anatomic landmarks created by the ring of fascial attachments of the breast.

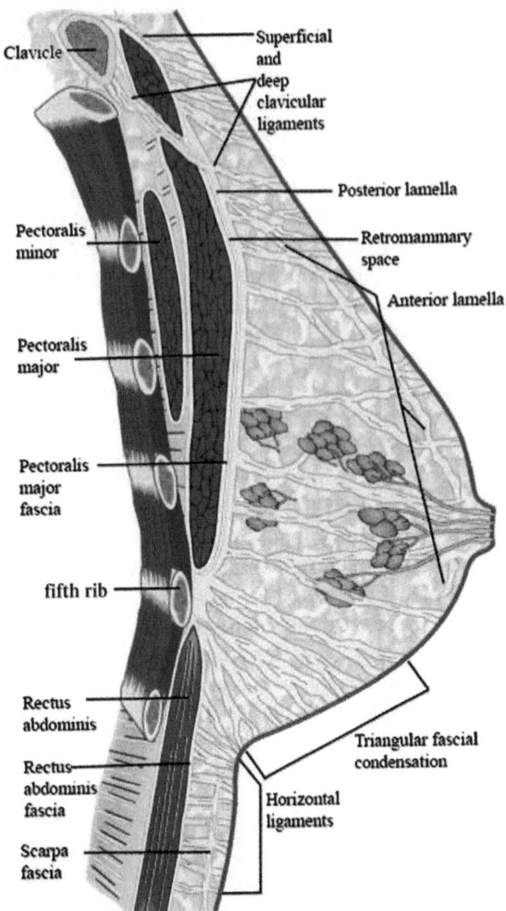

Fig. 3. Diagram of a sagittal section through the nipple, demonstrating the anterior and posterior breast capsule, ligaments, and triangular fascial condensation.

lowest inferior origin of the pectoralis was found at the fifth rib in 12%, sixth rib in 68%, and seventh rib in 20%. The IMF was noted to rest 1 rib level below the pectoralis in 36% of patients and at the same level in 61%. The implications for the anatomic location of the IMF to the pectoralis origin are of particular relevance for breast reconstructive surgery. Here, the fourth wise man who believes the 2 structures have no relationship other than proximity. The structures are considered to exist independently, yet with both breast augmentation and reconstruction the 2 structures have an intimate relationship.

LAMINATED NATURE OF PECTORALIS

Crescent-Shaped Origin of Muscle

The pectoralis muscle is a flat fan-shaped muscle on the anterior chest wall that acts to adduct and rotate the arm. The muscle has a crescentic origin from the medial half of the clavicle, the manubrium and body of the sternum, the costal cartilages of the second to sixth ribs, and the aponeurosis of the external oblique muscle (**Fig. 4**). All fibers converge toward the axilla to merge and insert on the lip of the bicipital groove of the humerus. The medial and inferior origins have the most clinical significance to the breast surgeon.[9]

The muscle is elevated and separated from the pectoralis minor for both augmentation and breast reconstruction to allow submuscular placement of the implant. With dual-plane augmentation and breast reconstruction the inferior origin of the pectoralis is divided.[10,11] Much controversy exists regarding the extent and degree of inferior and medial division. Underdissection can result in undesirable shape and projection.[12] Overdissection can result in symmastia, window shading, and implant malposition.[13]

Dual Layer of Pectoralis

The inferior border of the pectoralis is released off the chest wall to initiate breast reconstruction and with dual-plane augmentation. However, it is in the reconstructive arena where one is able to visualize the transected end of the muscle. In both partial submuscular and acellular dermis-based reconstructions, the free end of the muscle is sutured. After several years of manipulation, it was finally appreciated that the free edge represented only a portion of the muscle. Through serendipitous observation, the retracted edge of the undersurface of the muscle was retrieved to reveal the smooth undersurface of the pectoralis (**Fig. 5**). This observation spawned the hypothesis that the pectoralis muscle actually represents a laminated structure at the inferiormost level. When the inferior edge of the muscle is secured, one is traditionally only manipulating the superficial layer, while the deeper layer retracts superiorly. The significance of an incompletely controlled pectoralis muscle is addressed later.

Careful review of the pectoralis anatomy reveals an inferior origin from the fifth and sixth ribs.[9] Cadaveric dissection into the substance of the muscle identified a deep layer coming off the fifth rib and a superficial layer from the sixth. Blunt dissection easily separates the layers, with the deeper plane representing approximately 30% of the muscle volume (**Fig. 6**). When the inferior border of the pectoralis is manipulated, only the superficial layer is being secured, unless the retracted deeper layer is deliberately retrieved and included with the superficial layer. The fifth wise man only appreciates the pectoralis major as a solid unit.

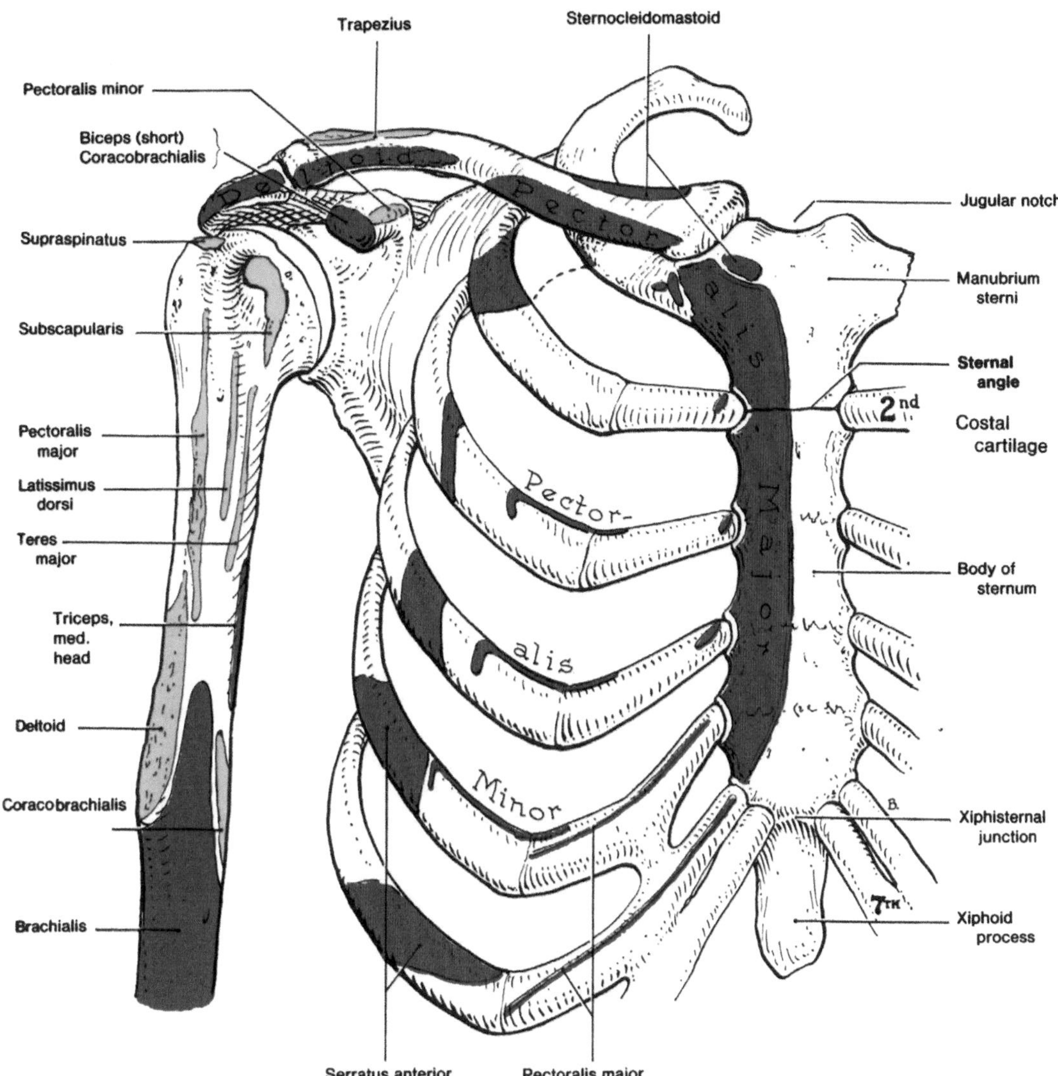

Fig. 4. Bones of the anterior chest wall showing the origin and insertion of pectoralis major. (*From* Moore KL, Agur AR, Dalley AF. Clinically oriented anatomy. Baltimore: Lippincott, Williams and Wilkins/Wolters Kluwer, 2013; with permission.)

Relationship to Inframammary Fold

Medial inflection point

The IMF is a critical landmark and essential feature of the aesthetically pleasing breast.[1] The exact limit of the IMF varies with the size of the breast and the size of the patient. The medial IMF and the lateral IMF may not be easily identified. In larger patients, the medial extent can seem to connect with the opposite breast and laterally may appear to go into the back. Most experienced surgeons have learned that manipulation of the breast is helpful to identify the medial and lateral extents of the IMF. The authors propose the terms medial inflection point (MIP) and lateral inflection point (LIP), as they more accurately represent the distal ends of the IMF when the breast is folded in on itself (**Fig. 7**). The MIP and LIP likely represent external manifestations of the medial and lateral triangular fascial condensation[6] (see **Fig. 2**). The MIP-LIP plane represents the base diameter of the breast footprint.[14]

The relationship of the IMF with the chest wall has been long sought and debated. It has been described to rest below the inferior pectoralis origin at the midaxial region of the breast.[7] The exact relationship of the IMF with pectoralis has not been previously described. However, the relationship with the chest wall becomes relevant after mastectomy whereby the removal of the breast tissue separates the breast envelope from the

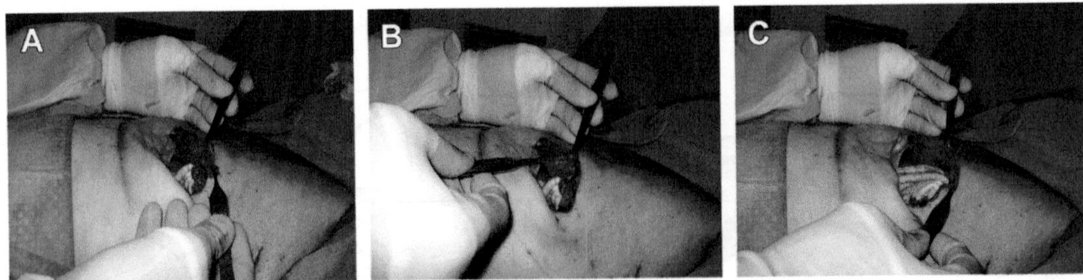

Fig. 5. Intraoperative view of the cut surface of the inferior border of the pectoralis major. (*A*) Superficial layer, (*B*) superficial and deep layer, and (*C*) deep layer with smooth undersurface.

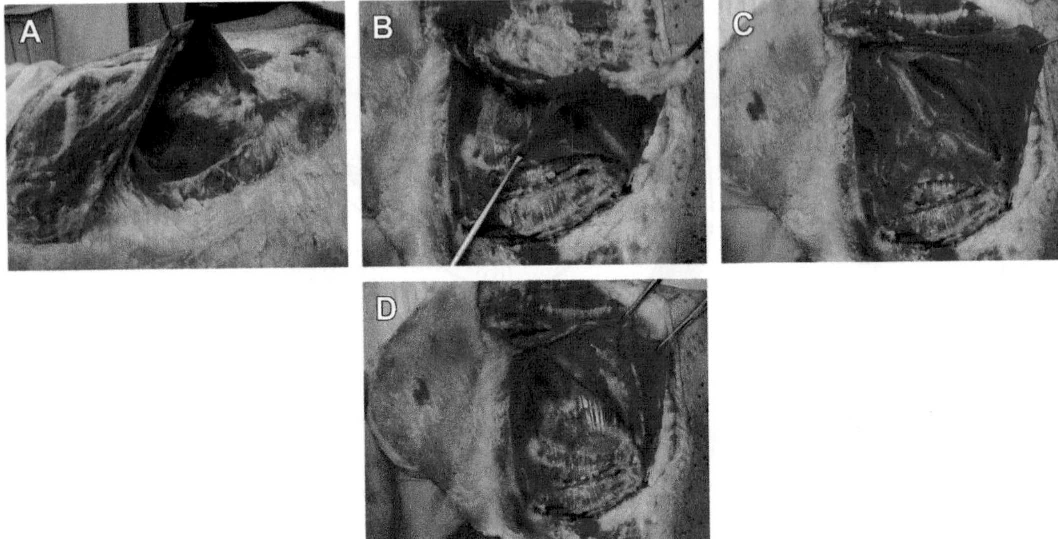

Fig. 6. Cadaver dissection of anterior chest wall. (*A*) Lateral approach to subpectoral space with origin from fourth, fifth, and sixth ribs, (*B*) separation of superficial and deep layers with rib origins marked, (*C*) deep layer bluntly separated and exposed, (*D*) deep layer retracted to reveal smooth undersurface of muscle.

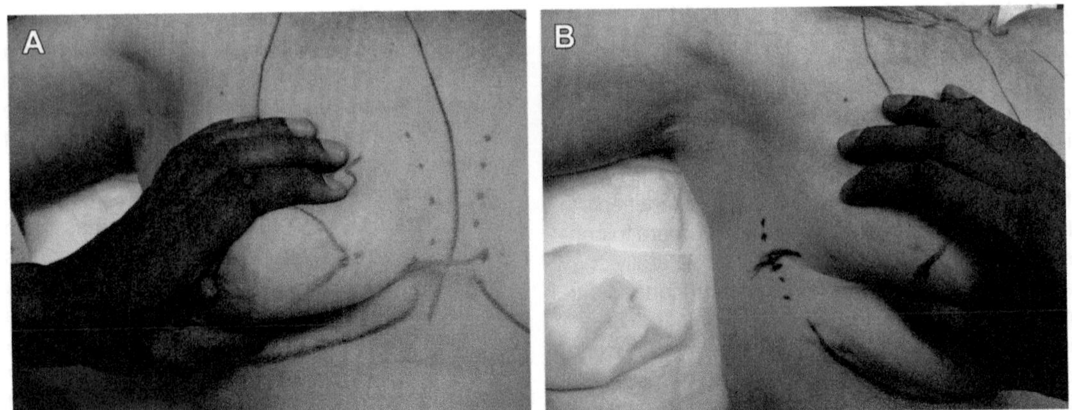

Fig. 7. Medial and lateral inflection points with folding of the breast. (*A*) MIP-medial and (*B*) LIP-lateral.

chest wall. Reestablishing this relationship is a priority in breast reconstruction. Various attempts to mark the natural position of the IMF with the chest wall have included sutures, staples, and dyes. The transcutaneous infiltration of methylene blue has been most useful in the authors' practice. It is here the relationship of the medial IMF with the pectoralis has unfolded. Routine use of this technique has demonstrated a consistent relationship of the MIP with the junction of the sternal and costal attachments of the pectoralis (**Fig. 8**). The value of this landmark is discussed in both aesthetic and reconstructive surgeries.

Lateral inflection point

The lateral extent of the IMF can be difficult to identify and can vary by the size of the breast and the size of the patient. However, the LIP can be identified in the same way as the MIP, by folding the breast on itself. It rests along the anterior axillary line but can seem to vary in larger patients. It is at the same level of the MIP and the 2 points form a horizontal plane with the nipple in patients without significant ptosis (**Fig. 9**). The plane of the MIP-LIP is not suggested as a reference point for ideal nipple position in individuals with ptosis at this time; however, it may represent a useful landmark in the future. Other than its location on the serratus anterior, no clinically significant reproducible internal anatomic relationship of the LIP and the chest wall could be identified. Skin attachments or zones of adherence of the lateral breast above the IMF have yet to be described. The lateral end of the triangular fascial condensation[6] may be the structure responsible for the external LIP, but it is not easily identified intraoperatively.

Central inflection point

The central or midaxial portion of the IMF is simple enough to appreciate. It rests at the lowest part of the breast on the chest wall in line with the nipple. Yet its position can ride up onto the lower pole after breast augmentation or reduction. The authors have chosen to define and designate this difference between the resting fold and the true fold anatomically (**Fig. 10**).[15] When marking a patient for any breast procedure, surgeons mark the resting fold where the skin of the breast touches the skin of the abdomen, creating a natural crease. Under tension the true fold is revealed, which ultimately becomes the final fold after augmentation. The authors have used the term central inflection point (CIP) because a similar folding technique is used to identify it, like the MIP and LIP. The CIP rests on the true fold in line with the nipple on average 1.5 cm below the resting fold. The CIP likely represents the lower limit of the horizontal ligaments.[6]

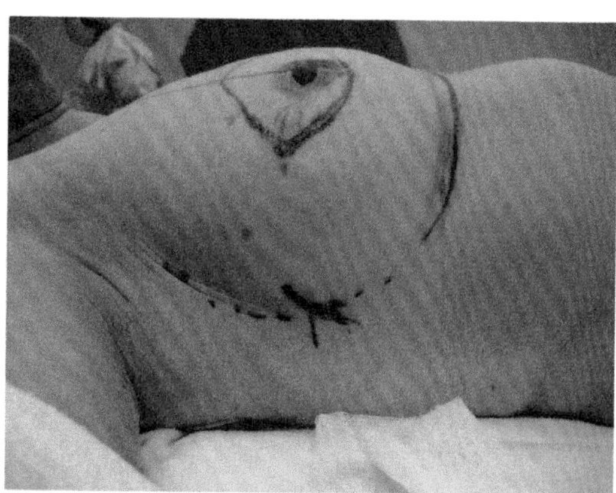

Fig. 9. Lateral inflection point on the anterior axillary line.

The CIP, like the LIP, thus far has not been visualized to have an easily identifiable internal anatomic landmark. As previously discussed, the IMF is known to rest superficially at or below the level of the pectoralis origin. Therefore, the CIP also rests at, or below, the inferior pectoralis origin at the level of the sixth or seventh rib.[2] There is, however, a significant variability in how the IMF relates to the inferior pectoralis origin.[8] In the authors' experience, internally the CIP has been visualized to lie approximately 5 cm below the MIP-LIP plane over the sixth rib.

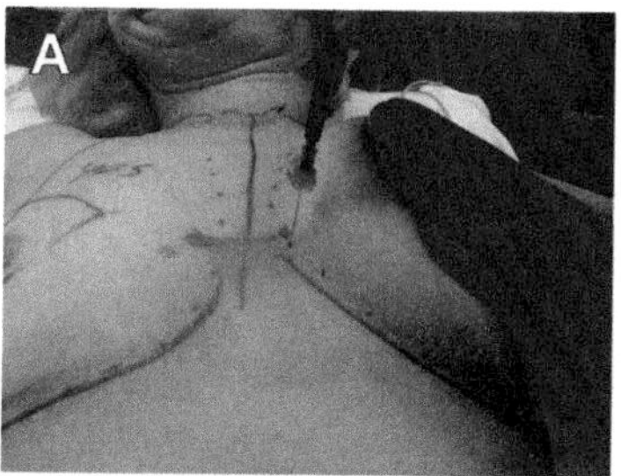

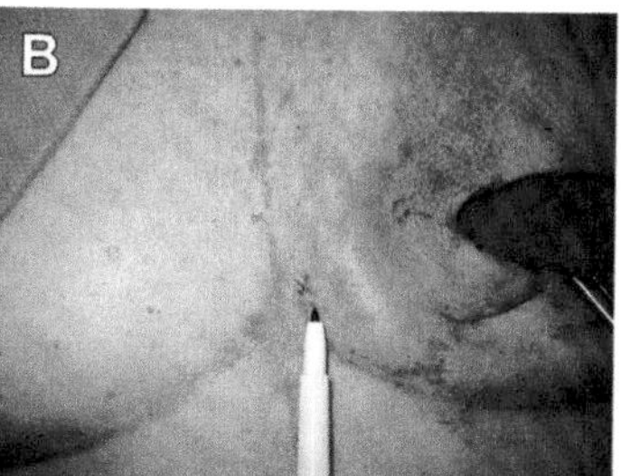

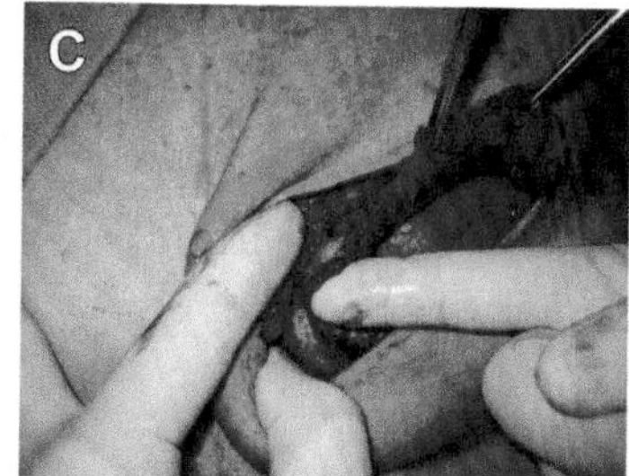

Fig. 8. Transcutaneous marking of the inframammary fold with methylene blue. (*A*) Intraoperative technique, (*B*) external MIP, and (*C*) internal MIP at the junction of the sternal and inferior origins of the pectoralis major.

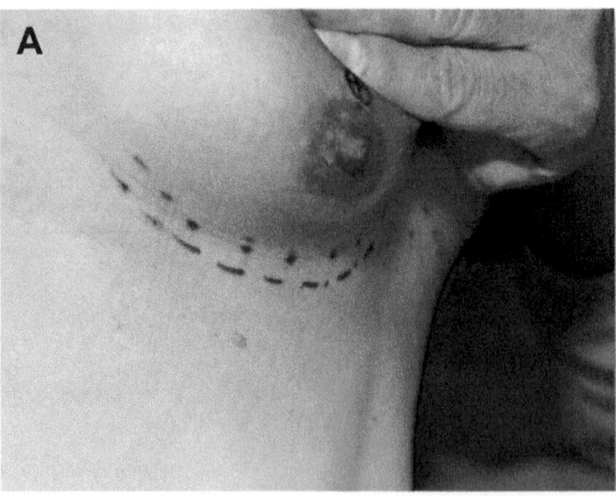

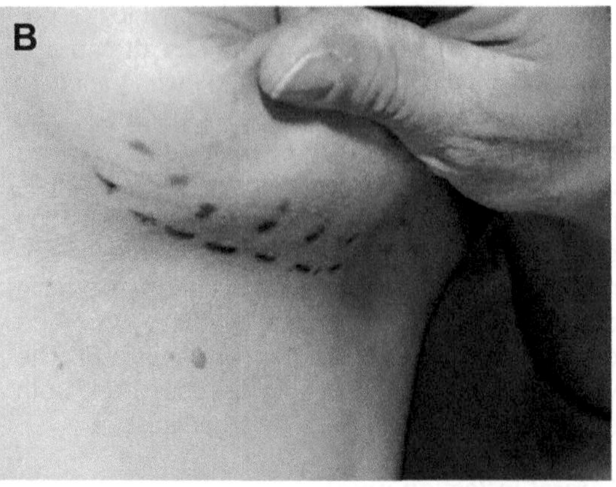

Fig. 10. Inframammary fold. (*A*) Resting fold; (*B*) true fold/central inflection point.

It is easy to see when one understands these anatomic boundaries how an incision may ride up onto the lower pole after breast reduction or augmentation with an IMF incision if the true fold is not taken into account. The final position of the breast, or the device, is the true fold. Most experienced surgeons have learned to appreciate the difference in the positions of the resting fold and the CIP on the true fold in breast surgery and incorporate it into their surgical planning.

In breast reconstruction, when superficial anatomy has been retained, reconstruction is straightforward. This CIP reference point is useful in immediate breast reconstruction where the anatomy has been poorly preserved, in delayed breast reconstruction where useful landmarks no longer exists, and in bilateral cases where a contralateral template is unavailable. The IMF can be successfully restored as an arc by marking a curvilinear line from MIP-CIP-LIP (**Fig. 11**).

CURRENT CONCEPT OF PECTORALIS ANATOMY AND ITS IMPLICATIONS

Right Angle Insertion of Inferior Origin to Vertical Sternal Origin

The pectoralis major is manipulated not only for breast aesthetics but also for head and neck, chest, breast, and upper extremity reconstructions. Yet it is almost universally perceived as having an L-shaped origin from the sternum and ribs (**Fig. 12**).[16] This perception influences the surgeon's behavior when manipulating the muscle inferiorly for breast surgery, leading to stopping short and incompletely releasing the muscle medially. The accepted standard for breast augmentation is to limit release of the pectoralis off the sternal origin. The perception of an L-shaped inferior origin prompts most surgeons to stop short at its medialmost horizontal extent. The muscle, however, continues to curve obliquely along the cartilaginous portion of the sixth rib until it meets the sternum, which leaves 1 to 2 cm of unclaimed territory medially. This misconception is the perception of the sixth wise man.

Consequences with Augmentation

Lateral misidentification

The value of understanding the laminated nature of the pectoralis major muscle is an increased intraoperative appreciation of the anatomy. Once the muscle is understood to arise inferiorly from the fourth, fifth, and sixth ribs the muscular fibers encountered are better understood. Experienced

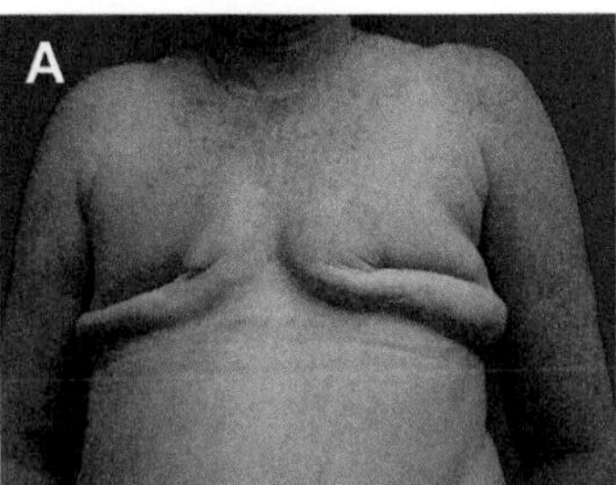

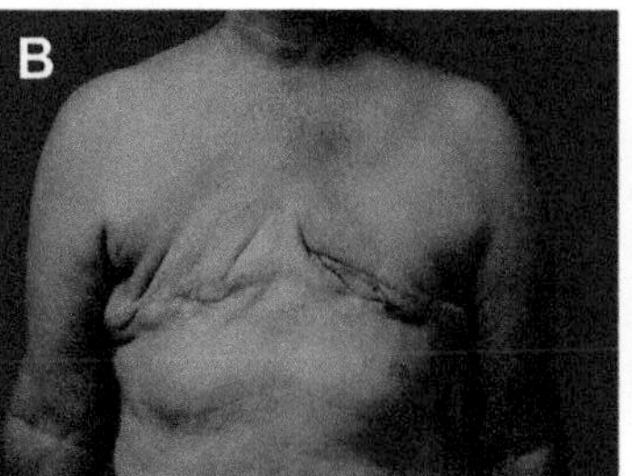

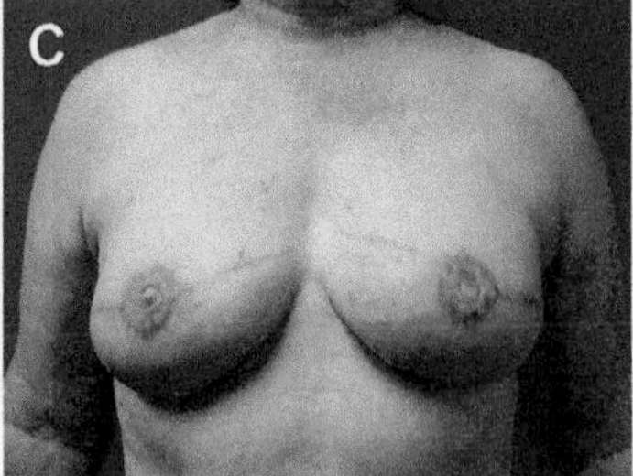

Fig. 11. Inframammary fold with delayed breast reconstruction. (*A*) Well-preserved IMF structure, (*B*) poorly preserved IMF, before (*C*) completed reconstruction with acellular dermis matrix and silicone implants, after.

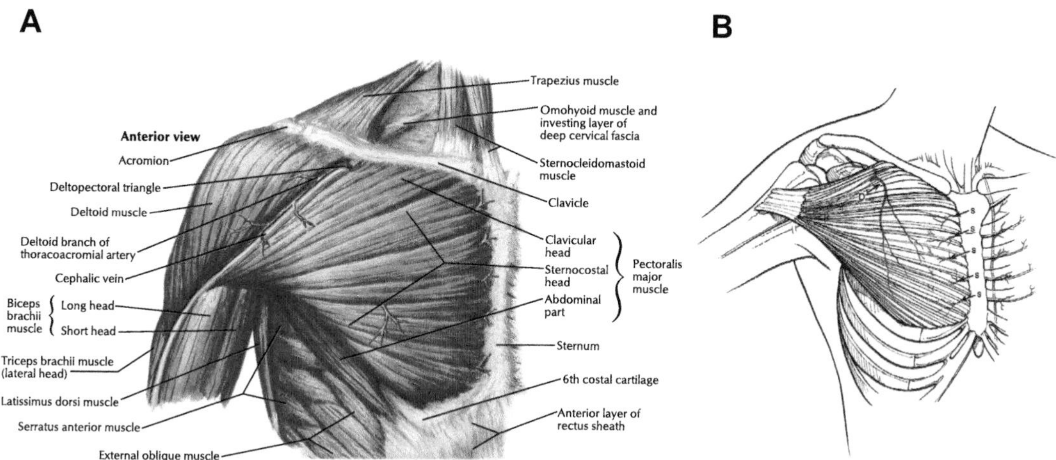

Fig. 12. Anterior chest wall demonstrating L-shaped inferior pectoralis origin. (*A*) Netter (Netter illustration from www.netterimages.com. © Elsevier Inc. All rights reserved) and (*B*) Mathes and Nahai. (*From* Mathes SJ, Nahai F. Reconstructive surgery: principles, anatomy, and technique. New York: Churchill Livingstone; 1997; with permission.)

surgeons have visualized the accessory fibers encountered with dissection in the submuscular plane.[17]

The lateral edge of the muscle is approached with the goal to access the avascular submuscular plane. Difficult access to this plane has been attributed to misidentification and dissection of the serratus.[18] However, from typical access points (periareolar or central IMF), the serratus is located at least 5 cm laterally. The surgeon has likely found the dense interface in the pectoralis origin between the fifth and sixth ribs, which is not easily bluntly dissected (**Fig. 13**). Reorientation of dissection a few centimeters superiorly allows for entry into the correct plane. This maneuver is simply bringing the level of dissection above the fifth rib, where the avascular plane can be approached with ease. The sixth wise man without an understanding of the laminated nature of the pectoralis believes he is disorientated and lost.

Underdissection

The subpectoral space is sufficiently developed to allow precise placement of the device. Internally, accessory fibers encountered medially are divided to develop the subpectoral space. Cadaveric dissection reveals that these internal accessory fibers arise from the fourth and fifth ribs and contribute to the deep layer of the pectoralis major. Release of these fibers does not completely separate the pectoralis from its inferior origin, with the remaining superficial layer from the sixth rib. With preservation of the superficial layer, the pocket remains completely submuscular. Disadvantages to complete submuscular device

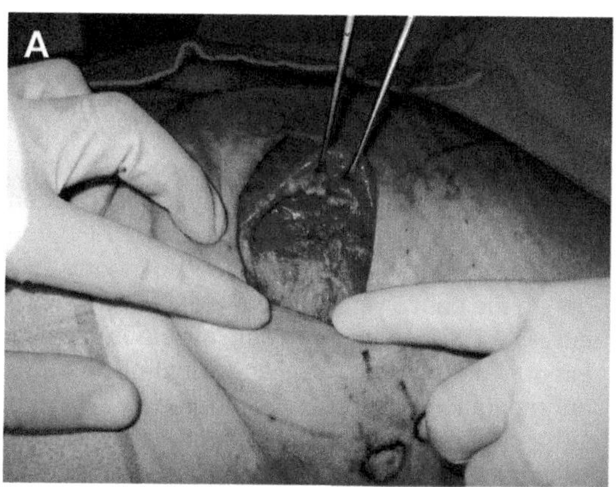

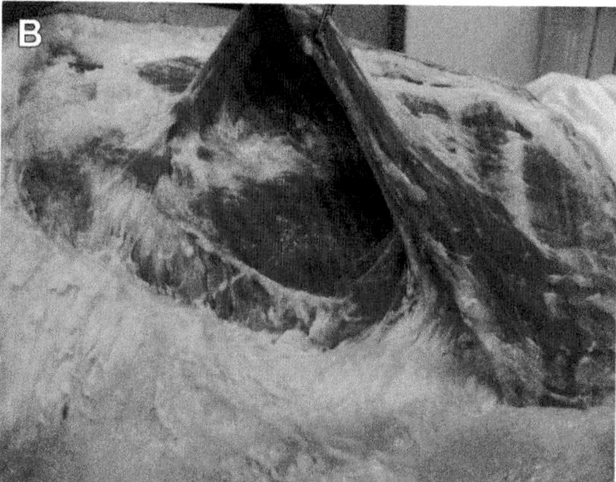

Fig. 13. Lateral border of pectoralis major at its inferior origin. (*A*) Intraoperative view of the fifth and sixth rib origin; (*B*) cadaveric view.

placement are prominent superior pole, tight lower pole, and potential snoopy deformity.[17]

Division of the superficial layer inferiorly is the key step in partial subpectoral placement of the device. The medial fibers of the superficial layer are approached with caution as their significance is debated. Preservation of medial fibers is advocated to avoid disinsertion of sternal attachments. A more liberal release is encouraged to promote medial pole fullness. It is generally agreed to limit dissection off the sternum; however, where to stop is nebulous. It is here the significance of the MIP landmark becomes relevant. The MIP is the surface landmark where the superficial fibers from the costal surface of the sixth rib travel obliquely and join the horizontal fibers from the sternum. Once the MIP is reached, further dissection should be terminated.

Overdissection medially

Medial dissection superior to the MIP is tempting to allow larger implant placement. The consequence of overzealous dissection beyond the MIP is division of the pectoralis off the sternum.[19] Division above the MIP can result in symmastia, window shading of the pectoralis, increased implant visibility, and traction rippling.[13]

Overdissection inferiorly

Inferiorly the superficial layer of the pectoralis major arises from the costal margin of the sixth rib and the aponeurosis of the external oblique muscle. Cadaveric and clinical dissection have shown the IMF to lie up to 2.0 cm below the inferior origin of the pectoralis.[7] When the inferior border is approached from the subpectoral plane, the deep fibers from the fifth rib, previously referred to as accessory fibers, are divided first. Superficial fibers are next visualized and are divided for partial subpectoral placement. Division of the superficial fibers directly off the rib surface places the plane of dissection in close proximity to the IMF. Continuing dissection along this vector risks dissection under the IMF, with potential for migration of the implant and bottoming out as a late consequence. Appreciation of pectoralis anatomy with division of the superficial fibers above the rib margin aids in protecting the integrity of the IMF as a support structure. Division of the superficial layer at least 1 cm above the rib margin leaves a sufficient cuff of soft tissue to avoid retraction of muscular perforators and vector away from the horizontal ligaments of the IMF support structure.[6,10]

The inframammary approach to breast augmentation potentially risks overdissection inferiorly. When the IMF is understood to be a support structure, dissection down to the chest wall should be done with the intent of preserving as much of this structure as possible. Dissection from the inframammary incision toward the chest wall goes through part of the triangular fascial condensation.[6] Directing the vector of dissection superiorly protects the horizontal ligaments, thus maintaining the support structure of the IMF. When a new IMF incision is required to achieve adequate lower pole projection, its position should not be below the CIP or no more than 1 cm below the resting fold.[10] Below this level, dissection risks disruption of the horizontal ligaments and at minimum should be repaired to maintain its support mechanism.

Consequences with Implant-Based Reconstruction

Complete submuscular reconstruction

Cosmetic breast surgery and reconstructive breast surgery are frequently thought of as separate entities by the seventh wise man; however, both surgeries share the same goal: to provide an aesthetically pleasing breast. The reconstructive arena has special challenges because of alterations in the soft-tissue envelope and chest wall structure. Implant-based reconstruction can be especially challenging in getting the patient and the implant to cooperate with one another. Complete submuscular placement of the implant can provide an acceptable breast mound, but limitations in soft-tissue compliance can restrict ultimate shape and projection. Tight lower pole, blunted IMF angle, and superior displacement of the implant have fueled enthusiasm for the combination of acellular dermis matrix (ADM) with partial submuscular placement of the implant. This technique has allowed for improved and more consistent shape and projection of breast reconstruction.[20–23] This approach is similar to partial submuscular breast augmentation with division of the pectoralis muscle off the chest wall inferiorly. The difference between the 2 is where the lower pole is supported with ADM in breast reconstruction and with breast soft tissue in augmentation.

Acellular dermis matrix-based reconstruction

Since the advent of acellular dermis-based reconstructions such as AlloDerm, the rate of reconstructions with ADM has increased nearly 25% during the past 5 years (**Fig. 14**) (data from LifeCell survey). The pectoralis major muscle is released inferiorly in a manner similar to dual-plane breast augmentation. Although the approach is internal (subpectoral) with augmentation and external with reconstruction, the goal is the same. Here the misconception of an L-shaped lower pectoralis border can be misleading.

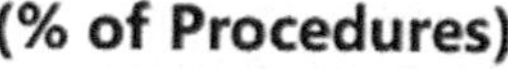

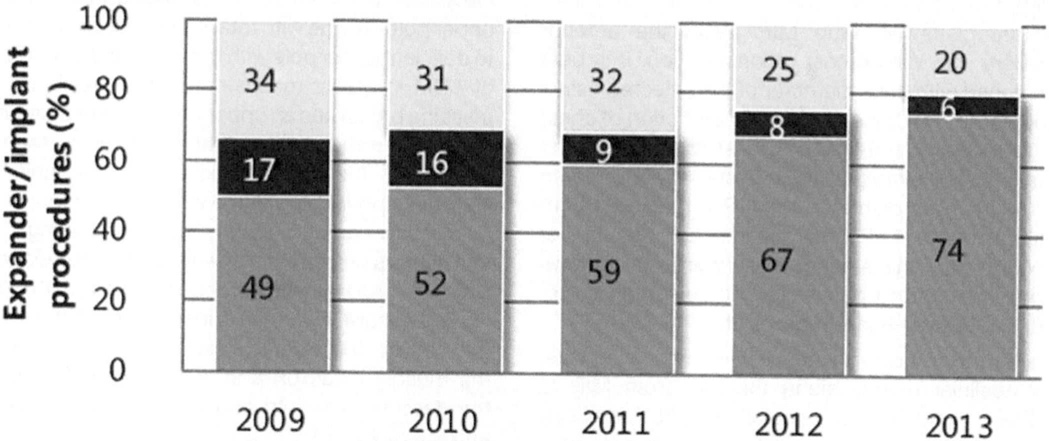

Fig. 14. Surgical technique used for tissue expander/implant procedures from 2009 to 2013.

With ADM-based reconstruction, the pectoralis is released up to its medial extent.[20,21] The medial limit of the inferior pectoralis is confused with the L-shape frequently pictured.[16] However, as shown with cadaveric dissection, inferiorly the superficial layer of the pectoralis continues obliquely along the sixth costal margin up to its sternal attachments at the MIP; this can be demonstrated with the surgical finger admitted to the medial limit of the pectoralis. When completely released up to the MIP, the finger is not restricted inferiorly and medial placement of the tissue expander is increased by 1 to 2 cm (**Fig. 15**). This procedure avoids lateral implant placement and poor medial pole definition; this can take the appearance of an inverted dog ear medially. When fully appreciated, the pectoralis is released up to the MIP and the ADM is inset into the chest wall at this point.

The MIP, CIP, and LIP can be thought of as surface landmarks to the breast footprint described by Blondeel and Hijjawi.[14] The ADM is inset onto the chest wall at the MIP, continues in a curvilinear manner along the IMF to the CIP then up to the LIP. The LIP has been visualized to rest on the serratus anterior in line with the anterior axillary line. As previously mentioned, a specific corresponding

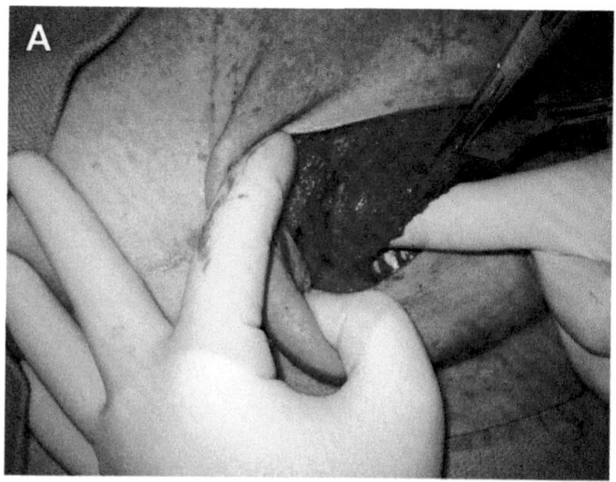

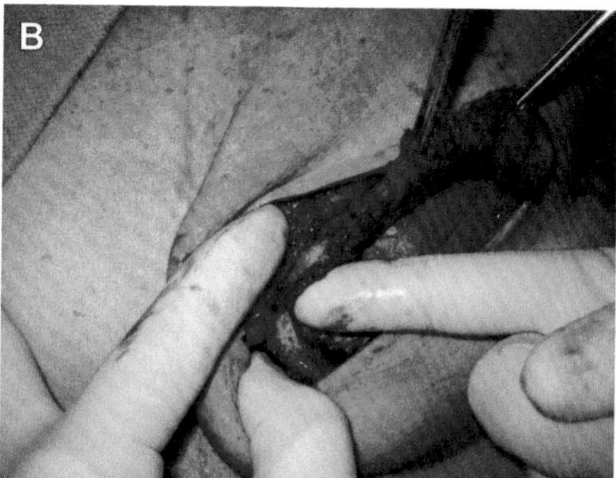

Fig. 15. Intraoperative approach to the MIP following release of the pectoralis inferiorly. (*A*) Incomplete release with inferior descent of the surgical finger restricted; (*B*) full release up to the MIP.

internal landmark for the LIP has yet to be identified, but it can be located. The LIP lies on a horizontal plane with the MIP along the anterior axillary line. With breast reconstruction, it is best matched with base diameter of the selected tissue expander. The base diameter is a function of chest wall anatomy, not size of breast or weight of the patient. For example, for a tissue expander with a 14 cm base diameter, the LIP is marked 14 cm lateral to the MIP. The marked LIP should not extend past the anterior axillary line; this allows for a customized pocket for the selected device, for the desired hand-in-glove fit.

Failure to resecure the deep layer Following inset of acellular dermis along the IMF from MIP to LIP, a precise submuscular pocket has been created. Surgery is completed with enclosure of the tissue expander under the newly created pectoralis/acellular dermis pocket. The inferior border of the pectoralis is approximated to the superior border of the ADM. As previously described, the pectoralis is a laminated structure with both a superficial and a deep layer. Typically, the free edge of the pectoralis is grasped; however, this represents only the superficial layer. The deeper layer has retracted superiorly, and unless deliberately retrieved is not secured with the superficial layer (see **Fig. 5**).

The significance of an uncontrolled deep layer is difficult to appreciate without first understanding its existence and its volume. It represents approximately 30% to 50% of the muscle volume and when not under sufficient tension atrophies, thus reducing the volume of tissue for upper pole coverage. The pendulum has swung from excess upper pole volume with total submuscular coverage to deficient upper pole with the increasing popularity of ADM in breast reconstruction. An aesthetically pleasing breast has an upper pole to lower pole ratio of 45:55, with a slope that is linear or slightly concave.[24] Multiple techniques are available to augment upper pole volume with shaped breast implants, intracapsular ADM,[22] and fat grafting.[15,23] The authors propose that the simplest and cheapest technique is to retrieve the deeper layer from the fifth rib and secure it with the superficial layer (**Fig. 16**); this can be appreciated when the undersurface of the muscle takes on a smooth appearance after the deep layer is retrieved and maintains tension and prevents partial muscle atrophy.

An additional consequence of an unsecured deep layer is a thin muscle junction with ADM; this increases the risk of delayed implant exposure at the muscle/ADM junction following inflation of the tissue expander. After separation of this thin junction, the expander rests directly under thin mastectomy flaps. If the junction is near the incision line, exposure of the expander may be imminent (**Fig. 17**). The risks are particularly magnified in patients requiring postoperative radiation. The need for secondary procedures such as latissimus flap coverage, although not completely eliminated, has been significantly reduced in the authors' practice, and their experience with this simple adaptation has been most favorable with no increase in operative time, expense, or risk.

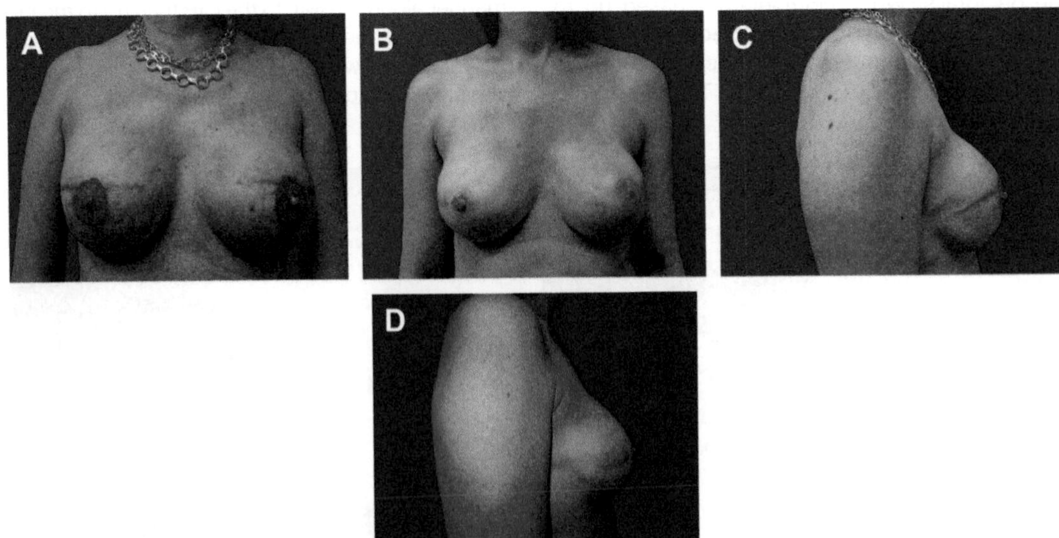

Fig. 16. Final breast reconstruction outcome with ADM and high-profile silicone implants. (*A, C*) Reconstruction with superficial layer control of the pectoralis with poor upper pole volume and slope; (*B, D*) reconstruction with dual-layer control of the pectoralis with improved upper pole volume and slope.

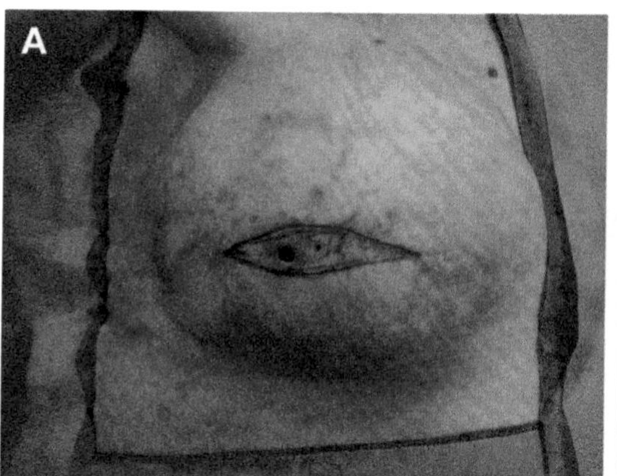

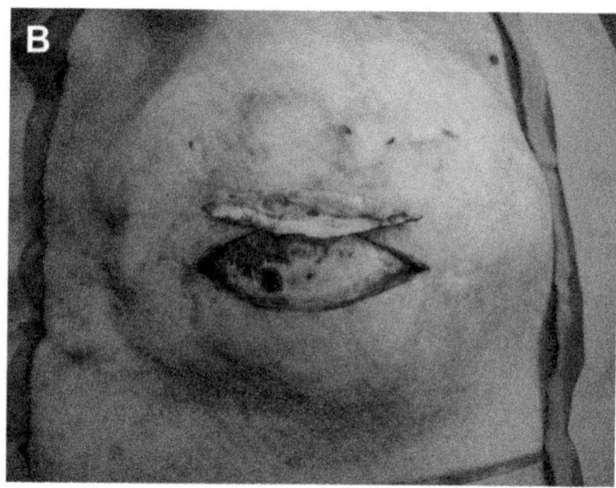

Fig. 17. Threatened exposure of tissue expander at incision line occurring at the junction of pectoralis and ADM. (*A*) Exposure through scar, (*B*) Exposure at pectoralis/AlloDerm junction.

Clinical Applications to Mastopexy and Reduction

Mastopexy and breast reduction techniques seek to reduce the skin envelope and reshape the breast conus for improved shape, size, and projection of the breast.[15] Although there is significant debate regarding the specific technique, there is less controversy than implant-based surgery. In both procedures, the skin envelope is reduced to match the final size of the breast conus. The IMF is marked for operative planning, regardless of the specific technique chosen. In smaller patients and with smaller breasts, markings are straightforward. However, in larger patients or breasts, the distal ends of the IMF can be difficult to pinpoint. It is here the value of the MIP, LIP, and CIP can be appreciated as reproducible external landmarks.

The medial end of the IMF when marked too short may result in a dog ear and in very large reductions risk crossing the midline. The MIP is a useful reference point to terminate the surgical incision. Similarly, the lateral end of the IMF may result in a dog ear if marked too short. A particular challenge in patients with BMI greater than 35 is where to stop with the lateral incision as it blends with the patient's lateral axillary lipodystrophy. As the LIP terminates at the anterior axillary line, the lateral incision should be limited to this point (**Fig. 18**). The additional challenge of achieving symmetry with bilateral surgery can be reduced with availability of reproducible landmarks.

Scars are an unavoidable consequence to any surgery. Plastic surgeons strive to minimize scar appearance by placing the scar in a favorable location. A most frustrating element to breast surgery is the mobility of IMF scars and their tendency to ride up. With breast augmentation, the CIP is identified and the incision is preemptively placed on the true fold in anticipation of a final acceptable position of the scar. The tension created by the implant exposes the true fold, which ultimately becomes the final fold. The same mechanism is at play after mastopexy/reduction. When closed under excessive tension, the pressure of the conus on the skin envelope exposes the true fold, which ultimately becomes the final fold. Thus, the incision appears to ride up. Adequate preoperative planning for a sufficient skin envelope should balance with judicious reduction of the breast such that tension on the lower IMF is minimized. The CIP when marked during mastopexy/reduction can serve as a useful tension meter.

DISCUSSION

All surgeons equally desire to avoid unintended outcomes. The reasons for unintended outcomes are multifactorial and can be due to patient selection, technique, and experience. The surgeon never expects to be the direct cause. Yet something as simple as a narrow perspective has been made by many learned men. The anatomy of the breast from the skin envelope, breast tissue, underlying musculature, and chest wall are all intimately related. Regardless of the various techniques for cosmetic, functional, and reconstructive breast surgery, the goals and principals are the same.

Appreciating the dynamic nature of the breast and these new insights into muscle and breast anatomy allows the plastic surgeon to also appreciate the surface structure and how it relates to the IMF and the chest wall and their clinical implications. Folding the breast on itself reveals the MIP, CIP, and LIP along the IMF. These are valuable reproducible surface landmarks, which have both useful internal and external significance in augmentation, mastopexy, reduction, and reconstruction.

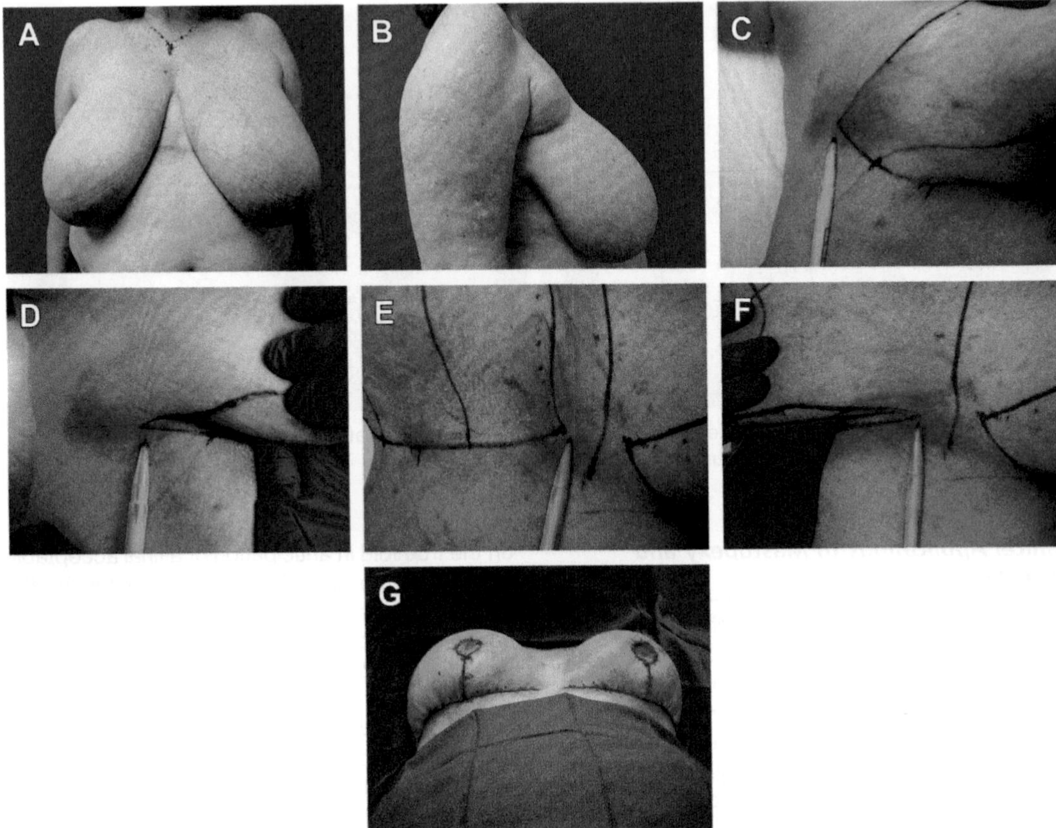

Fig. 18. Breast reduction of 1300 g in a patient with body mass index 35 kg/m^2. (*A, B*) Preoperative images. (*C, D*) LIP at rest and with folding; (*E, F*) MIP at rest and with folding. (*G*) Intraoperative image.

Further appreciation of the dynamic nature of the pectoralis has been heretofore underappreciated. It is well known that the pectoralis major is a type V flap and can be split segmentally when based off its medial perforators.[25] Less well known is the laminated nature of the pectoralis muscle with a superficial layer and a deep layer, arising from the fifth rib and sixth rib, respectively. Most experienced surgeons have visualized portions of this layered muscle in some manner and from various approaches but never understood its full and true nature. With pure submuscular augmentation, often the deep layer only is separated, whereas both layers are divided with dual-plane augmentation techniques. In ADM-based breast reconstruction, only the superficial layer heretofore has been secured to the ADM. A dual-layer closure is recommended to fully control the pectoralis to maintain muscle tension, upper pole volume, and enhanced coverage of the device.

The authors have tied multiple observations and practices, much like observations of the learned men of Indostan, into a more comprehensive animal. Understanding in one area will lead to greater understanding in another and to improved outcomes.

Editorial Comments by Bradley P. Bengtson, MD

The laminar anatomy of the pectoralis major muscle, the reflection points of the breast and the inframammary fold are anatomic structures we look at every single day, but do not really understand. The specific muscle and fascial anatomy, vectors, insertions and variability significantly affect outcomes in breast augmentation, revision and reconstruction. The muscles are not single uniform sheets of muscle but laminar in nature. If these individual layers are not taken into account and are overly released surgeons can create window-shading and minimize muscle coverage. If under-released they can create an implant position is too far lateral and/or too high. The fascial fiber of the lower portion of the breast insert at an oblique angle and the true fold of the breast is actually 1.5–2.0 cm lower than the resting fold or inferior skin reflection point. This true fold is where the base of the implant will rest unless the fold is otherwise sutured or set higher and is a common reason for fold malposition. These nuances in patient anatomy are vitally important for the plastic surgeon to understand and obtain consistent long-term results.

REFERENCES

1. Carlson GW, Grossl N. Preservation of the inframammary fold: what are we leaving behind? Plast Reconstr Surg 1996;98(3):447–50.
2. Muntan CD, Sundine MJ. Inframammary fold: a histologic reappraisal. Plast Reconstr Surg 2000; 105(2):549–56 [discussion: 557].
3. Boutros S, Kattash M. The intradermal anatomy of the inframammary fold. Plast Reconstr Surg 1998; 102(4):1030–3.
4. Maillard GF, Garey LJ. An improved technique for immediate retropectoral reconstruction after subcutaneous mastectomy. Plast Reconstr Surg 1987; 80(3):396–408.
5. Bayati S, Seckel BR. Inframammary crease ligament. Plast Reconstr Surg 1995;95(3):501–8.
6. Matousek SA, Corlett RJ. Understanding the fascial supporting network of the breast: key ligamentous structures in breast augmentation and a proposed system of nomenclature. Plast Reconstr Surg 2014; 133(2):273–81.
7. Nanigian BR, Wong GB. Inframammary crease: positional relationship to the pectoralis major muscle origin. Aesthet Surg J 2007;27(5):509–12.
8. Madsen RJ Jr, Chim J. Variance in the origin of the pectoralis major muscle: implications for implant-based breast reconstruction. Ann Plast Surg 2015;74(1):111–3.
9. Moore KL. Clinically oriented anatomy. 2nd edition. Baltimore (MD): Williams & Wilkens; 1985.
10. Tebbetts JB. Dual plane breast augmentation: optimizing implant-soft-tissue relationships in a wide range of breast types. Plast Reconstr Surg 2001; 107(5):1255–72.
11. Spear SL, Parikh PM. Acellular dermis-assisted breast reconstruction. Aesthetic Plast Surg 2008;32(3):418–25.
12. Pacik PT. Augmentation mammaplasty: enhancing inferomedial cleavage. Aesthet Surg J 2005;25(4): 359–64.
13. Lindsey JT. The case against medial pectoral releases: a retrospective review of 315 primary breast augmentation patients. Ann Plast Surg 2004;52(3): 253–6 [discussion: 257].
14. Blondeel PN, Hijjawi J. Shaping the breast in aesthetic and reconstructive breast surgery: an easy three-step principle. Plast Reconstr Surg 2009;123(2):455–62.
15. Bengtson B. Acellular dermal matrices in secondary aesthetic breast surgery: indications, techniques, and outcomes. Plast Reconstr Surg 2012;130(5 Suppl 2):142S–56S.
16. Mathes SJ, Nahai F. Reconstructive surgery: principles, anatomy and technique. Baltimore (MD): Churchill Livingstone; 1997.
17. Hammond DC. Atlas of aesthetic breast surgery. Edinburgh (United Kingdom): Saunders; 2008.
18. Khan UD. Muscle-splitting breast augmentation: a new pocket in a different plane. Aesthetic Plast Surg 2007;31(5):553–8.
19. Sanchez ER, Howland N. Anatomy of the sternal origin of the pectoralis major: implications for subpectoral augmentation. Aesthet Surg J 2014;34(8): 1179–84.
20. Breuing KH, Warren SM. Immediate bilateral breast reconstruction with implants and inferolateral AlloDerm slings. Ann Plast Surg 2005;55(3): 232–9.
21. Breuing KH, Colwell AS. Inferolateral AlloDerm hammock for implant coverage in breast reconstruction. Ann Plast Surg 2007;59(3):250–5.
22. Maxwell GP, Gabriel A. Revisionary breast surgery with acellular dermal matrices. Aesthet Surg J 2011;31(6):700–10.
23. Spear SL, Sher SR. Focus on technique: supporting the soft-tissue envelope in breast reconstruction. Plast Reconstr Surg 2012;130(5 Suppl 2): 89S–94S.
24. Mallucci P, Branford OA. Concepts in aesthetic breast dimensions: analysis of the ideal breast. J Plast Reconstr Aesthet Surg 2012;65(1):8–16.
25. Tobin GR. Pectoralis major segmental anatomy and segmentally split pectoralis major flaps. Plast Reconstr Surg 1985;75(6):814–24.

Weight Measurement and Volumetric Displacement of Breast Implants and Tissue Expanders

Why Port and Shell Volumes Matter in Breast Reconstruction, Augmentation, and Revision

Chad G. Wenzel, MD[a], William F. Wacholtz, PhD[b], David A. Janssen, MD[c,*], Bradley P. Bengtson, MD[d,e]

KEYWORDS

- Saline breast implants • Silicone gel breast implants • Breast tissue expanders
- Volumetric displacement of implants • Weight measurements of breast implants • Saline density
- Silicone gel density

KEY POINTS

- There are significant differences in weight and volumetric characteristics between silicone and saline breast implant of which most plastic surgeons are unaware.
- Plastic surgeons need to be aware of these differences for both in-breast implant exchange from saline to silicone conversions and 2-stage breast reconstruction.
- Until now, measuring the volume created by the expander has been solely reliant on using the volume of injected saline into the expander.
- The volume occupied by the tissue expander shell and filling port have been largely estimated or disregarded.
- In addition, these differences are commonly ignored in saline to silicone gel implant exchanges.

INTRODUCTION AND BACKGROUND

The aesthetic results and outcomes following breast augmentation and reconstruction with implants and tissue expanders continue to improve and are becoming increasingly accurate. With the advent of 3-dimensional imaging and simulation, very specific volumes of the breast may be calculated, simulated, and compared. Many plastic surgeons continue to be unaware of the differences between saline and silicone devices, and fail to consider the additional weight and displaced volume that the saline shell and expander components add to the weight and volume of the overall device. In addition, saline is more dense than silicone and adds slightly to the volume differences. These differences in volume are becoming more

Disclosure: See last page of article.

[a] Medical College of Wisconsin, Milwaukee, WI, USA; [b] Department of Chemistry, University of Wisconsin, Oshkosh, WI, USA; [c] Fox Valley Plastic Surgery, 2400 Witzel Avenue, Oshkosh, WI 54904, USA; [d] Bengtson Center for Aesthetics and Plastic Surgery, 555 MidTowne Street, NE Suite 110, Grand Rapids, MI 49503, USA; [e] Department of Surgery, Michigan State University, East Lansing, MI, USA

* Corresponding author. Bengtson Center for Aesthetics and Plastic Surgery, 555 MidTowne Street, NE Suite 110, Grand Rapids, MI 49503.

E-mail address: Djanssen@fvpsurgery.com

Clin Plastic Surg 42 (2015) 481–491
http://dx.doi.org/10.1016/j.cps.2015.06.010
0094-1298/15/$ – see front matter

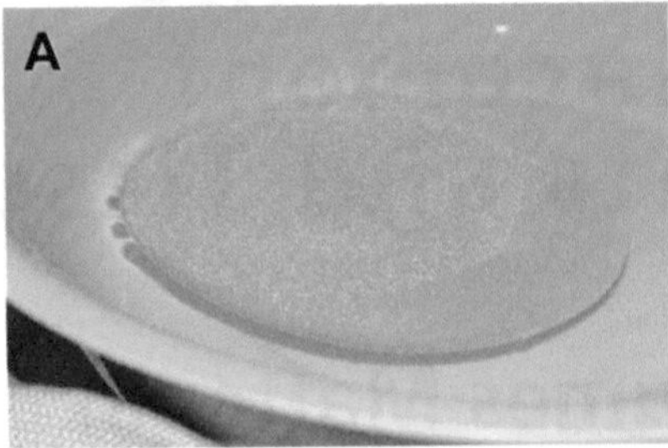

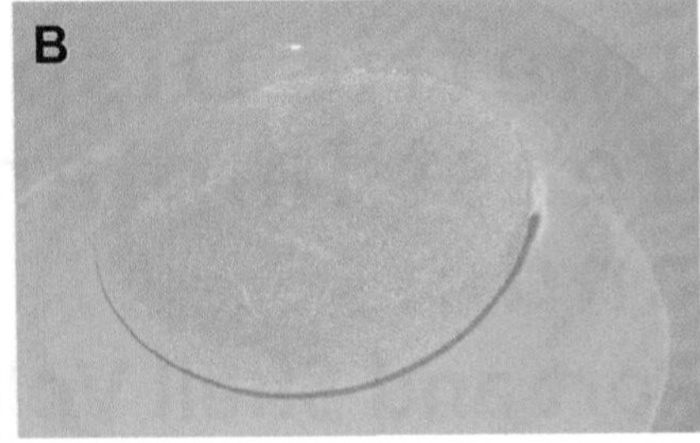

Fig. 1. (*A, B*) Silicone implants float when placed in a saline bath.

important in achieving optimal outcomes and symmetry. Finally, saline implants are filled in situ, so their weight and displaced volume does not include the implant shell. Silicone implants, however, are constructed, weighed, and volumetrically measured, including the shell weight and total displaced volume, by the manufacturer.

So what weighs more, saline or silicone? Silicone implants will float when placed in a saline bath because silicone is less dense than saline (**Fig. 1**). Saline implants hover just beneath the surface, because they are isodense with the saline bath (**Fig. 2**).

The relative densities of saline and silicone shells are:

- Density of silicone elastomer = 1.10 to 1.17 g/cm^3
- Density of silicone gel filler = 0.93 to 0.97 g/cm^3
- Density of normal saline = 0.99 to 1.05 g/cm^3

Because of the density difference between saline and the inner gel filler, even 0.1 to 0.2 g/cm^3 may make a difference in weight and volume, especially in larger devices.

Additionally, one of the most common procedures in plastic surgery for breast reconstruction is the use of a temporary breast tissue expander followed later by the permanent placement of a breast implant in a 2-step process.[1,2] According to 2012 statistics, silicone implants are the most common type of permanent implant selected by most plastic surgeons.[3] In numerous studies, this approach has been shown to be safe, and produces high rates of aesthetic satisfaction and effective reconstruction after mastectomy.[4–6] The 2-step reconstruction has been practiced for many years, with surgeons using tissue expanders to develop the breast, and later selecting an appropriate implant that best matches breast volume, height, and projection to fill the defect. A common practice within this surgery involves overexpanding the breast pocket with the tissue expander to create more volume than the final implant actually occupies.[1,7–9] This action is taken to develop an expanded skin envelope and create a higher degree of lower pole stretch and ptosis of the permanent implant for improved aesthetics and reconstruction. With this in mind, the size of the pocket to be created is preoperatively assessed and determined by approximating the volume occupied by the empty tissue expander plus the added volume of saline anticipated to be injected into the expander. Although this is a clinically proven approach, this study aims to consider the issue that tissue expanders comprise more than the fluid injected into them. By simple visual inspection, an expander's fill port and shell both occupy volume. To the best of the authors' knowledge, this is only the second study to address the issue that these physical components occupy a significant volume in the breast pocket, with the first being a study of Mentor Corporation (Santa Barbara, CA, USA) products by McCue and colleagues in 2010.[10] Although this unknown volume is compensated for by

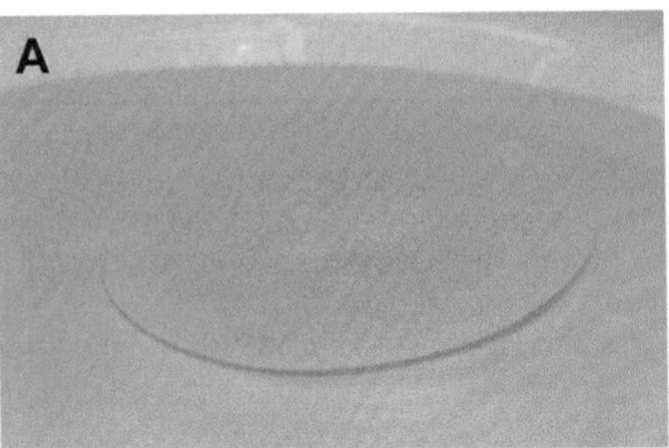

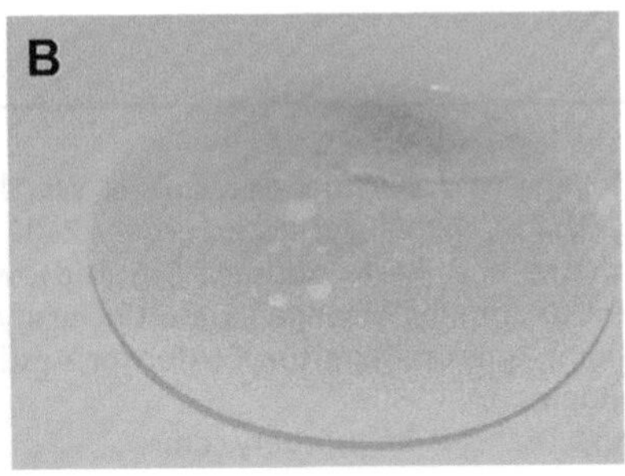

Fig. 2. (*A, B*) Saline implants hover in a saline water bath because they are isodense.

surgeons approximating the volume the total tissue expander occupies, the exact process is imprecise. The purpose of phase II of this study is to compare the actual volume of tissue expanders that are injected with specific amounts of fluid with both the volume of fluid injected into them and the potential final implants of similar stated volumes. Future applications of this research are numerous, given the high frequency that 2-step reconstructions are performed, the great emphasis on surgical accuracy, and the significant psychological and aesthetic impact it has on a large population of patients.

METHODS

For phase I of this study, serial weights of empty and saline-filled devices, specifically the Natrelle Style 68 and 168 textured devices, were compared. These devices were weighed both empty and filled with the clinical formulation of injectable normal saline. For the volumetric phase II study, volumes of both breast implants and tissue expanders were measured on 3 trial days, with each trial including 3 separate measurement tests of each expander and implant for a total of 9 trials. Twenty-three Natrelle silicone gel Style 20 high-profile type implants, which varied in volume from 120 to 800 mL, acted as controls.[11] Six Style 133MV textured tissue expanders, which varied in maximal inflations from 250 to 700 mL, were also tested.[12] The tissue expanders were first evacuated of any air via vacuum to prevent residual air, which is inherent in the production process, from affecting the experimental results. While structural change from overinflation was not an anticipated issue,[13] the expanders were just filled to their stated capacity with a 50-mL syringe in 50-mL aliquots with distilled water. All tissue expanders were filled to their stated capacity to establish the lower bound of percent influence of their physical components. An apparatus, shown in **Fig. 3**, was constructed to measure the total volume of the tissue expanders and breast implants. First, a hole was drilled near the top of a large plastic container, which was placed on an elevated pedestal. A flexible Tygon tube was fitted and sealed into the hole with silicone caulk. The tubing was run downward toward a second container, which was placed on a calibrated balance. The first container was filled with distilled water over the top of the hole with the tube in it. The excess water drained out until the water level rested just below the hole's opening. The apparatus was constructed in this manner so that any object placed into the upper container would cause all of the water displaced by the object to run down into the second

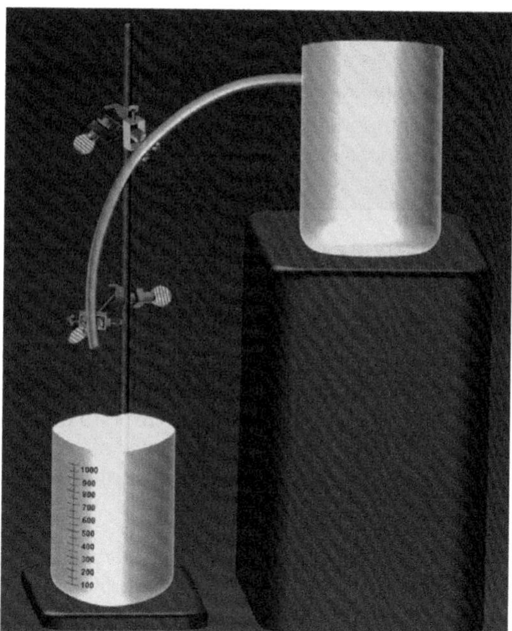

Fig. 3. Apparatus for measurement of the volume of tissue expanders.

container. The second container was dried and tared on the balance before each trial so that all water that entered it could be accurately measured. To measure either a tissue expander or implant, each was placed into the upper container and was allowed to fully submerge itself below the surface of the water. The mass of the displaced water and the temperature of the water were recorded, the latter because the density of water is very specific at given temperatures.[14]

Computational Methodology

The calculation of the volume of the water displaced in each experiment by a tissue expander or implant was based on the mass and temperature of the displaced water. These amounts were calculated using Equation 1.

$$\text{Density}_{\text{water}} = \text{Mass}_{\text{Total}}/\text{Volume}_{\text{Total}} \quad (1)$$

Equation 1 was solved for total volume to give Equation 2. The temperature of the water, which yielded its density, and the mass displaced by each object was measured during each trial.

$$\text{Volume}_{\text{Total}} = \text{Mass}_{\text{water}}/\text{Density}_{\text{Total}} \quad (2)$$

Once the total volume of the object was known, Equation 3 was used to discover the effect of the port and shell of each tissue expander on the amount of water displaced.

$$\text{Volume}_{\text{Total}} = \text{Volume}_{\text{Physyical Components}} + \text{Volume}_{\text{Injected Water}} \quad (3)$$

This equation was solved for the volume of the physical components, which yielded Equation 4, which was possible as the total volume of each expander had been derived and the injected water had previously been measured and recorded.

$$\text{Volume}_{\text{Physical Components}} = \text{Volume}_{\text{Total}} - \text{Volume}_{\text{Injected Water}} \quad (4)$$

Finally, the percent influence of the port and shell on the total volume of each tissue expander was calculated using Equation 5. Equation 6 outlines the additional percentage of volume created by the physical components of the expanders.

$$\text{Percent influence} = ((|\text{Volume}_{\text{Injected Water}} - \text{Volume}_{\text{Total}}|)/\text{Volume}_{\text{Total}}) \times 100 \quad (5)$$

$$\text{Percent of additional volume} = ((\text{Volume}_{\text{Total}} - \text{Volume}_{\text{Injected Water}})/\text{Volume}_{\text{Injected Water}}) \times 100 \quad (6)$$

All data, figures, and tables were statistically analyzed and generated using Microsoft Excel 2008.

RESULTS

Phase I results evaluated a series of saline breast implant shells. Dry saline implant shells, depending on implant size and style, ranged from 10 to 40 g in weight. The more common implant sizes are shown in **Table 1**.

Tissue expanders, owing to their thick backing and infusion port, which weigh 10 g, adds 40 to 90 g depending on expander size (**Fig. 4**). For example, a 450-mL smooth saline implant filled to 450 mL of saline actually weighs 500 g and would require a 500-mL silicone implant to replace volume for volume (see **Fig. 4**), and likely more if the saline device is overfilled, as is common practice. Expanders weigh even more; for example, if a 400-mL Style 133MV expander is partially filled with 350 mL of saline, it actually weighs 425 g (see **Fig. 4**). The expander port weighs 10 g (see **Fig. 4**).

Table 1
Weights of varying saline implant shells

Volume (mL)	Weight (g)
270	~15
300	~16
330	~18
360	~20
420	~22
450	~23
500	~26

In phase II, the first experiment compared the stated volume of breast implants with their actual measured volume. The trials with the implants showed that the manufacturer's stated volume for each implant was within 2.8 mL or less for every breast implant tested. **Table 2** articulates these data in full detail. Moreover, the percent difference between the stated and measured volumes of each implant was 1% or less in every volume of implant.

In the same manner, tissue expanders were examined. The injected volume of distilled water, which represented injected saline, was compared with the total displaced volumes of the tissue expanders. **Table 3** displays these results. The volume of injected solution and the total volume occupied by each tissue expander varied significantly across all volumes of tissue expanders examined. The difference between the fill volume of the smallest expander and actual displacement was 41.6 mL. This trend generally and steadily increased up to the largest expander of 700 mL, which differed by 72.9 mL between fill volume and total measured volume. The column in **Table 3** describing the percent influence is of particular importance, as it shows how much the volume of the shell and fill port affected the total volume displaced by each tissue expander. Even at the largest injected volume of 700 mL, the percent of total volume affected by the expander's physical components was 9.4%. **Fig. 5** shows the trend of the implants' fill volumes compared with the actual volumes they occupied. With the exception of the 500-mL tissue expander, the expander volumes increased in an almost exactly linear fashion. The trend line fitted to the tissue expander total volumes resulted in an *r* value of 0.99. The physical components of the 400-mL and 500-mL tissue expanders, as measured, occupied almost the same volume. However, the apparent deviation in linearity that this presumes is within 2 standard deviations of the regression line for each measured tissue expander.

Finally, **Fig. 6** and **Table 4** demonstrate the difference between the measured volume displaced by each breast implant and that of a corresponding tissue expander, which was filled to the same volume as an implant. **Fig. 6** articulates that there is a significant difference between the two, and that the expander's displaced volume greatly

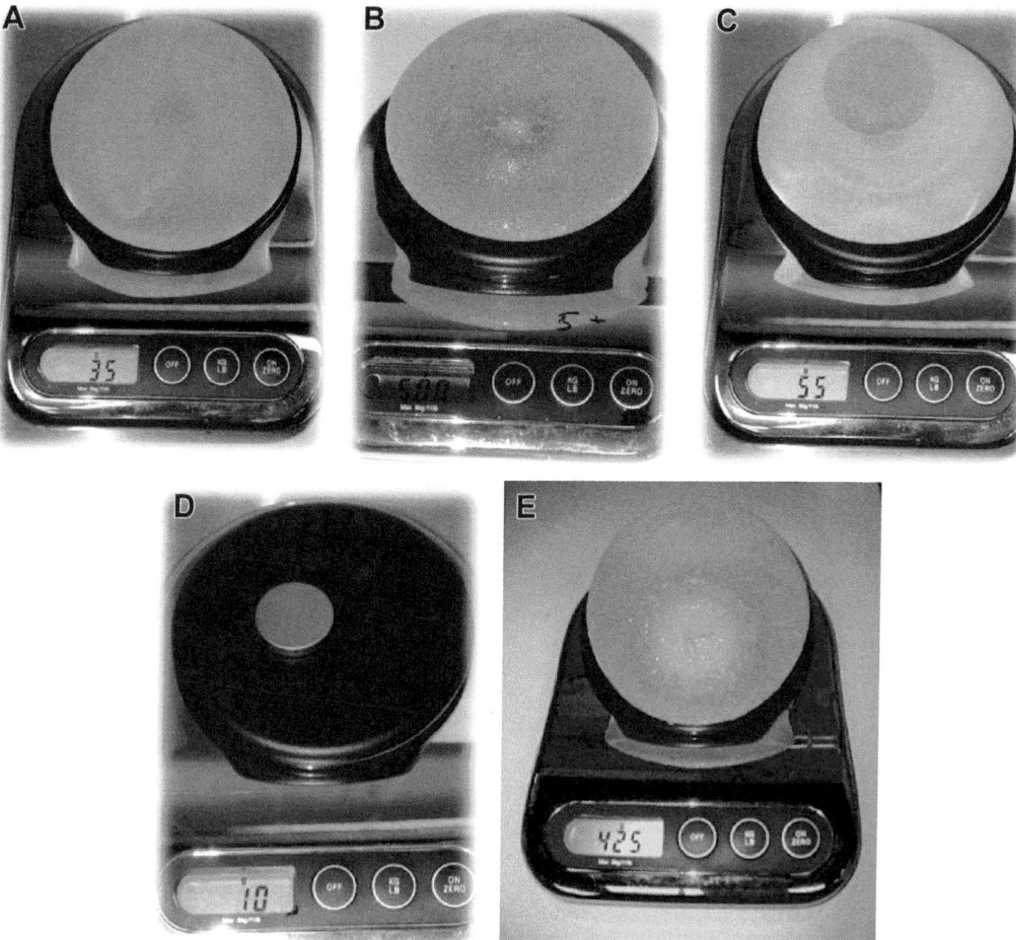

Fig. 4. (*A*) A 450-mL saline implant shell with a weight of 35 g. (*B*) A 450-mL textured implant filled to 450 mL of saline, which weighs 500 g. (*C*) A Natrelle Style 133FV 400-mL expander shell, which weighs 55 g. (*D*) An expander port from a 133FV expander weighing 10 g. (*E*) The Style 133FV 400-mL expander partially filled with 350 mL of saline, weighing 425 g.

exceeds the volume of each associated implant. For the smallest tissue expander and implant paring, the tissue expander occupied an additional 58.5 mL. This trend continued up to the largest tissue expander, which displaced an extra 71.4 mL of fluid compared with its corresponding implant.

DISCUSSION

The main findings of this 2-phase study were:

- The overall weight of a saline breast implant or tissue expander is significantly greater than the instilled volume alone, and in fact averages 1 or 2 implant sizes larger in volume than the instilled volume alone.
- Current expanders add even more weight to the overall device because of its thicker backing and metal port.
- There are differences in physical properties between saline and silicone.
- Saline implant shells can add 5% to 10% to the overall weight of the implant because saline devices are filled into an empty shell, whereas the factory measurements of weight and displacement of silicone devices include their inherent shell weight.
- Displaced volumes of physical components of tissue expanders had a significant impact on the total volume they occupy in comparison with the instilled saline alone.
- Displaced volumes of water are similar to weight differentials.

It is clear that saline implants weigh and displace significantly more volume than most surgeons recognize. After inspection of the results presented here, it can clearly be observed

Table 2
Stated and average measured volume of breast implants

Stated Implant Volume (mL)	Average Displacement of Implant (mL)	Standard Deviation	Average Difference Between Stated and Measured Volumes (mL)	Percent Influence of Difference (%)
120	120.2	2.78	0.2	0.2
140	139.7	2.99	0.3	0.2
160	160.8	2.66	0.8	0.5
180	181.2	3.12	1.2	0.7
200	200.3	2.23	0.3	0.1
230	232.4	3.33	2.4	1.0
260	258.8	2.99	1.2	0.5
280	280.5	3.33	0.5	0.2
300	299.4	3.60	0.6	0.2
325	326.2	4.25	1.2	0.4
350	352.0	3.31	2.0	0.6
375	376.1	4.48	1.1	0.3
400	402.1	2.02	2.1	0.5
425	427.8	2.00	2.8	0.7
450	452.2	4.36	2.2	0.5
475	477.3	3.52	2.3	0.5
500	500.8	2.90	0.8	0.2
550	551.3	3.70	1.3	0.2
600	600.4	3.96	0.4	0.1
650	651.6	3.75	1.6	0.2
700	701.5	4.13	1.5	0.2
750	751.2	3.73	1.2	0.2
800	802.8	4.66	2.8	0.4

Data articulate the close match between the stated volume of each implant and its corresponding measured volume.

Table 3
Influence of physical components of tissue expanders

Tissue Expander Injected Volume (mL)	Volume Displaced by Tissue Expander (mL)	Standard Deviation	Average Difference of Stated vs Observed Expanders (mL)	Percent Influence of Physical Components on Total Volume (%)	Additional Percentage of Volume Created (%)
250	291.6	2.72	41.6	14.3	16.7
300	357.9	3.16	57.9	16.2	19.3
400	467.1	3.60	67.1	14.4	16.8
500	564.2	2.44	64.2	11.4	12.8
600	670.0	2.99	70.0	10.4	11.7
700	772.9	4.32	72.9	9.4	10.4

Significant difference was observed between expander fill volume and displaced volume. Furthermore, there is a striking effect of the physical components on the total volume of each expander, both in their percent influence on total volume and the additional volume that they create.

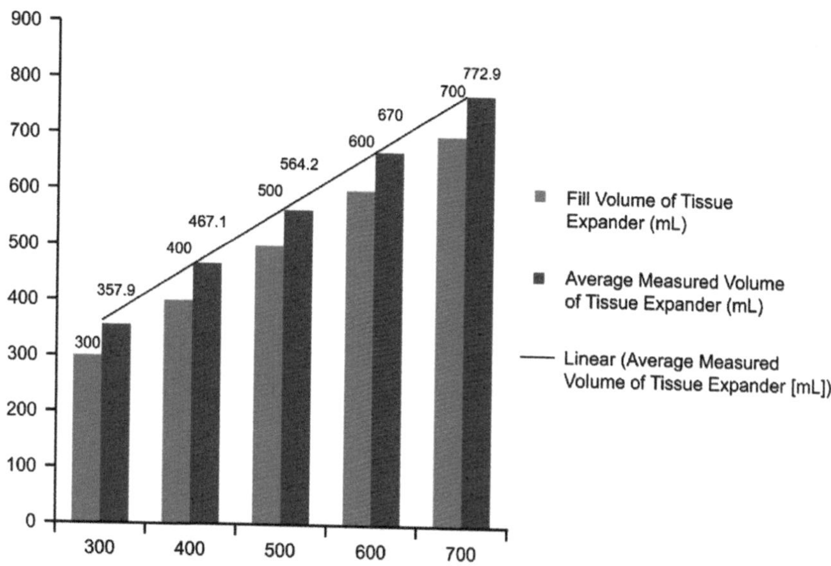

Fig. 5. Comparison of tissue expander fill volume and average measured volume. The key feature depicted is the difference between the fill volume of each tissue expander and the total measured volume of the expander. The difference is due to the tissue expanders' physical components. The linear trend line fitted to the "Measured Volume of Tissue Expander" bars (*red*) had an *r* value of 0.99, which showed high statistical correlation.

that the fill port and shell dramatically affect the total volume of the tissue expanders, and must be taken into account by the surgeon when developing the breast for future placement of a permanent implant. For all of the different tissue expanders measured, the port and shell added significant volume. The concept that the physical components of expanders possess noteworthy volume, while previously hypothesized or clinically estimated, now has a concrete value for

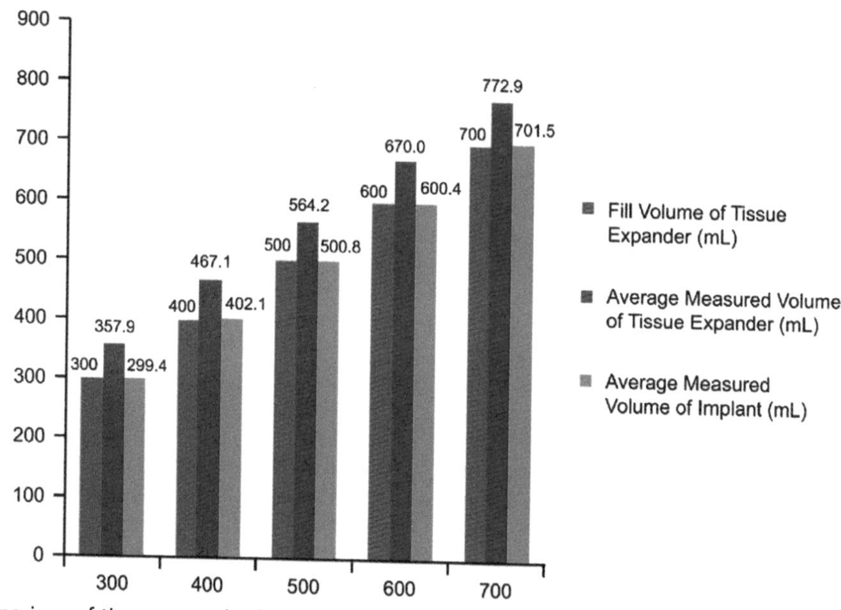

Fig. 6. Comparison of tissue expander fill volume, actual volume, and corresponding implant volume. The graph shows the volume theoretically created with a tissue expander (*blue*), the volume actually created by the same tissue expander (*red*), and the volume occupied by a corresponding permanent implant (*green*).

Table 4
Comparison of tissue expanders with implants

Fill Volume of Tissue Expander (mL)	Volume of Tissue Expander (mL)	Average Measured Volume of Corresponding Implant (mL)	Difference Between Average Measured Implant and Tissue Expander (mL)
300	357.9	299.4	58.5
400	467.1	402.1	65.0
500	564.2	500.8	63.4
600	670.0	600.4	69.6
700	772.9	701.5	71.4

Data indicate a significant difference between the volume created for the breast pocket and the volume occupied by the permanent implant.

the Allergan model measured. These data will allow for precise assessment of the volume these tissue expanders create for a corresponding amount of injected saline used for inflation. The knowledge of the volume created will further allow for accurate matching of an implant into the created breast, and should remove a significant amount of previously associated approximation. In addition, although the implants measured in this study were not anatomically shaped, the issue of understanding the exact volume created by an expander comes under sharp focus when considering anatomic implants, including the Allergan 410 textured implant. Because these types of implants require a "hand-in-glove" fit with the volume created by the preceding expander, it is paramount that these 2 volumes correlate precisely to prevent implant rotation or malpositioning.[15] Clearly the physical components of tissue expanders increase the total pocket size beyond the volume injected. Therefore, not taking this into account will necessitate either additional procedures during implant placement, such as a capsulorrhaphy to decrease or restructure the final pocket size,[16] or require an increase in the size of the planned implant needed to fill the developed volume. In addition, many surgeons are transitioning from a volumetric-only view of implants to a "biodimensional" or "tissue-based planning" approach. This approach takes into consideration the actual implant dimensions, with breast and implant base width, height, and projection now coming into play. When considering breast reconstruction with shaped implants, surgeons must give particular consideration to using shorter height devices than the expander height, the same or a slightly more narrow expander width compared with the final shaped device, or even underfilling the expander at least by 50 to 75 mL to make up for the shell and port weight and certainly avoiding overexpansion.

In evaluating these results, it is important to note that the physical components of the expander had less of a percent influence on the total volume as the expander size increased. This result was an expected one because there was a significant increase in injected fluid volume for each increase in tissue expander capacity. Compared with the port and shell size, which increased only to minor degrees, there was a significant comparative increase in fluid volume, which caused the percent influence of the physical components to trend downward with increasing expander inflation size. However, whereas the percentage of total volume that was affected by the port and shell was greater in the small-sized tissue expanders, a greater volumetric impact was seen in the larger-sized expanders. Both of these findings are significant clinically because they affect the sizing of tissue expanders differently, and must be taken into account.

The results of this study can further be applied to 2 additional practices associated with the 2-step reconstruction after mastectomy. The first concerns the overexpansion of submuscular tissue for the breast pocket. This approach has become common for developing the breast pocket for better ptosis of the final implant. This aspect is especially important if the contralateral breast is devoid of surgery, and matching native anatomy is of the utmost priority. Depending on the surgeon's preference, the volume created by the tissue expander may exceed the final implant volume by up to 20% to 30%.[1,5,8,17,18] However, given that this study shows that the physical components provide an additional 10.4% to 19.3% of volume, the developed breast pocket could be significantly larger than anticipated if they are not accounted for. Therefore, it is crucial to take these findings into consideration when inflating the expander, and also during selection of a final implant.

Additionally, tissue expander volume displacement correlates with expander weight differentials and is nearly identical to volume displacement of water with the proximity of volume and density (1 mL = ~1 g). Because of the expander's thick backing and infusion port, which weigh 10 g, the total added weight is 40 to 90 g depending on the expander size (see **Fig. 4**). For example, if a 400-mL Style 133FV expander is partially filled with 350 mL of saline it actually weighs 425 g (see **Fig. 4**). The expander port alone weighs 10 g (see **Fig. 4**).

As an example of standard saline devices, a 450-mL smooth saline implant filled with 450 mL of saline, has a total actual weight of 500 g. Volume for volume it would take a 500-mL silicone implant to replace a saline device filled to 450 mL (see **Fig. 4**), and incrementally more if the saline device is overfilled, as is common practice.

Furthermore, the common use of AlloDerm, other acellular dermal matrices, or biological scaffolds for breast reconstruction is also affected by these findings. AlloDerm, which is an acellular dermal matrix that is free of antigens, has become an important tool for plastic surgeons.[19,20] Many investigators have provided approaches for its use and for assessment of the amount of dermal matrix needed for inferior pole coverage for implants, sling creation for an implant, or a combination of these and other additional applications.[21–25] In fact, Haddock and Levine[20] have previously created equations to compare fill volume and AlloDerm surface area and height. Given the significant consideration currently being given to this subject, it is essential to also consider the additional volume created by the physical components of the tissue expander. This additional volume also then affects the surface area that the AlloDerm will need to cover and support. Although the assessment of the added surface area created by the physical components of expanders was beyond the scope of this study, the conclusion can be drawn that the difference is not inconsequential.

While these results prove that the shell and port of tissue expanders dramatically affect their total volumes across the board, they also present 2 interesting fragments of data, the first of which is that the volumes displaced by the breast implants were not precise according to the manufacturer's stated volumes. This variability was hypothesized to be due to slight variability between implants produced, and is consistent with prior data analysis on the variability between production batches.[26] However, the overall variability observed was statistically insignificant. The second observation is that the rate at which the port and shell affected the total volume of the tissue expanders did not follow an exact logarithmic scale as was initially suspected. The 400-mL and 500-mL expanders had almost identical physical component volumes. However, as stated previously, the results for these 2 tissue expander volumes fell within 2 standard deviations of the regression line fitted from the smallest to largest tissue expander.

Through these experiments, it is evident that there is a significant need for future study in this arena. This study assessed only one specific style of tissue expander and compared it with one style of implant from the same company. Additional testing of multiple tissue expanders and implants of the same sizes needs to be done to confirm these findings. However, variability between batch productions is minimal, so an initial conclusion can be drawn that these findings are indeed accurate. Furthermore, although the notion that the physical components of tissue expanders do indeed occupy statistically significant volume compared with the total volume of inflated tissue expanders, the exact volumes found in this study are not necessarily applicable across styles of tissue expanders, much less between companies. Initial support of this is evident from the study of Mentor products by McCue and colleagues[10] in 2010. Because of the variability in the size of ports and shells for different styles of tissue expanders, it is apparent that today's plastic surgeons must have a database from which they can quickly reference the impact of the physical components of tissue expanders to make appropriate and precise adjustments when inflating an expander to develop a breast in both the clinic and operating room settings. This pilot study provides a stepping-stone for future investigation. Ultimately, the most important goal to be achieved by creating a database is that patients might have better surgical results and outcomes. With an increasing number of women choosing breast reconstruction because of either mastectomy after cancer occurrence or prophylactic mastectomies,[27] adding proficiency and accuracy to this specific surgical approach is essential. Early and superior breast reconstruction has a significant influence on patient psychology and sexuality.[28,29] A future database would simplify reconstruction, enhance aesthetics, reduce complication rates, and thereby help women cope and persevere after surviving a difficult health ordeal.

Lastly, as a result of this research, the authors hope that surgeons will weigh or displace removed expanders or saline implants, document these data, and use them to direct the choice of the new devices. With the high demand for aesthetics and quality outcomes in both breast revision and reconstruction, surgeons will require immediate access to this additional knowledge to help choose the best option and create the best possible symmetric outcome for every patient.

Materials used for volumetric displacement studies

- 1000-mL glass beaker
- Balance (accurate to nearest gram)
- Flexible Tygon tubing
- 2000-mL plastic beaker
- Silicone caulk
- Twenty-three silicone gel Style 20 (Allergan, Inc, Irvine, CA, USA) high-profile type implants (120–800 mL)
- Six Style 133MV tissue expanders (Allergan) (maximal inflations ranging from 250 to 700 mL)
- Distilled water

Materials used for weight measurement studies

- Standard operating room scale
- Smooth saline Style 68 Implants
- Style 133MV tissue expanders

DISCLOSURE

None of the authors have any financial compensations or specific financial interests or holdings to report. The breast implants and tissue expanders were product samples, and were provided by Allergan free of charge to be used to advance knowledge in the field of plastic surgery. Dr B.P. Bengtson is an Allergan consultant, but has no conflicts with the topics of this research. Writing and editorial assistance was provided to the authors by Peloton Advantage of Parsippany, NJ and funded through a publication grant by Allergan Inc, Irvine, CA. Allergan was not involved in the writing of this article, and neither honoraria nor payments were made for authorship by Allergan.

Editorial Comments by Bradley P. Bengtson, MD

There are differences between saline and silicone implants that the majority of plastic surgeons do not fully recognize. A number of factors may contribute to this including an increased density of saline over silicone gel, the added weight of the implant shell, expander port weights, routine overfilling of saline devices and the potential inaccuracies in saline filled implants. These differences must be taken into account particularly when exchanging saline implants or tissue expanders out for silicone devices. These differences may be documented with displacement techniques or also by weight utilizing standard scales available in the operating rooms. Volume and weight are just one of the dimensions when considering Tissue Based Planning solutions in breast procedures. Regardless, it is very important to displace or weigh all saline devices and expanders and keep the potential volume and weight differences in mind particularly during implant or expander exchanges.

ACKNOWLEDGMENTS

The authors would like to thank the University of Wisconsin, Oshkosh for the use of their laboratory space and equipment. The authors would also like to thank Allergan, Inc for their contribution in supplying the devices for use in this study, and Dr Chris Wichman of Creighton University for his help with statistical analysis and project planning.

REFERENCES

1. Spear SL, Spittler CJ. Breast reconstruction with implants and expanders. Plast Reconstr Surg 2001; 107:177–87.
2. Radovan C. Breast reconstruction after mastectomy using the temporary expander. Plast Reconstr Surg 1982;69:195–206.
3. American Society of Plastic Surgeons. 2012 plastic surgery statistics report. Available at: http://www.plasticsurgery.org/Documents/news-resources/statistics/2012-Plastic-Surgery-Statistics/full-plastic-surgery-statistics-report.pdf. Accessed June 24, 2014.
4. Eriksen C, Lindgren EN, Frisell J, et al. A prospective randomized study comparing two different expander approaches in implant-based breast reconstruction: one stage versus two stages. Plast Reconstr Surg 2012;130:254e–64e.
5. Cordeiro PG, McCarthy CM. A single surgeon's 12-year experience with tissue expander/implant breast reconstruction: Part II. An analysis of long-term complications, aesthetic outcomes, and patient satisfaction. Plast Reconstr Surg 2006;118:832–9.

6. Spear SL, Majidian A. Immediate breast reconstruction in two stages using textured, integrated-valve tissue expanders and breast implants: a retrospective review of 171 consecutive breast reconstructions from 1989 to 1996. Plast Reconstr Surg 1998; 101(1):53–63.
7. Cordeiro PG. Breast reconstruction after surgery for breast cancer. N Engl J Med 2008;359:1590–601.
8. Pusic AL, Cordeiro PG. An accelerated approach to tissue expansion for breast reconstruction: experience with intraoperative and rapid postoperative expansion in 370 reconstructions. Plast Reconstr Surg 2003;111:1871–5.
9. Castelló JR, Garro L, Nájera A, et al. Immediate breast reconstruction in two stages using anatomical tissue expansion. Scand J Plast Reconstr Surg Hand Surg 2000;34:167–71.
10. McCue JD, Lacey MS, Cunningham BL. Breast tissue expander device volume: should it be a factor? Plast Reconstr Surg 2010;125:59–61.
11. Allergan, Inc. The Natrelle product catalog. Available at: http://www.natrelle.com/professional/pdf/natrelle_product_catalog.pdf. Accessed June 24, 2014.
12. Allergan, Inc. Directions for use: Style 133V series tissue expander matrix with magna-site® injection sites. Available at: http://www.allergan.com/assets/pdf/M724-B_133V_TE_DFU.pdf. Accessed June 24, 2014.
13. Hallock GG. Maximum overinflation of tissue expanders. Plast Reconstr Surg 1987;80:567–9.
14. Pidwirny M. Physical properties of water. In: Fundamentals of physical geography. 2nd edition. 2006. Available at: http://www.physicalgeography.net/fundamentals/8a.html. Accessed June 28, 2014.
15. Brown MH, Shenker R, Silver SA. Cohesive silicone gel breast implants in aesthetic and reconstructive breast surgery. Plast Reconstr Surg 2005;116:768–79.
16. Loustau HD, Mayer HF, Sarrabayrouse M. Pocket work for optimising outcomes in prosthetic breast reconstruction. J Plast Reconstr Aesthet Surg 2009;62:626–32.
17. Engel H, Huang J-J, Lin C-Y, et al. Subcutaneous tissue expansion and subsequent subpectoral implantation for breast reconstruction in Asian patients: safety and outcome. Ann Plast Surg 2012;70:135–43.
18. Fan J, Raposio E, Wang J, et al. Development of the inframammary fold and ptosis in breast reconstruction with textured tissue expanders. Ann Plast Surg 2002;26:219–22.
19. LifeCell. AlloDerm tissue matrix defined. Available at: http://www.lifecell.com/health-care-professionals/lifecell-products/allodermr-regenerative-tissue-matrix/allodermr-tissue-matrix-defined/. Accessed June 24, 2014.
20. Haddock N, Levine J. Breast reconstruction with implants, tissue expanders and AlloDerm: predicting volume and maximizing the skin envelope in skin sparing mastectomies. Breast J 2010;16:14–9.
21. Zienowicz RJ, Karacaoglu E. Implant-based breast reconstruction with allograft. Plast Reconstr Surg 2007;120:373–81.
22. Gamboa-Bobadilla GM. Implant breast reconstruction using acellular dermal matrix. Ann Plast Surg 2006;56:22–5.
23. Spear SL, Parikh PM, Reisin E, et al. Acellular dermis-assisted breast reconstruction. Aesthetic Plast Surg 2008;32(3):418–25.
24. Salzberg CA. Nonexpansive immediate breast reconstruction using human acellular tissue matrix graft (AlloDerm). Ann Plast Surg 2006;57:1–5.
25. Breuing KH, Warren SM. Immediate bilateral breast reconstruction with implants and inferolateral AlloDerm slings. Ann Plast Surg 2005;55:232–9.
26. Brandon JH, Young VL, Jerina KL, et al. Variability in the properties of silicone gel breast implants. Plast Reconstr Surg 2001;108:647–55.
27. Serletti JM, Fosnot J, Nelson JA, et al. Breast reconstruction after breast cancer. Plast Reconstr Surg 2011;127:124e–35e.
28. Stevens LA, McGrath MH, Druss RG, et al. The psychological impact of immediate breast reconstruction for women with early breast cancer. Plast Reconstr Surg 1984;73:619–26.
29. Al-Ghazal SK, Sully L, Fallowfield L, et al. The psychological impact of immediate rather than delayed breast reconstruction. Eur J Surg Oncol 2000;26:17–9.

Teaching Breast Augmentation

A Focus on Critical Intraoperative Techniques and Decision Making to Maximize Results and Minimize Revisions

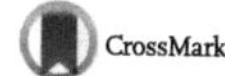

Michael Bradley Calobrace, MD[a,b,*]

KEYWORDS

• Breast augmentation • Complications • Incisions • Pocket • Capsular contracture
• Operative approach • Inframammary fold • Dual plane

KEY POINTS

- Preoperative assessment should determine choice of implant, breast pocket, incision, and need to lower inframammary fold.
- Surgical approach, implant choice, and operative technique can affect the incidence of capsular contracture.
- Inframammary fold positioning is critical to establishing optimal implant placement in the pocket.
- Creating a controlled pocket minimizes the risk of implant malposition or rotation.
- The dual plane maximizes coverage and support of the breast implant while minimizing the negative attributes of submuscular placement.

Video of the intraoperative steps of breast augmentation surgery accompanies this article at http://www.plasticsurgery.theclinics.com/

INTRODUCTION

The operative approach in breast augmentation begins with careful and thoughtful consideration preoperatively to the many variables that ultimately affect the final result. Most decisions are made during preoperative evaluation and require expert operative execution to minimize the risks of unsatisfactory outcomes.

PREOPERATIVE PLANNING

One of the most critical steps in achieving excellence in breast augmentation is the preoperative evaluation. Such an evaluation should identify not only the appropriate implant to achieve optimal results but also the location of the incision, the implant pocket, asymmetries of the breast, chest wall, and nipple-areolar complex,

Disclosure: Dr M.B. Calobrace has been a speaker for Mentor, Allergan, and Sientra with no financial disclosure. He is also a stockowner and general partner of Strathspey Crown Advisory Board, of which Alphaeon Corporation is a wholly owned subsidiary.

[a] Division of Plastic Surgery, Department of Surgery, University of Louisville, Louisville, KY, USA; [b] Division of Plastic Surgery, Department of Surgery, University of Kentucky, Lexington, KY, USA
* Calobrace Plastic Surgery Center, 2341 Lime Kiln Lane, Louisville, KY 40222.
E-mail address: drbrad@calobrace.com

Clin Plastic Surg 42 (2015) 493–504
http://dx.doi.org/10.1016/j.cps.2015.06.005

and the potential need to lower and manage the inframammary fold (IMF). The preoperative markings create a roadmap for the planned procedure (**Fig. 1**). Evaluation of the soft-tissue coverage, including quality of skin and breast tissue, amount of breast parenchyma present, and the level of ptosis, is essential in determining the optimal pocket for implant placement. Precise pocket creation and appropriate implant choice are the best safeguards against postoperative implant malposition issues. Likewise, one of the major drivers of revision surgery after a breast augmentation is capsular contracture.[1,2] There is significant evidence that contamination with biofilm development is a significant causative component in the development of capsular contracture.[3–6] Therefore, the surgical approach, implant choice, and operative technique can all affect the development of capsular contracture. At the preoperative planning stage, every effort should be made to minimize this risk. **Box 1** summarizes some of the implant and surgical technique options that have been associated with lower capsular contractures.[7–23]

Box 1
Characteristics associated with incidence of reduced capsular contracture

No-touch technique

Nipple shields

Pocket irrigation with triple antibiotics

Insertion sleeve

Submuscular implant pocket

Textured implants

Inframammary incision

Cohesive shaped implants

PATIENT POSITIONING

Patients are placed on the operating room table in the supine position. The arms are secured to the armboard at 45° to stabilize the patient in the upright position (**Fig. 2**). This positioning allows access for the surgeon to stand and yet relaxes the pectoralis muscle, providing a more accurate assessment of the implant position and the redraping of the breast tissue overlying it. Placing the arms by the patient's side is a useful alternative, but assessing the patient with the arms outstretched at 90° should be avoided.

INFILTRATION OF LOCAL ANESTHETIC

Before surgical preparation, 50 mL of a local field block of 1/4% lidocaine, 1/8% bupivacaine, and 1:400,000 epinephrine is injected (**Table 1**). The injection is placed in the dermis along the planned incision line, deep to the dermis along the IMF, the medial pectoral border, the anterior axillary line, and deep to the breast parenchyma, in a fanning fashion throughout the area of planned pocket creation (**Fig. 3**). These injections provide assistance not only in operative hemostasis but also in the management of postoperative pain.

SURGICAL PREPARATION AND STERILE DRAPING

After local infiltration, nipple shields (created by placing a small piece of Tegaderm over each nipple-areolar complex) provide a barrier against potential bacterial contamination[8] (**Fig. 4**). The patient is prepped with chlorhexidine and draped to provide a sterile field with the entire chest and bilateral breasts visible for assessment during the procedure. The sterile dressings must be secured

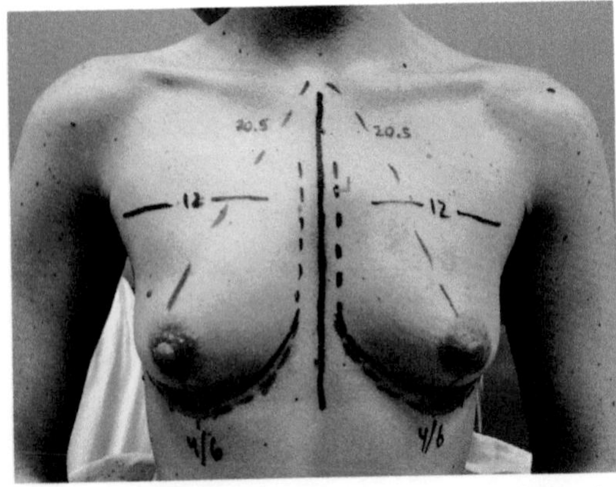

Fig. 1. Preoperative markings create a roadmap for the planned procedure.

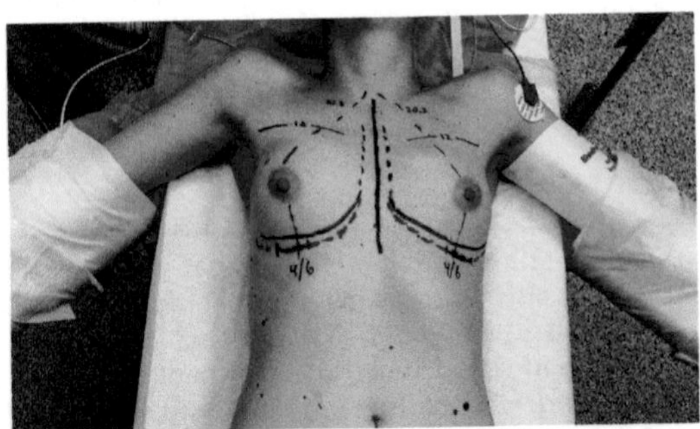

Fig. 2. The arms are secured to the armboard at 45° to allow appropriate evaluation of breast implant placement in the upright position.

Table 1
Breast local anesthetic formula

1/2% lidocaine plain	25 mL
1/2% lidocaine/1:200,000 epinephrine	25 mL
1/2% bupivacaine/1:200,000 epinephrine	25 mL
Injectable saline	25 mL
1/4% lidocaine, 1/8% bupivacaine, 1:400,000 epinephrine	100 mL

to prevent disruption in the sterile field while placing the patient in the upright position.

INCISION

The decision on incision placement is based on a variety of variables, including patient and surgeon preferences, anatomic considerations, and implant type and size. The size of the incision depends on the location, but in general should be as small as possible and yet large enough to safely dissect the pocket and place the implant without distortion or injury to the device. In general, the length of the incision would be smaller with saline than with silicone implants, and longer when placing more cohesive implants, larger implants, or textured implants. Implant fractures of form-stable cohesive implants and rupture or distortion of silicone implants has been associated with attempting to place implants through incisions

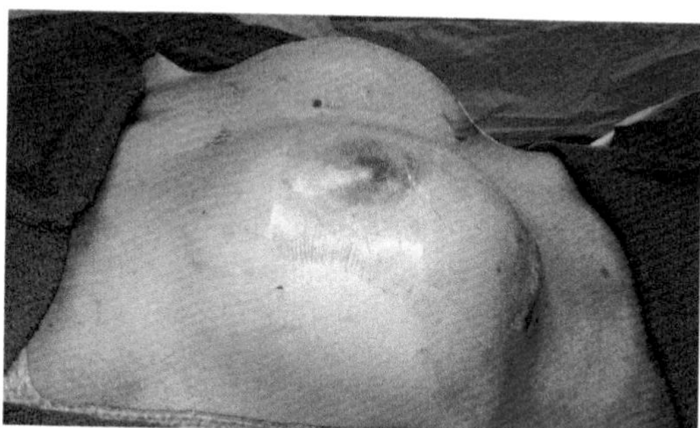

Fig. 4. Nipple shields are placed to provide a barrier against potential bacterial contamination.

inadequate to accommodate the implant. In addition, the quality of the scar is often better if a slightly larger scar is created, reducing the stretch and retraction injury placed on the scar. Incision length ranges include 3–4.5 cm for saline implants, 4–6 cm for silicone round implants, and 4.5–7 cm for shaped cohesive silicone implants.

Inframammary Fold Positioning

Predicting the final position of the IMF is critical to determining the placement of all breast incisions, but especially the inframammary incision. This task can be challenging, as so many variables contribute to the final position of the fold. The IMF is formed by the fusion of the anterior and posterior leaves of the superficial fascia, which is intimately associated with the dermis at the lowest

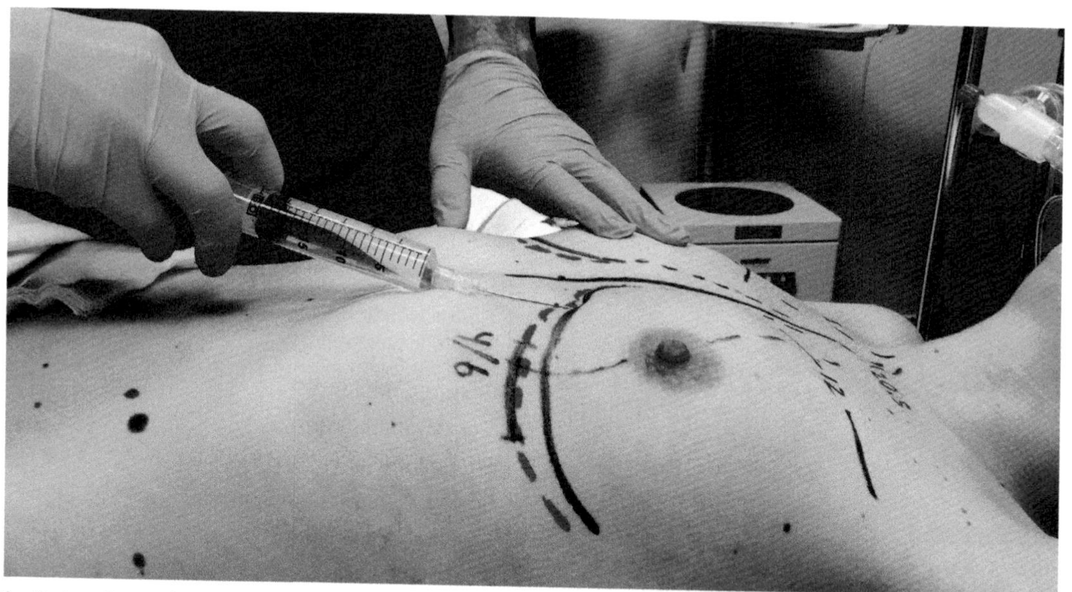

Fig. 3. Local anesthetic is injected into each breast to assist in intraoperative hemostasis and postoperative pain control.

aspect of the inferior pole of the breast.[24] Before surgery, the IMF is identified and marked in the sitting position. The true IMF position is actually determined by performing an IMF expansion test. The breast is grasped and autorotated inferiorly to identify the inferior extent of the attachments of the IMF (**Fig. 5**): this is the best predictor of where the fold will naturally sit after breast augmentation. The amount of lower pole skin required and the ultimate position of the fold is a function of many factors, including the type of implant (saline versus silicone, round versus shaped), size of implant, pocket location, and the strength and stability of the soft tissue of the lower pole. The distance measured from the nipple to the true fold under maximal stretch assesses the amount of lower pole skin available to accommodate the selected implant. An acceptable standard that has been used states that an implant with a base diameter of 11 cm requires 7 cm, a base diameter of 12 cm requires 8 cm, and a base diameter of 13 requires 9 cm.[25] A more comprehensive evaluation has been described using tissue-based planning principles.[26] In the High Five System analysis, variables are analyzed including implant volume, patient's base width, implant base width, anterior pulled skin stretch, and nipple to fold distance under maximal stretch. Based on the selected implant, a reference chart provides the desired nipple to fold distance, which, if longer than the measured distance, will require IMF lowering. In determining fold position, the author has found an extremely useful alternative method. This calculation takes into consideration implant selections that may fall outside the limits of appropriate tissue-based planning. The required distance from nipple to fold is calculated as a function of implant height and implant projection, which is useful for both round and shaped implants.

Optimal N-IMF distance = $\frac{1}{2}$ implant projection + $\frac{1}{2}$ implant height

IMF Lowering = Optimal N-IMF distance − measured N-IMF distance (maximal stretch)

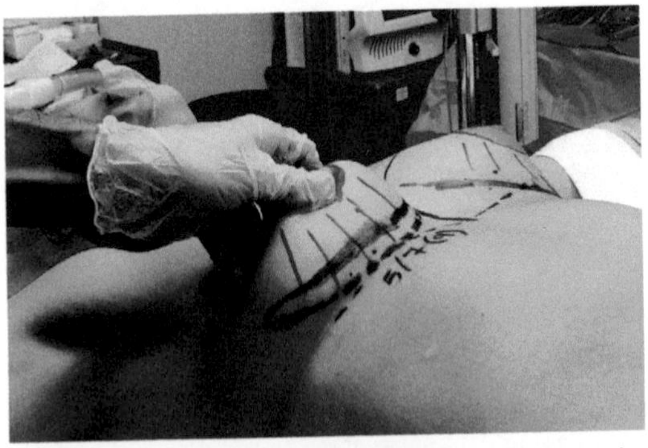

Fig. 5. The true fold, the best predictor of where the fold will lie postoperatively, is assessed by autorotation of the breast inferiorly to identify the inferior extent of the fascial attachments at the fold.

If the desired N-IMF distance is equal to or less than the measured N-IMF distance, the fold does not require lowering. The distance can be adjusted based on expectation for lower pole stretch postoperatively. This observation has become increasingly important as more textured round and shaped implants are being used. It is important to recognize that IMF lowering is less often required when placing a smooth silicone implant, especially if higher-profile or larger-sized implants are used secondary to lower pole stretch over time.[27,28] However, when placing textured implants, IMF lowering may be required more often than smooth implants, owing to less lower pole stretch and inferior implant descent created by the frictional component or adherence of the texture in the implant pocket.[13,29] Likewise, shaped implants are not only textured but also have a greater volume of a more cohesive gel present in the lower pole of the implant, thus requiring more lower pole skin to accommodate the implant.[20–23,30,31] **Box 2** identifies some implant and soft-tissue characteristics that may be associated with a greater need to lower the IMF because of the lesser postoperative stretching of the lower pole.[13,20–23,26–31]

Box 2
Characteristics associated with less stretching of the lower pole

- Textured implants
- Cohesive implants
- Shaped implants
- Silicone versus saline implants
- Lower profile implants
- Smaller implants
- Tight, firm breast skin

Inframammary Incision

The inframammary incision is the most commonly used, owing to its direct access and visualization of the pocket with the least injury to surrounding structures. After determining the IMF position (either the native true fold position or the planned lowered position), a paramedian line is drawn through the center of the breast and bisects the newly drawn IMF. The incision's medial extent begins 1 cm medial to the paramedian line and extends laterally for the appropriate distance, as previously described (**Fig. 6**). The incision is made with a #15 blade through the skin to the mid-dermis. Dissection is then carried out with electrocautery through the skin and subcutaneous tissue, beveling upward while rotating the breast off of the chest wall. Once dissection has been carried superiorly for 1 cm, the dissection is carried through the superficial fascia and toward the lateral pectoral border deep on the chest wall. This beveling maneuver preserves a small cuff of superficial fascia at the incision, which ensures the fold is not inadvertently lowered and also provides a cuff of fascia that will prove useful during closure (**Fig. 7**).

Periareolar Incision

Although used less often in the past few years, this incision can be very useful for avoidance of a scar

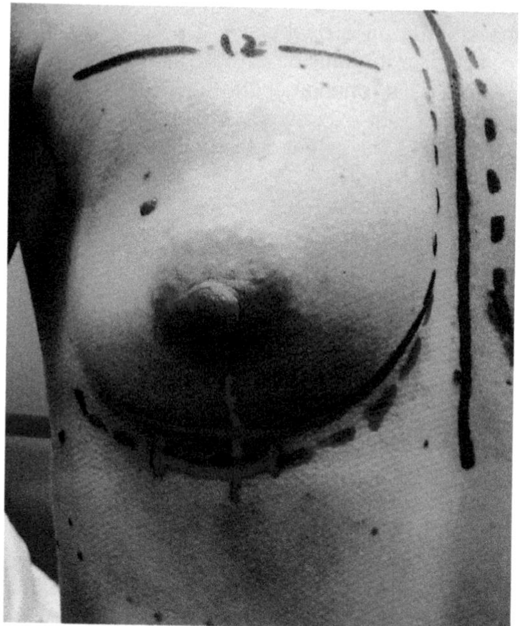

Fig. 6. The incision is made starting 1 cm medial to the paramedian line of the breast and extending laterally for the appropriate distance.

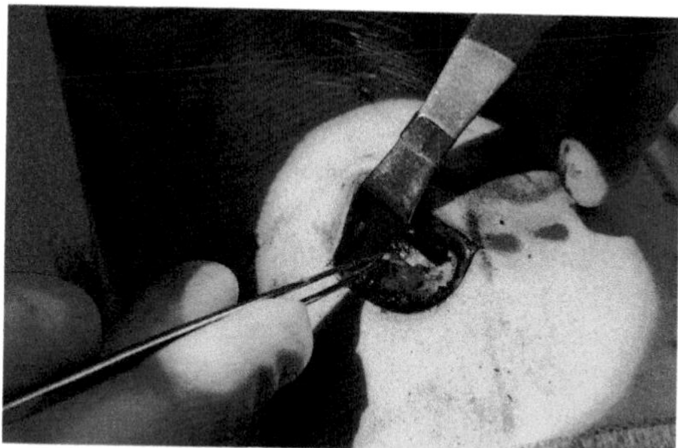

Fig. 7. Preservation of a small cuff of Scarpa fascia during initial dissection avoids inadvertent lowering of the IMF and assists in anchoring the fold during closure.

in the fold of the breast. It is most inconspicuous when there is a distinct border and a marked color contrast between the areolar skin and surrounding breast skin. Patients with smaller areolar complexes also may be inappropriate because of difficulty in implant placement, especially with larger, textured, or shaped implants, as injury to the implant can occur while trying to place an implant through the longer breast tunnel associated with these incisions. The incision is made between 3 o'clock and 6 o'clock through the skin with a #15 blade directly on the border between areola and adjacent breast skin. Dissection is carried through the inferior aspect of the breast directly through the breast tissue to the retroglandular plane until the lateral pectoralis border is identified. Care should be taken not to carry the dissection superiorly and inadvertently devascularize the nipple-areolar complex. Dissection inferiorly in the subcutaneous plane down to the IMF has been described but may not be optimal, as it can create significant distortion and stretch deformities in the lower pole of the breast.

IMPLANT POCKET

Pocket Decision

There continues to be divergence of opinion as to the optimal pocket for breast implants. The subglandular/subfascial pocket is the most natural for the implant, with avoidance of animation deformities seen with submuscular implants, enhanced correction of constricted breast or ptotic breasts, ease of dissection, and less postoperative discomfort for the patient.[32–35] The advantages of the submuscular pocket have included lower capsular contracture rates, enhanced coverage of the implant, minimal issues of wrinkling, and provision of a more natural upper pole and enhanced support for the breast implant.[11–13,32–34,36]

Undoubtedly, the issues of wrinkling and need for enhanced coverage with saline implants provided the impetus for submuscular pockets becoming the preferred pocket by surgeons in the United States.[29,37,38] It has been widely accepted that an upper pole pinch test of 2 cm is required to place an implant in the subglandular/subfascial pocket to reduce the risk of upper pole implant visibility or wrinkling. With the availability of silicone implants, both round and shaped, and simultaneous fat grafting, the optimal pocket choice may be even more elusive.

Pocket Control

No matter which pocket is selected, it is helpful during the marking process to identify as accurately as possible the pocket size necessary to accommodate the selected implant. This precaution will provide a pocket that maintains the implant in a control position and minimizes the risk of postoperative implant malposition. In breast augmentation with round implants, the accurate placement of the IMF and control of the medial and lateral extent of the pockets provide ideal implant positioning to achieve the desired cleavage and minimize lateral migration of the implant.[29] When using a shaped implant, a controlled pocket is even more essential to minimize the risk of implant rotation postoperatively.[23,30,31] This outcome requires not only controlling the pocket similarly to a round implant, but additionally limiting the dissection of the superior pocket to snugly accommodate the height of the shaped implant.

Dual-Plane Pocket

Maximizing soft-tissue coverage whenever possible has been one of the most important guiding principles in the success in breast augmentation. Inadequate coverage, often combined with heavy, oversized implants, leads to soft-tissue parenchymal atrophy, skin stretching resulting from the pressure and weight of the implant, and ultimate wrinkling and palpability of the implants and associated breast deformities.[27,28] The dual plane, initially described by Tebbetts,[36] maximizes coverage and support of the breast implant while minimizing the distractors of submuscular placement, including animation deformities and pseudoptosis of the breast tissue overlying the submuscular implant (ie, Snoopy deformity).

When performing a dual-plane pocket, the lateral pectoral border is identified and fascia incised to expose the underlying muscle. Upward retraction of the breast tissue will usually elevate the lateral border, allowing further dissection and placement of the retractor beneath the overlying pectoralis muscle (**Fig. 8**). It is an extremely important principle to never cut through the muscle if you cannot tent the muscle upward. Inability to elevate the muscle may indicate that the muscle fascia is extremely adherent, or more likely that the identified muscle is actually not the pectoralis, but rather the serratus, rectus, or an intercostal muscle. Continuing the dissection through an intercostal could inadvertently penetrate the pleural space with a resultant pneumothorax. Once the edge of the pectoralis is safely elevated and the subpectoral space is identified, dissection is carried upward centrally to the superior extent of the pocket. Dissection is then carried laterally to identify the pectoralis minor, and is continued superficial to it until the lateral border of the pocket is reached. Dissection is then continued along the lateral border of the pocket, identifying and staying superficial to the serratus muscle until the inferior extent of the pocket at the IMF is reached. The muscle is then released along the planned IMF, staying 1 cm superior to the fold to account for caudal muscle descent (**Fig. 9**). Dissection directly at the fold will often lead to a fold that is lower than planned as the muscle retracts inferiorly. In performing a dual-plane approach, great care should be taken to stop the dissection along the fold at the most medial extent along the sternum. Dissection should absolutely not be continued superiorly along the sternum, as has been previously taught. Preservation of the most caudal attachment of the pectoralis muscle along the sternum in a dual-plane approach is critical to minimize the chance of windowshading of the pectoralis, a phenomenon that often leads to medial implant exposure and unsightly animation deformities. The extent of the pocket is completed

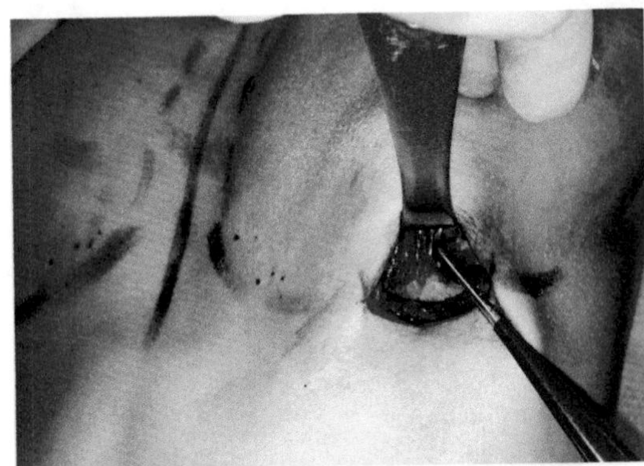

Fig. 8. Upward retraction on the breast tissue elevates the lateral border of the pectoralis muscle, allowing further dissection and placement of the retractor under the muscle.

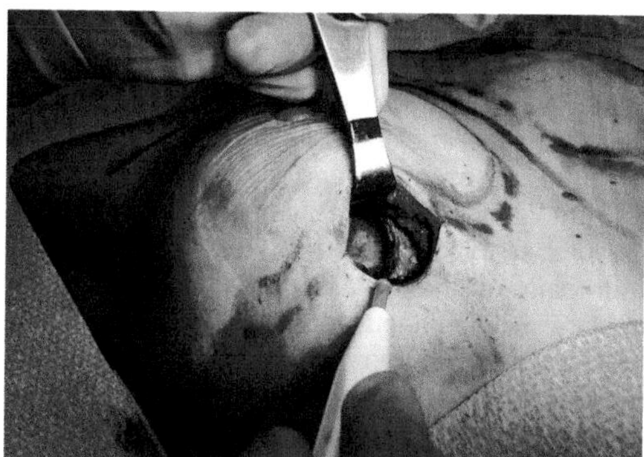

Fig. 9. The pectoralis muscle is released along the IMF staying 1 cm superior to the fold to account for caudal muscle descent.

by defining the medial pectoral border by dividing the accessory slips of pectoralis muscle that insert along the ribs, preserving the main body of the muscle as it inserts along the sternum. Dividing these muscles with electrocautery and not depending on blunt dissection improves postoperative cleavage and maintains prospective hemostasis.

The final maneuver in the dual-plane approach is creating the subglandular pocket inferiorly. The levels of dual plane represent the amount of muscle released from the inferior breast tissue and resultant inferior subglandular pocket (**Fig. 10**). Division of the inferior pectoralis muscle just above the IMF during initial pocket dissection created a level-1 dual plane. The level of dual plane required varies, and each surgery can be tailored to provide the optimal level based on soft-tissue requirements and implant selection. In general, creating a subglandular pocket inferiorly is required to either redrape the skin and breast tissue more accurately over the implant or for expansion and exposure of the lower pole, such as in a tuberous or constricted breast. The levels of dual plane are a continuum and not fixed points. The release of the caudal edge of the muscle is performed incrementally, creating the least amount of release that will adequately address the lower pole (**Fig. 11**). When creating a dual plane to address the laxity of the lower pole, placement of a retractor into the breast pocket and elevating superiorly while rocking the breast tissue over the retractor will assist in assessing the effects of the implant on the skin and breast tissue once placed in the pocket. When a dual plane is created for expansion and exposure, the level will depend on the need to access the parenchyma for radial scoring. This action usually requires at least level-2 and often level-3 dual plane to expose the retroareolar tissue.

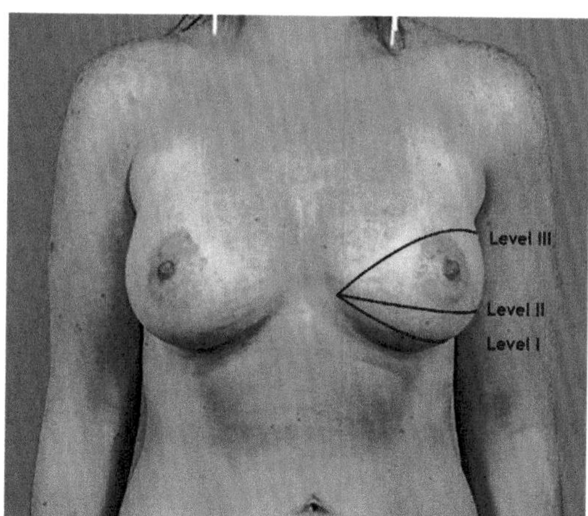

Fig. 10. The dual-plane pocket includes a submuscular pocket superiorly and a subglandular pocket inferiorly, based on the extent of muscle release off the overlying breast tissue. The dual-plane levels include: level 1, the caudal edge of the muscle is present in the lower pole below the areola; level 2, the caudal edge is at the inferior areola; and level 3, the caudal edge is at the superior areola.

If required, IMF lowering must occur in the subglandular pocket, as the attachments creating the fold are superficial to the deep pectoral fascia.[39] Thus, a subglandular or dual-plane approach provides the necessary subglandular plane in the lower pole of the breast. Dissection to the deep pectoral fascia will likely result in maintenance of the fold structure, resulting in a double-bubble deformity.

IMPLANT PLACEMENT

Once dissection is complete, the pocket is prepared for the implant. The pocket is irrigated with

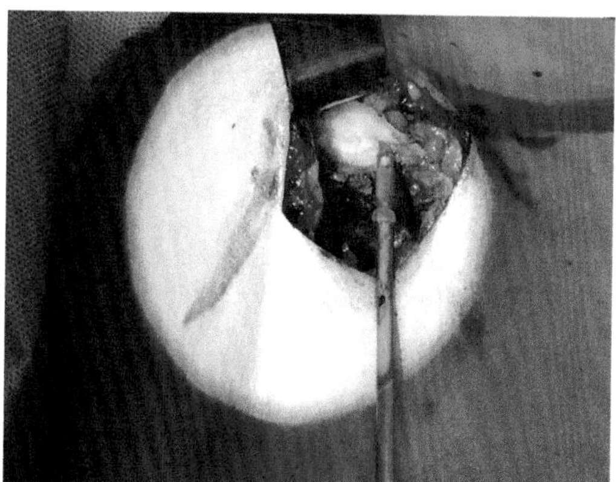

Fig. 11. The dual plane is created by exposing the caudal edge of the pectoralis muscle and incrementally releasing off the overlying breast tissue, creating a subglandular pocket inferiorly.

modified Adams formula of triple antibiotic solution/betadine solution (50 mL of povidone-iodine, 1 g of cefazolin sodium, 50,000 units of bacitracin mixed in 500 mL of normal saline) and hemostasis is assessed.[10] It is the goal during the operation to achieve prospective hemostasis with minimal blood staining; however, a final assessment is mandatory before implant placement. The implants are soaked in the irrigation solution before insertion. Gloves are changed and rinsed with the irrigation solution to remove any lint or powder.

The implant is then placed either manually or with the assistance of an insertion sleeve such as the Keller funnel[9] (**Fig. 12**). The opening of the funnel should be cut large enough to allow easy egress of the implant through the funnel, easily confirmed by passing the implant with irrigation solution through the funnel before insertion. The implant orientation is then confirmed in the funnel, and a maneuver of squeezing the implant through the funnel with pressure exerted on the back of the funnel allows the implant to slip into the breast pocket. These maneuvers provide a "no-touch" technique, which has been associated with lower capsular contracture rates.[7] The funnel allows for easier implant placement with potentially smaller incision requirements in comparison with manual placement. It has proved especially helpful with textured implants, which can be much more challenging and require larger incisions compared with smooth implants.[29] Whereas many of the shaped implants can be placed with the funnel, the firmer and larger cohesive shaped implants may pose a challenge because of the lack of implant and gel flexibility, and may not be appropriate for the funnel. Once the implant is in the pocket, a finger-assisted assessment and manipulation of the implant within the pocket is necessary to confirm its proper placement and assure appropriate redraping of the breast parenchyma over the implant. This maneuver is especially important with textured devices, as these implants are less mobile and less likely to stretch the pocket and, thus, a distortion or wrinkling of the implant in a tight pocket may be permanent if not resolved before closure. Repeated removal and insertions of the implant should be avoided to minimize implant or incision damage, potential contamination, and pocket overdissection. This approach is especially important with shaped implants, as a stretched pocket from overmanipulation could lead to implant rotation postoperatively.

CLOSURE

Before incision closure, the patient should be placed in the upright position to assess implant position, fold position, symmetry, and the adequacy of the dual plane (**Fig. 13**). Any additional adjustments of the dual plane can be accomplished after the patient is replaced in the recumbent position by simply retracting the breast tissue superiorly off the implant, identifying the

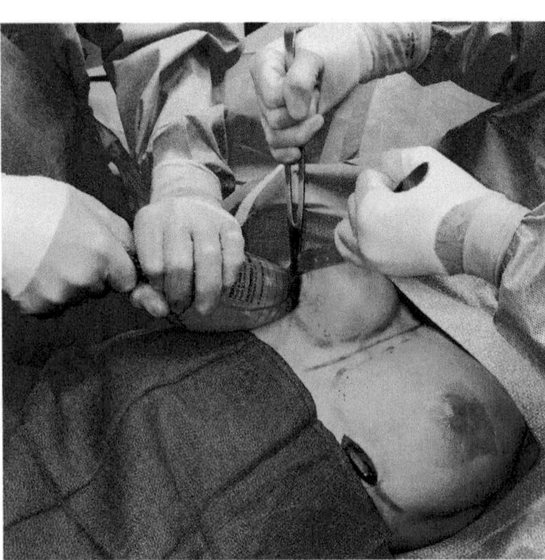

Fig. 12. An insertion sleeve such as the Keller Funnel can facilitate implant placement. The implant should be oriented appropriately in the funnel before placement, and the funnel opening must be adequate to allow a smooth and gentle passage of the implant through it.

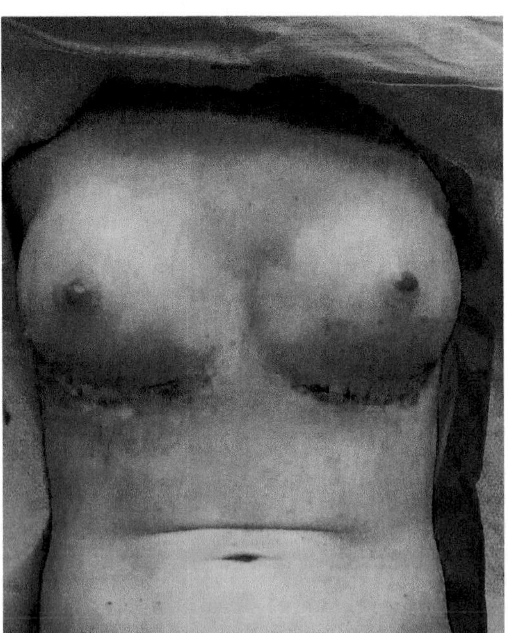

Fig. 13. The patient is placed in the upright position to assess implant position, fold position, symmetry, and the adequacy of the dual plane before closure.

caudal edge of the muscle, and releasing it incrementally off the overlying breast tissue to the desired level. Reassessment in the upright position after appropriate adjustments is advisable to confirm position of implants and the optimal relationship between the implant and the overlying breast tissue.

A significant advantage of the inframammary approach that is often underappreciated is the ability to accurately and effectively control the fold position during closure of the incision. The cuff of superficial Scarpa fascia that was preserved during the initial incision is used to secure the fold during closure. In general, if the IMF structure is well developed and stable, and has not been violated or lowered during the procedure, then reapproximation of the superficial fascia during closure is usually adequate. However, when the fold is unstable from either inherent weakness in the fold structure or its disruption with fold lowering, closure should include stabilization of the fold structure. This maneuver is accomplished by securing the caudal edge of the Scarpa fascia present on the lower incisional edge to the underlying deep fascial structures with an absorbable suture such as 2-0 Vicryl or permanent suture (**Fig. 14**). This suturing is usually done by simply incorporating the superficial and deep fascia together during closure, but can be also performed by first placing 3 sutures on the lower flap, securing the Scarpa fascia to the underlying deep fascia followed by closure of the incision. Unique to both round and shaped textured devices, the implant must be seated accurately at the base of the breast pocket, as it is less likely to settle in the breast pocket postoperatively as can be seen with smooth breast implants. Thus, special care must be taken during closure not to inadvertently injure the breast implants. The incision is closed in 3 layers: Scarpa fascia superiorly to Scarpa fascia (with or without deep fascia) inferiorly, deep dermis, and subcuticular.

The periareolar incision lacks the ability to control the fold structure during closure. Closure includes closing the breast tissue deep to the incision, followed by deep dermal interrupted suture and a running subcuticular with absorbable sutures (Video 1).

POSTOPERATIVE MANAGEMENT

The management of breast augmentation is variable among surgeons, and the type of device

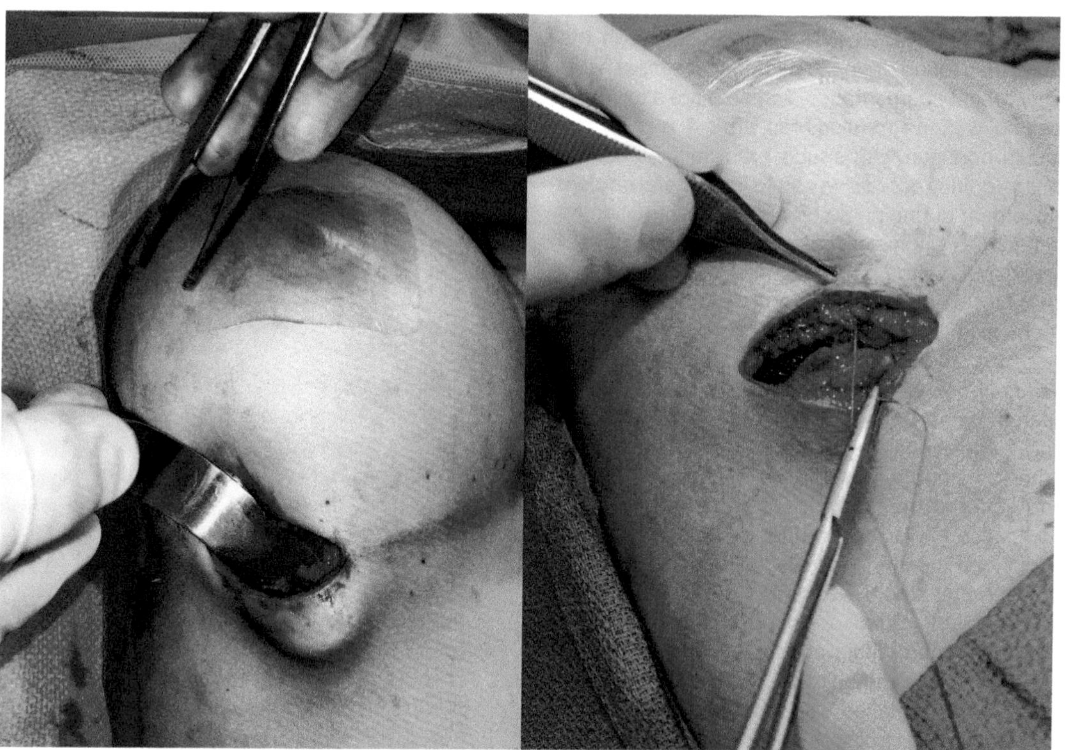

Fig. 14. When stabilization of the IMF is required because of inherent weakness in the fold structure or secondary to fold lowering (*left*), closure requires incorporating deep fascial structures into the Scarpa fascia closure to secure the fold position (*right*).

used can alter the postoperative protocols. In the author's practice, all patients are wrapped in an ace wrap for the first 24 hours followed by a sports bra to be worn 23 hours per day for the next 4 weeks. Early range of motion, beginning in the recovery room, is initiated for all patients, which includes shoulder rolls in both directions in addition to elevation of the arms outward to the sides and over the head. With smooth devices, implant massage begins postoperatively on day 4 and includes displacing the implant upward and downward in the pocket, crossing the arms and pulling the implants inward to create cleavage, and downward pressure on the implants to stretch the lower pole. With textured implants, both round and shaped, limited arm movement other than range of motion is recommended for the first week. Implant massage is contraindicated, as the textured surface can irritate the pocket and potentially create serous fluid around the implant. Likewise, the implants are placed in a controlled pocket with the implant positioned appropriately at the base of the pocket; displacement could lead to implant malposition or, in the case of shaped devices, rotation of the implant. The different types of texture available vary considerably in terms of texture aggressiveness and implant adherence, and the exact postoperative protocol and decision on drain placement should be based on these considerations, although the author has found drains to be unnecessary in a primary breast augmentation. Patients are allowed to resume wearing regular bras after 4 weeks, but should continue with sports bras during bedtime for an additional 2 to 4 weeks to limit lateral implant movement during pocket formation. Normal activity resumes within a few days after surgery, but exercise and high-impact activity should be delayed for 3 to 4 weeks. Whereas smooth implants often seem high initially and often require downward massage and the use of breast bands or bandeaus, textured devices that are appropriately seated in the base of the breast pocket should only occasionally require such maneuvers. Whereas smooth implants will seem more mobile and softer in the first few weeks after surgery in comparison with textured devices, the textured implants will soften with modest movement often present after 4 to 6 weeks. If a variety of smooth and textured (round or shaped) breast implants are being used within a practice, it is extremely important to communicate to ancillary staff the type of device placed with each patient to initiate the appropriate postoperative protocol, as inappropriate instructions can lead to postoperative problems such as seromas, malposition, and rotational deformities.

SUMMARY

The successful outcome of breast augmentation begins with careful preoperative and intraoperative decision making (Video 1). These decisions often affect the final outcome and the long-term success of the operation. Consideration of the patient's desired outcome, soft-tissue and chest wall characteristics, and the degree of ptosis provide important information in determining the optimal implant, incision, and pocket. The availability of a wide array of implant shapes and sizes has allowed surgeons a greater ability to tailor the breast augmentation to meet these requirements. The ability to create an accurate and symmetric pocket that allows for appropriate breast tissue redraping and placement, and management of the IMF, are hallmarks of a reproducible and successful breast augmentation procedure.

Editorial Comments by Bradley P. Bengtson, MD

Dr Calobrace has done a great deal to advance our specialty and advance our techniques and outcomes in Breast Plastic Surgery. Recognizing the critical importance of preoperative planning, this chapter combines planning as well as critical intraoperative technical steps and precise surgical execution to produce predictable, consistent outcomes to maximize patient outcomes and minimize adverse events and subsequent revisions.

SUPPLEMENTARY DATA

Supplementary data related to this article can be found online at http://dx.doi.org/10.1016/j.cps.2015.06.005.

REFERENCES

1. Spears SL, Murphy DK, Slicton A, et al. Inamed silicone breast implant core study results at 6 years. Plast Reconstr Surg 2007;120:8S–16S.
2. Cunningham B, McCue J. Safety and effectiveness of Mentor's MemoryGel implants at 6 years. Aesthetic Plast Surg 2009;33:440–4.
3. Araco A, Caruso R, Araco F, et al. Capsular contracture: a systematic review. Plast Reconstr Surg 2009;124:1808–19.
4. Virden CP, Dobbke MK, Stein P, et al. Subclinical infection of the silicone breast implant surface as a possible cause of capsular contracture. Aesthetic Plast Surg 1992;16:173–9.
5. Pajkos A, Deva AK, Vicery K, et al. Detection of subclinical infection in significant breast implant capsules. Plast Reconstr Surg 2003;111:1605–11.

6. Rieger UM, Mesina J, Kalbermatten DF, et al. Bacterial biofilms and capsular contracture in patients with breast implants. Br J Surg 2013;100:768–74.
7. Mladick RA. "No-touch" submuscular saline breast augmentation technique. Aesthetic Plast Surg 1993;17:183–92.
8. Wixtrom RN, Stutman RL, Burke RM, et al. Risk of breast implant bacterial contamination from endogenous breast flora, prevention with nipple shields, and implications for biofilm formation. Aesthet Surg J 2012;32:956–63.
9. Moyer HR, Ghazi B, Saunders N, et al. Contamination in smooth gel breast implant placement: testing a funnel versus digital insertion technique in a cadaver model. Aesthet Surg J 2012;32(2):194–9.
10. Adams WP, Rios JL, Smith S. Enhancing patient outcomes in aesthetic and reconstructive breast surgery using triple antibiotic breast irrigation: six-year prospective clinical study. Plast Reconstr Surg 2006;118(Suppl 7):46S–52S.
11. Stevens WG, Nahabedian MY, Calobrace MB, et al. Risk factor analysis for capsular contracture: a 5-year Sientra study analysis using round, smooth and textured implants for breast augmentation. Plast Reconstr Surg 2013;132(5):1115–23.
12. Schaub TA, Ahmad J, Rohrich RJ. Capsular contracture with breast implants in the cosmetic patient: saline versus silicone. A systematic review of the literature. Plast Reconstr Surg 2010;126:2140–9.
13. Namnoum JD, Largent J, Kaplan HM, et al. Primary breast augmentation clinical trial outcomes stratified by surgical incision, anatomical placement and implant device type. J Plast Reconstr Aesthet Surg 2013;66(9):1165–72.
14. Barnsley GP, Siigurdson LJ, Barnsley SE. Textured surface breast implants in the prevention of capsular contracture among breast augmentation patients: a meta-analysis of randomized controlled trials. Plast Reconstr Surg 2006;117:2182–90.
15. Hakelius L, Ohlsen L. Tendency to capsule contracture around smooth and textured gel-filled silicone mammary implants: a 5-year follow-up. Plast Reconstr Surg 1997;100:1566–9.
16. Burkhardt B, Eades E. The effect of biocell texturizing and povidone-iodine irrigation on capsule contracture around saline-inflatable breast implants. Plast Reconstr Surg 1995;96:1317–25.
17. Coleman DJ, Foo IT, Sharpe DT. Textured or smooth implants for breast augmentation? A prospective controlled trial. Br J Plast Surg 1991;44:444–8.
18. Malata CM, Felderg L, Coleman DJ, et al. Textured or smooth implants for breast augmentation? Three year followup of a prospective randomized controlled trial. Br J Plast Surg 1997;50:99–105.
19. Weiner RC. Relationship of incision choice to capsular contracture. Aesthetic Plast Surg 2008; 32:303–6.
20. Hammond DC, Migliori MM, Caplin DA, et al. Mentor Contour Profile Gel implants: clinical outcomes at 6 years. Plast Reconstr Surg 2012;129:1381–91.
21. Maxwell GP, Van Natta BW, Murphy DK, et al. Natrelle style 410 form-stable silicone breast implants: core study results at 6 years. Aesthet Surg J 2012;32:709–17.
22. Jewell ML, Jewell JL. A comparison of outcomes involving highly cohesive, form-stable breast implants from two manufacturers in patients undergoing primary breast augmentation. Aesthet Surg J 2010;30:51–65.
23. Caplin DA. Indications for the use of MemoryShape breast implants in aesthetic and reconstructive breast surgery: long-term clinical outcomes of shaped versus round silicone breast implants. Plast Reconstr Surg 2014;134(3S):27S–37S.
24. Muntan CD, Sundine MJ, Rink RD, et al. Inframammary fold: a histological reappraisal. Plast Reconstr Surg 2000;105:549–56.
25. Teitelbaum S. The inframammary approach to breast augmentation. Clin Plast Surg 2009;36:33–43.
26. Tebbetss JB, Adams WP. Five critical decisions in breast augmentation using five measurements in 5 minutes: the high five decision support process. Plast Reconstr Surg 2005;116:2005–16.
27. Adams WP. The process of breast augmentation: four sequential steps for optimizing outcomes for patients. Plast Reconstr Surg 2008;122:1892–900.
28. Tebbetts JB, Teitelbaum S. High- and extra-high-projection breast implants: potential consequences for patients. Plast Reconstr Surg 2010;126:2150–9.
29. Calobrace MB, Kaufman DL, Gordon AE, et al. Evolving practices in augmentation operative techniques with Sientra HSC round implants. Plast Reconstr Surg 2014;134(Suppl 1):57S–67S.
30. Hammond DC. Technique and results using MemoryShape implants in aesthetic and reconstructive breast surgery. Plast Reconstr Surg 2014;134(Suppl 3):16S–26S.
31. Schwartz MR. Algorithm and techniques for using Sientra's silicone gel shaped implants in primary and revision breast augmentation. Plast Reconstr Surg 2014;134(Suppl 1):18S–27S.
32. Strasser EJ. Results of subglandular versus subpectoral augmentation over time: one surgeon's observations. Aesthet Surg J 2006;26:45–50.
33. Goes JCS, Landecker A. Optimizing outcomes in breast augmentation: seven years of experience with the subfascial plane. Aesthetic Plast Surg 2003;27:178–84.
34. Serra-Renom J, Garrido MF, Yoon T. Augmentation mammoplasty with anatomic soft, cohesive silicone implant using the transaxillary approach at a subfascial level with endoscopic assistance. Plast Reconstr Surg 2005;116:640–5.
35. Graf R, Pace DT, Damasio RC, et al. Subfascial breast augmentation. Chapter 50. In: Eisenmann-Klein M,

Heuhann-Lorenz C, editors. Innovations in plastic and aesthetic surgery. New York: Springer; 2008. p. 406–13.
36. Tebbetts JB. Dual plane breast augmentation: optimizing implant-soft-tissue relationships in a wide range of breast types. Plast Reconstr Surg 2001; 107:1255–72.
37. Maxwell GP, Gabriel A. The evolution of breast implants. Plast Reconstr Surg 2014;134(Suppl 1): 12S–7S.
38. Maxwell GP, Gabriel A. The evolution of breast implants. Clin Plast Surg 2009;36:1–13.
39. Schusterman MA. Lowering the inframammary fold. Aesthet Surg J 2004;24:482–5.

Strategies and Challenges in Simultaneous Augmentation Mastopexy

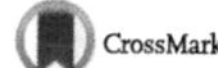

Michelle A. Spring, MD[a,*], Emily C. Hartmann, MD, MS[a,b], W. Grant Stevens, MD[a]

KEYWORDS

• Augmentation mastopexy • Breast augmentation • Mastopexy • Breast implants
• Combined augmentation mastopexy • Simultaneous augmentation mastopexy • Breast lift

KEY POINTS

- Identify pertinent anatomy and indications for simultaneous augmentation mastopexy.
- Discuss operative strategies for simultaneous augmentation mastopexy.
- Identify how to avoid and treat potential complications of simultaneous augmentation mastopexy.

INTRODUCTION

Plastic surgeons have been performing simultaneous breast augmentation with mastopexy for decades.[1–20] Although staging procedures remains the safest option in certain situations, in many cases these procedures are now being performed together, with excellent results and low complication rates. Proper patient evaluation and tissue-based planning is important, and it is critical to evaluate these patients carefully when planning this challenging procedure. Breast measurements, chest wall contour and breast footprint, breast tissue density, skin laxity, nipple and parenchymal ptosis, and the patient's expectations must be considered. The goals include creating a pleasing breast shape with symmetry of the breast mound and nipple position, upper breast fullness, tightening of loose skin, and an increase in overall breast size, with longevity of results and a low rate of capsular contracture or other implant complications. Many types of skin incisions can be used: a superior crescent, circumareolar ("donut"), circumvertical ("lollipop" or "owl"),[21,22] circumvertical with small inframammary fold extension ("owl with feet"), full Wise pattern ("anchor"), an inframammary fold incision only to improve pseudoptosis ("smile"), or an inverted T pattern without circumareolar component if the nipple and areola in good position ("sailboat") (**Fig. 1**). Implants can be placed in a variety of tissue planes through mastopexy incisions, including a subpectoral, subglandular, or subfascial placement. Some surgeons may prefer to stage breast augmentation and mastopexy as 2 separate procedures, and this is sometimes the safest option in certain situations. However, these procedures are commonly performed simultaneously, with excellent results and low complication rates.[3–6]

BREAST VASCULAR ANATOMY

Nipple blood supply is an important consideration in augmentation mastopexy surgery. The effect of implant placement and tissue undermining on the blood supply must be considered. If the implant is placed in the subglandular plane and significant tissue undermining is performed, the blood supply may be severely compromised. Subpectoral

Disclosures: See last page of article.
[a] Keck School of Medicine of University of Southern California, Los Angeles, CA 90033, USA; [b] Marina Plastic Surgery, 4644 Lincoln Boulevard, #552, Marina del Rey, CA 90252, USA
* Corresponding author.
E-mail address: drmichellespring@gmail.com

Clin Plastic Surg 42 (2015) 505–518
http://dx.doi.org/10.1016/j.cps.2015.06.008
0094-1298/15/$ – see front matter

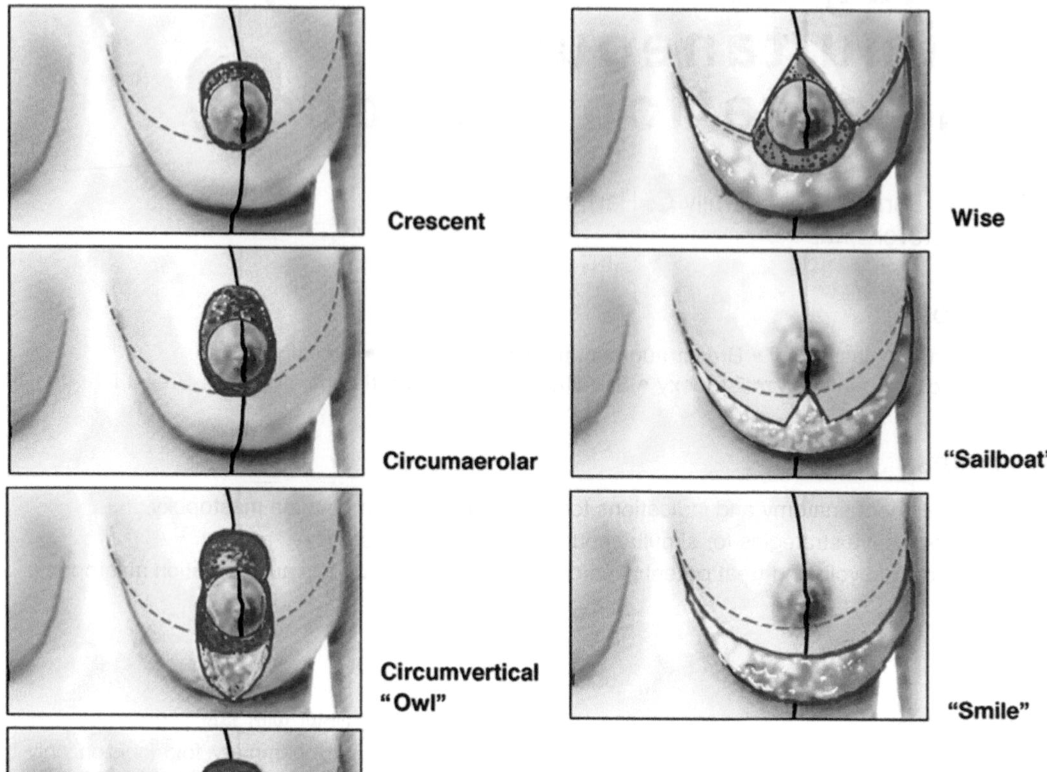

Fig. 1. Types of mastopexy incisions.

placement of the breast implants does not disrupt the musculocutaneous perforators and is less likely to interfere with blood supply. In addition, the placement of large implants in any plane that results in undue tension on the mastopexy closure can cause vascular compromise. In a recent updated review by the authors,[23] the average implant size placed in more than 1100 simultaneous augmentation mastopexies was 323 mL.

There is variability and overlap between sources of blood supply to the breast. The most important arterial sources are the internal mammary (internal thoracic) artery perforators, which are the dominant vessels (**Fig. 2**). The second to fourth internal mammary perforators are the main blood supply for a superior or superomedial pedicle. The reader is referred to numerous articles for a more in-depth summary the breast vascular anatomy.[24–28]

INDICATIONS FOR AUGMENTATION MASTOPEXY

Patients requiring augmentation mastopexy are often older than those desiring enlargement with implants. Such patients may have lost weight or are postpartum, and the sequelae of increased tissue laxity, parenchyma loss, striae, and nipple ptosis require a mastopexy to create an aesthetic breast shape. Women with Regnault grade 1 ptosis who desire enlargement are frequently treated with breast augmentation alone; however, nipple position alone is often inadequate to determine whether a simultaneous mastopexy would benefit the patient. There is a challenging subset of women who present with "in-between" breasts. These patients may benefit from a dual-plane breast augmentation.[29] Patients who have grade 1, mild grade 2, or grade 4 ptosis in the setting

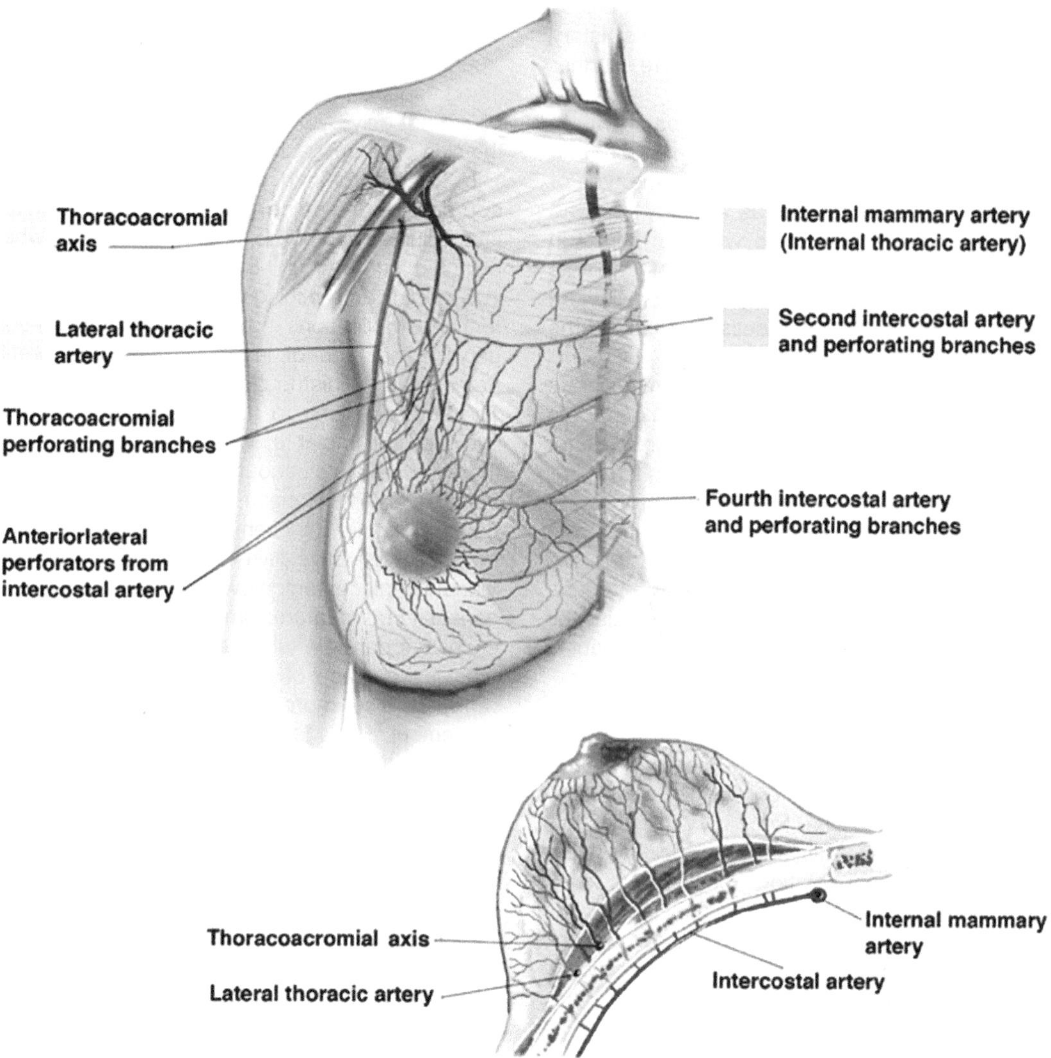

Fig. 2. Breast vascular anatomy.

of surrounding skin laxity pose another challenge. Placing an implant without removing excess tissue can result in skin and glandular tissue hanging off the implant. Another example of a challenging situation is women with mild constriction, with a short nipple to inframammary fold (IMF) distance, mild parenchymal herniation into the areola, or both. Patients without obvious significant breast ptosis often do not expect to hear that they may benefit from a breast lift, and may be unwilling to accept any additional scars. In addition, there is a common public perception that larger implants will suffice as a "lift" and that there is no need for additional scars. Patients often benefit from education about the role of breast augmentation and mastopexy, and the rationale for the surgeon's advice. Patients with significant grade 2 or 3 ptosis require mastopexy in addition to augmentation.

PREOPERATIVE PREPARATION

Preoperative planning is essential to a successful outcome with any breast surgery, and in particular for simultaneous augmentation mastopexy. A thorough personal and family breast history should be noted. According to the American Society of Plastic Surgeons published guidelines in accordance with the American Board of Internal Medicine, the use of routine mammograms before breast surgery should be avoided. Patients of specific age groups should undergo annual screening mammograms, and additional screening is not necessary unless there are concerning aspects of the patient's history or physical examination that require further investigation.[30]

Breast measurements including base width, sternal notch to nipple distance, and nipple to IMF distance are helpful when determining the type of mastopexy incision to use, as are the size and shape of implants. The base width is helpful in determining the appropriate range of implants that will fit the patient's anatomy, as the base width of the implant should not excessively exceed the breast base width. Planning excessively large implants at the same time as a mastopexy may create more postoperative complications, given the opposing forces on the tissues. If there is doubt about vascularity or the patient desires large implants, it may be prudent to stage the procedure. There may be pressure placed on the surgeon to perform simultaneous surgery, given that the public has an expectation of undergoing only 1 procedure, but the pressure of competition should not bias the surgeon's analysis and consideration for patient safety.

Patient characteristics such as native asymmetry, chest wall contour, amount of subcutaneous fat and breast tissue density, degree of nipple or parenchyma ptosis (ptosis grades can be categorized according to the Regnault classification) (**Fig. 3**), quality of the skin, any previous breast surgery, and patient expectations must all be considered when planning surgery. The goal is to create an aesthetically pleasing breast contour with an appropriately positioned nipple-areolar complex, upper pole fullness, tightening of the loose skin envelope, breast symmetry, and increased breast volume. Staging procedures is always an option when there is concern about tissue viability and blood supply. The volume of the implant is determined not only by the breast footprint but also by the skin envelope laxity and parenchyma volume. The Tebbett method describes a mathematical approach to determine ideal breast implant shape and volume, and these criteria are useful when planning surgery.[31,32] Soft-tissue dynamics are important in determining the final outcome and potential complications in breast augmentation surgery.[33] The type of implant shape and profile determines the distribution of fill within the breast. The authors prefer to use silicone implants and avoid saline implants, which lead to deflations, more complaints about implant visibility and palpability, and higher revision rates.[3–5,34] Subpectoral implant placement is associated with more postoperative pain in comparison with subglandular placement; however, the incidence of capsular contracture, implant palpability, and excess upper pole fullness is diminished with the muscle coverage of the implant.[35,36] Mammography is also more accurate with subpectoral placement.[37,38] Many women who present for augmentation mastopexy have thin, lax skin and tissue, and partial coverage of the implant results more naturally appearing breasts.

Circumareolar mastopexies have higher rates of revisions and patient dissatisfaction,[23] and the authors avoid them unless less than 2 cm of lift is needed without significant skin laxity or striae Some surgeons may successfully use a crescent mastopexy for minimal lifting with augmentation,

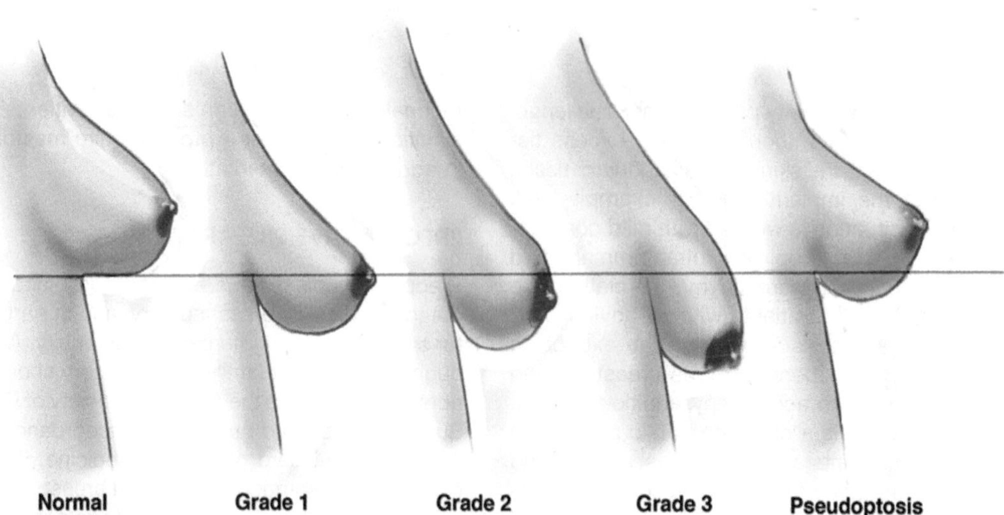

Fig. 3. Regnault classification of ptosis.

but the authors rarely find this as useful as a concentric or circumareolar mastopexy in terms of acceptable scarring.[20,23,39–41]

Managing patient expectations and well-documented informed consent are important components of preoperative preparation, as mastopexy surgery is a frequent source of litigation in plastic surgery.[42,43] Photo-documentation of the patient's breasts preoperatively is imperative. Patients rarely recognize their own preoperative breast asymmetry and are unaware of the difference in individual native breast and chest shape, an important aspect to point out to the patient before surgery. Many women have strong preferences for nipple position and upper pole fullness versus a more natural upper breast slope, in addition to size. It is important to discuss these issues with the patient preoperatively. Patients who are not counseled preoperatively are often surprised when they note differences in tissue fullness from the upper pole of the breast compared with the lower and lateral part of their breasts. Mild implant palpability or rippling when patients bend over is usually the consequence of having breast implants, particularly in thin patients or those without substantial breast tissue. Weight loss can exacerbate this issue. Patients may consider it a complication when they feel the implant edge laterally if they are not forewarned of this.

The authors find it helpful to remind the patient that no 2 sides of the body are mirror images of each other and that her breasts will never be completely symmetric. It is important to discuss in detail the type and extent of incisions planned so that the patient is not surprised by the resulting scars. It is also important to discuss that breast implants are not designed to be lifetime devices, and that the patient may need additional surgery on her breasts in the future, as well as the Food and Drug Administration recommendation for surveillance of silicone breast implants.

OPERATIVE STRATEGY

All augmentation mastopexy patients are marked preoperatively in the standing position. Patients are given a dose of preoperative antibiotics, and lower extremity sequential compression devices are placed. The arms are abducted and wrapped so that the patient can be positioned upright during the procedure. The areola is marked with a 42-mm diameter nipple marker, and the preoperative markings are measured and rechecked. The pocket for the implant is created through the vertical incision, unless a circumareolar incision is planned. The authors' preference is to use a subpectoral pocket, releasing the inferior and inferomedial fibers of the pectoralis major muscle. Patients with constricted breasts may benefit from subglandular breast implant position to create a more rounded breast,[44] although the authors prefer to use a dual-plane implant placement in this situation with aggressive scoring of the parenchymal bands of the inferior pole (**Fig. 4**). The position of the implants should be symmetric and in good position at the time of surgery. Meticulous hemostasis is ensured. Implant sizers with tailor tacking of the mastopexy incisions is a useful technique when dealing with breast asymmetry. The pockets are irrigated with triple antibiotic solution or betadine and rinsed, and once the implants are placed the deep tissue is closed completely. The mastopexy markings are then checked, and this portion of the procedure commences. The authors do not routinely use drains with primary augmentation mastopexy.

Borderline Ptosis

Patients with borderline ptosis and expectations of a nipple positioned over the most projecting part of the breast often benefit from a circumareolar mastopexy, as they require less than 2 cm of nipple-areolar complex elevation. A nonabsorbable interlocking wagon-wheel or purse-string suture is placed in the deep dermis with the knot buried deeply to avoid extrusion (**Figs. 5** and **6**). Caution must be taken to avoid a tight purse-string suture that can cause vascular compromise to the nipple as the areolar skin is pulled taut. There is often mild pleating of the skin that resolves postoperatively. Scar and areolar widening can still occur postoperatively, but the permanent suture (and choosing patients who do not require significant skin excision) helps reduce this consequence. With significant skin excision, the breast can also appear flattened without an aesthetic natural cone shape that results from horizontal tightening. This consequence should be discussed with patients if they insist on avoiding additional scars. If not warned preoperatively, some patients will complain of postoperative "puffiness," particularly when their body temperature is warm, as the purse-string suture restricts areolar spreading but the underlying tissue expands.

Deflated Ptosis Grades 2 and 3

Patients with ptosis grades 2 and 3 and skin laxity usually require a circumvertical or anchor-type skin excision. The inframammary incision is kept to a minimum, but the authors find that patients do not tolerate skin puckering or dog ears, and the IMF incision seems to be the most acceptable of all mastopexy scars. The implant is placed through the vertical skin and parenchymal incision.

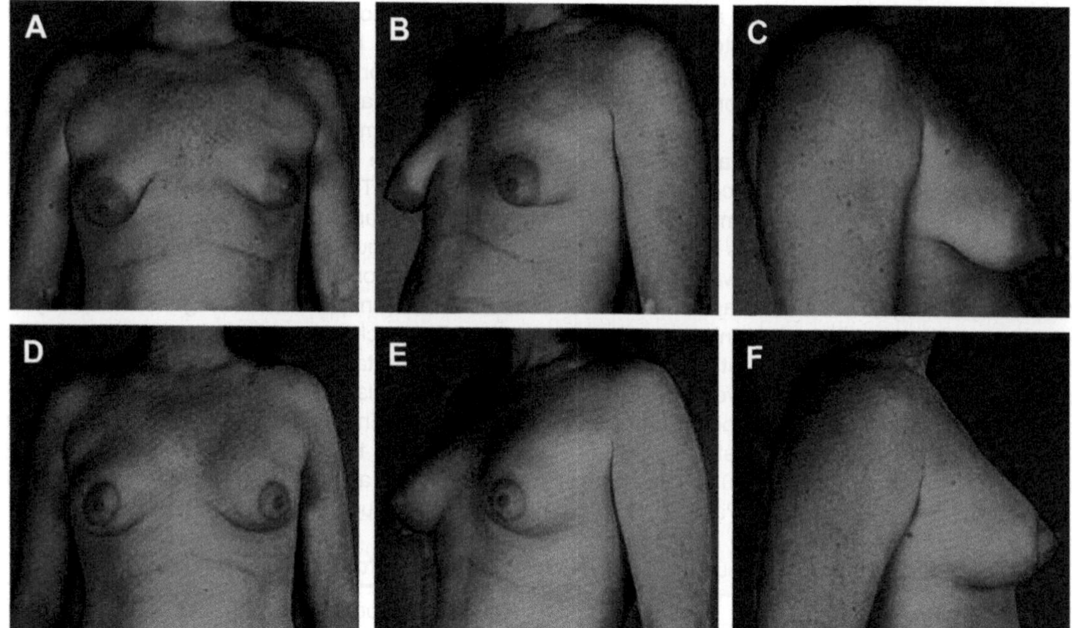

Fig. 4. Tuberous breast deformity. (*A–C*) An 18-year-old woman who presented with bilateral tuberous breast deformity and asymmetry. She underwent a single-staged primary augmentation with smooth round saline implants (right breast, 272 mL; left breast, 322 mL), circumvertical mastopexy on the right breast, and circumareolar mastopexy on the left breast. (*D–F*) Same views 17 months postoperatively.

This action offsets the plane of tissue healing from the T junction in the healing skin. This type of mastopexy offers the ability to better correct asymmetric nipples, wide breasts, and significant skin laxity. Invariably, the lower pole of the breast will stretch over time, which can lead to pseudoptosis. To accommodate this natural stretching, the inferior pole of the breast is closed with enough tension that it appears slightly flat on profile. Any irregularity of the areola shape is corrected at the time of surgery. A teardrop-shaped areola will not round out postoperatively. Inferior release of the dermis below the areola may be necessary to allow superior movement of the nipple complex without tethering. Appropriate positioning of the nipple over the implant must be planned and

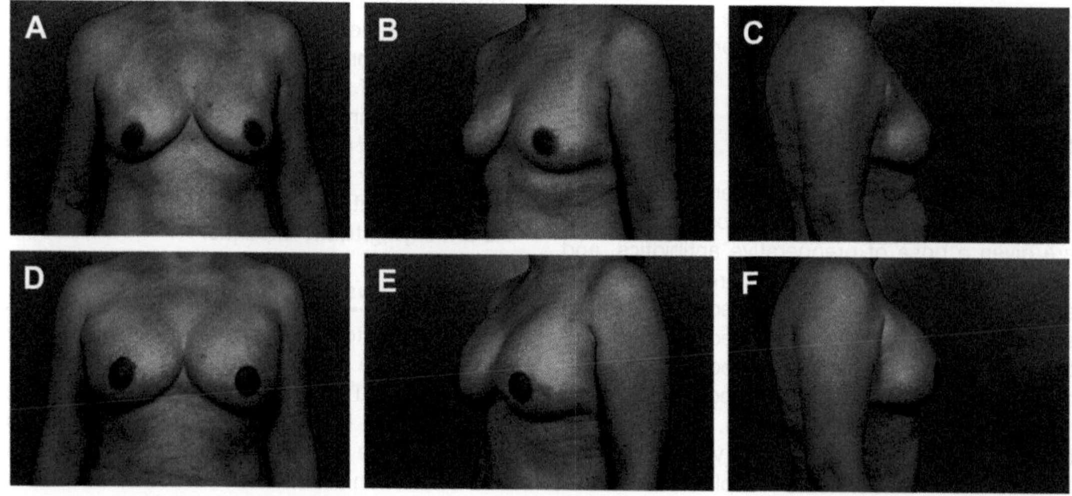

Fig. 5. Circumareolar mastopexy. (*A–C*) A 47-year-old woman with grade 2 ptosis. (*D–F*) Six months postoperatively following a circumareolar mastopexy augmentation.

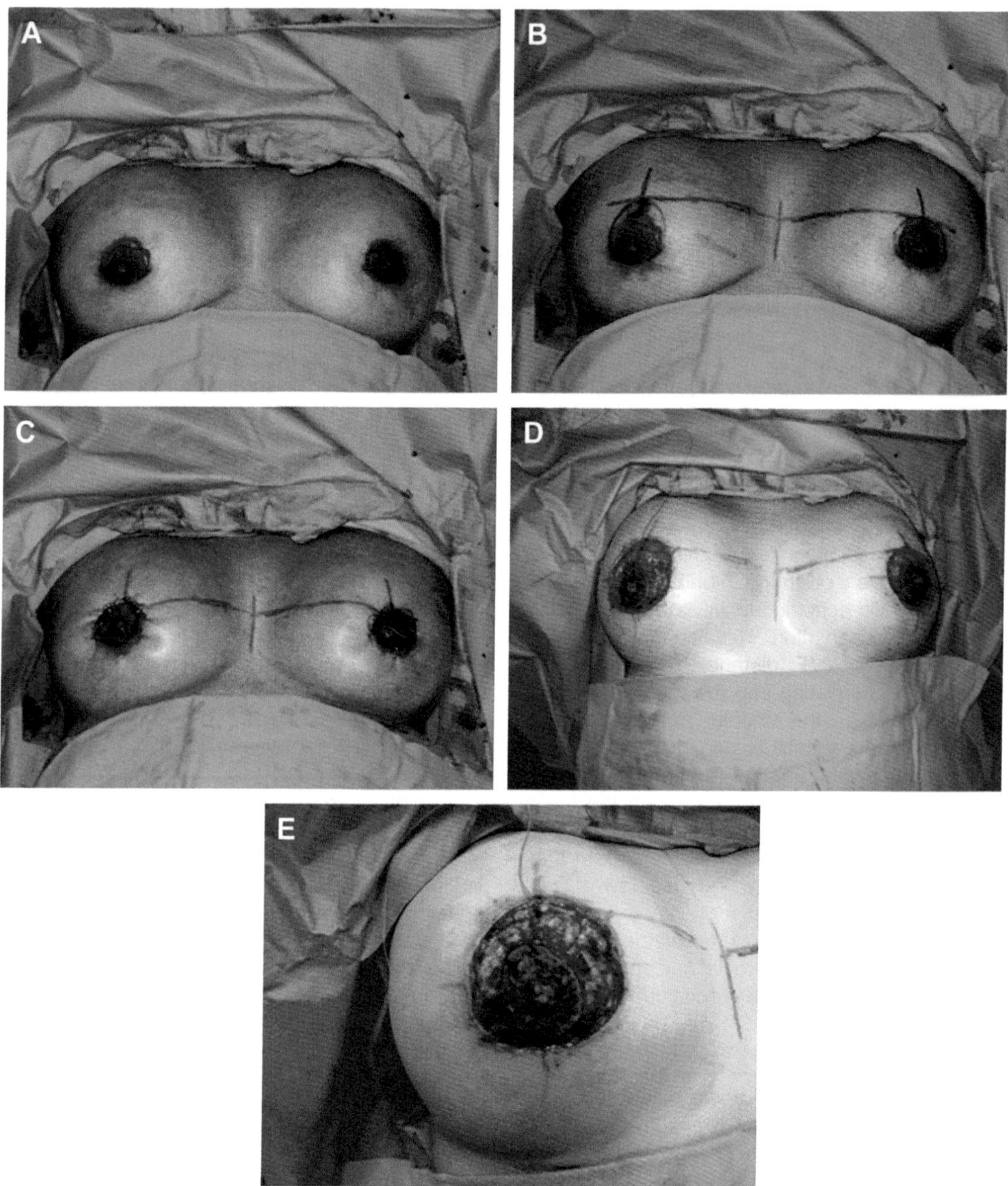

Fig. 6. Intraoperative view of circumareolar mastopexy. The areolar size is cut using the appropriately sized cookie cutter (*A*). The nipple position is determined (*B*), and tailor tacking may be used to double check the position (*C*). The circumareolar skin is de-epithelialized (*D*). A wagon-wheel closure is performed using a permanent suture (*E*), and the skin is closed using a running subcuticular suture.

checked intraoperatively to avoid nipples that are too high or too low.

Grade 4 Ptosis (Pseudoptosis)

Patients with grade 4 ptosis may have adequate nipple position and areolar size. This rare situation can be treated with only an inverted-T mastopexy, although the authors find that most patients benefit from slight repositioning of the areolas. Mild pseudoptosis can often be corrected with an augmentation alone; however, in the face of heavy pseudoptotic glandular tissue the authors find that a more pleasing breast shape is created by performing a mastopexy to elevate the parenchyma and excise redundant skin (**Fig. 7**).

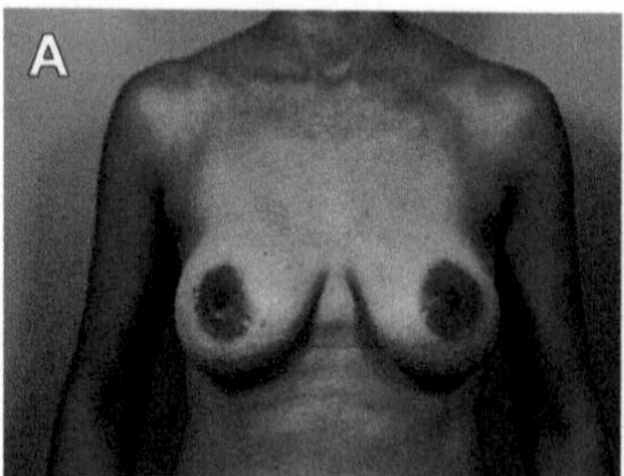

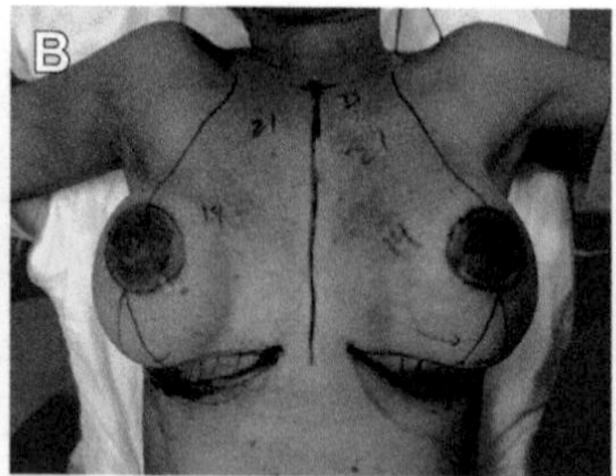

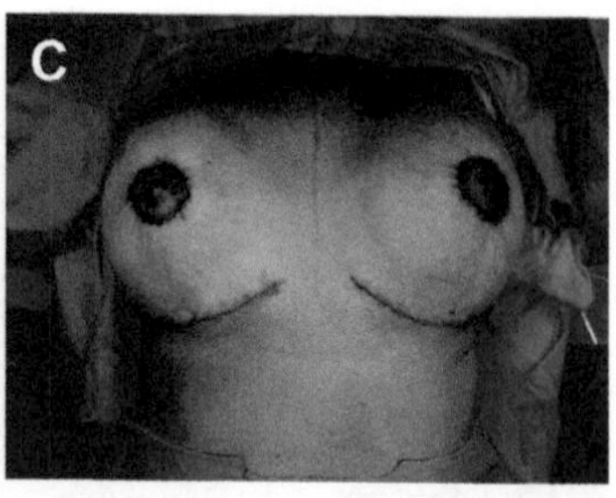

Fig. 7. Pseudoptosis. (*A*) This woman presented with widened areola and pseudoptosis following breast augmentation 6 years prior. Intraoperatively she was marked for a "sailboat" mastopexy to reduce both vertical and horizontal excess, and circumareolar excision of the widened areola. (*B*) She underwent removal of her old implants with capsulotomies and replacement with 547-mL silicone devices. (*C*) Once the implants were placed the vertical component of the mastopexy was not necessary, and she underwent a "smile" mastopexy to reduce the vertical excess.

Constricted or Tuberous Breast

It is estimated that 83.2% of women have a degree of breast constriction,[45] and this native breast shape can have a profound impact on postoperative shape. Mild constriction will only be identified with careful observation. Telltale signs include a short nipple to IMF distance, disproportional breast tissue herniating into the areola, or a lack of convexity to the medial breast contour. Teardrop-shaped implants can be useful in this patient population, as the form-stable silicone helps to differentially put pressure on the lower pole of the breast. Intraoperative release of inferior and inferior-medial parenchymal bands and tight tissue can create a more rounded lower pole. Often these patients do not have horizontal excess, and therefore are better candidates for a circumareolar mastopexy to reduce enlarged areolas and limit breast tissue herniation.

Native Breast Asymmetry

Patients with significant breast size asymmetry often benefit from a slight breast reduction on the larger side, and may also need different implant sizes because of variations in breast dimensions. Sterile implant sizers and mastopexy tailor tacking are useful in these challenging situations. Many patients are not aware of subtle size asymmetry, and this should be pointed out preoperatively as they will likely notice any discrepancy after surgery. When debating between placing the same size of implants or trying to correct a slight size asymmetry, the authors find that patients are most satisfied if postoperative asymmetry corresponds with what they are used to: that is, if the patient's right breast is slightly larger preoperatively, and placing a bigger implant on the contralateral side leads to a slightly larger left breast, patients will not tolerate this as well as when using the same-size implants, while accepting that they will have asymmetry based on their native breast tissue.

COMPLICATIONS

Published reviews of outcomes following 1-stage augmentation mastopexies have shown varying outcomes and complication rates.[7,8,11,12,46–48]

Hematoma

Meticulous hemostasis is of the utmost importance to decrease the incidence of hematoma. In a recently published meta-analysis encompassing 4856 cases of simultaneous augmentation-mastopexy cases, the pooled hematoma rate was 1.37%.[48] Direct visualization with cautery rather than blunt dissection has been described as a way to reduce hematoma formation.[49] Hematomas should be drained promptly not only to avoid excess pressure on the tissues and subsequent ischemia but also because blood collections can increase the risk for both infection and capsular contracture.[50]

Infection

Although an intraoperative sterile technique is paramount during any surgery, the addition of an implant should heighten the need to avoid contamination. Sequelae following infection include overt soft-tissue infection possibly leading to implant loss, in addition to the long-term effect of occult infection leading to capsular contracture.[51] The "no-touch" technique was first described in 1914 to minimize handling of metal for orthopedic procedures.[52] Once this method was adopted for the placement of breast implants, the incidence of infection decreased significantly.[53] The pooled risk of infection following simultaneous augmentation mastopexy is 2% (ranging from 0%–14% in the current literature).[48]

After simultaneous augmentation mastopexy, infection of the soft tissues must be treated aggressively with antibiotics and frequent follow-up to avoid wound breakdown and involvement of the implant.

Skin and Nipple Necrosis

Skin necrosis or breakdown can occur most commonly at the T zone of an anchor-type mastopexy. Nipple necrosis is a rare and potentially devastating complication. It is important to obtain any history of previous breast surgeries, and consider nipple blood supply when performing simultaneous augmentation mastopexy. The tissue should never be closed with excessive tension; it is better to place a smaller implant and close the tissue safely than risk partial or complete nipple necrosis.[4]

Implant Visibility or Rippling

Significant rippling of implants can have a variety of causes. Saline implants may ripple more than silicone, and textured shells more than smooth shells.[54] Over time, rippling can worsen as the implants put pressure on the parenchyma, and thin the tissue or create contour deformities in the rib cage, causing the implants to hold a different position in the chest. Correction is often difficult because the overlying tissue is usually thin. Exchanging textured shells to smooth, saline to gel-filled implants, and moving the implant from a subglandular to subpectoral pocket position can help improve this situation. Other methods to decrease implant visibility include creating a completely new pocket in the subfascial or subcapsular plane, using acellular dermal matrix to provide more implant coverage, or placing fat grafts to add additional support and volume to the area.

Pocket Asymmetry or Implant Malposition

Preventing malposition is easier than correcting it. Implant malposition may be a result of faulty or asymmetric pocket dissection or incomplete release of the pectoralis major muscle, and it is usually apparent early after surgery. In these cases, revisions require either further dissection, plication of an overly dissected pocket, or the creation of new pockets for the implants. The pocket can be reinforced with the patient's own capsular tissue, and a neosubpectoral or neosubcapsular pocket can be helpful in difficult cases.[14,15] If the pocket asymmetry is due to asymmetry of the native breast or chest wall or to capsular contracture, attention to the underlying cause is required.

Symmastia

Symmastia is a challenging problem to overcome, and is best avoided at the time of primary augmentation mastopexy. It may be due to aggressive dissection of the medial implant pocket, and can be exacerbated by ribcage abnormalities or closely positioned native breast footprints. The placement of large implants can increase the risk of symmastia.

Subpectoral Implant Movement

Implant motion with flexion of the chest muscles is expected after augmentation in the subpectoral plane, and is particularly evident in thin patients who lack breast parenchyma volume. Preoperative counseling is important to discuss this potential issue. Care is taken not to overdissect the pectoralis major muscle from the medial insertion to the sternum, as this can result in increased distortion.

Pseudoptosis: "Bottoming Out"

Pseudoptosis is a term used for when the nipple to IMF distance elongates, creating the appearance of nipples that are positioned too high on the breast. This condition can be due to the relatively thin inferior pole skin and tissue stretching under the weight of the implants, or actual violation of the IMF and displacement of the implants inferiorly. The authors strive to create a flattened lower pole at the time of surgery to allow for postoperative stretch. This action should be taken with maximum tension on the underlying parenchyma, and not by relying only on skin tension during closure. It is important to conservatively dissect the IMF region so as to leave supporting tissue for the implant. Some patients require lowering of the IMF, and in instances where it is considered that the fascia is not supportive, tacking sutures are used to reinforce the fold.

Capsular Contracture

Capsular contracture is a common reason for revision of breast augmentation, with or without mastopexy.[55] The etiology of capsular contracture is an enigmatic phenomenon made evident by the litany of studies.[36,56–60] Infection and bacterial contamination are linked to capsular contracture[56] and, therefore, meticulous attention to the avoidance of contamination intraoperatively is paramount. Intraoperative techniques such as reprepping the chest, changing gloves, avoiding multiple people handling the implants, placing an occlusive dressing over the nipple,[61,62] using a no-touch technique, irrigating the pocket with antibiotic solution[63] or Betadine solution and rinse,[57] and avoiding powdered gloves have all been used to help reduce risk. Placing the implants in the subpectoral plane has been shown to reduce the risk of capsular contracture.[36] The authors prefer to use textured implants to reduce capsular contracture, based on the lower rate of this complication.[3–5,16,18,55] Some data show that the inframammary incision may result in a lower contracture rate in comparison with the periareolar approach,[64] presumably because of less bacterial contamination from the ductal tissue.[17]

Hematoma formation has also been correlated with capsular contracture[50,65]; therefore, great care should be taken to achieve hemostasis. In addition, the avoidance of drains is associated with a low prevalence of capsular contracture.[56]

Malposition and Shape of the Nipple-Areola Complex

Malposition of the nipple-areolar complex can occur following augmentation mastopexy. As nipples can be positioned too high or too low at the time of surgery, it is important to take into account overall skin characteristics and implant size when planning nipple position. Normal postoperative implant settling and tissue stretching will alter the position of the nipple-areola complex relative to the breast mound over time. Planning the top of the areolar pattern conservatively and tailor-tacking during surgery with the patient upright can help avoid placing the nipples too high or asymmetrically. A mosque-pattern areola design is often used, although this does not guarantee a symmetric circular areola. If a teardrop-shaped areola is seen following inset, it is important to re-excise the skin, as this shape does not tend to improve with time postoperatively (**Fig. 8**).

Double Bubbles

Double bubble has been used to describe 2 different problems: ptosis of glandular tissue drooping over an implant, and a persistent inframammary crease on the lower breast pole. The former problem results from the breast tissue projecting over and hanging below the more superiorly located implant, creating a contour deformity. This condition can occur if the mastopexy is not aggressive enough in elevating the glandular tissue and tightening the skin, or if the initial implant pocket has not been released sufficiently to allow inferior displacement of the implant. In addition, it may be due to a breast base width/implant width mismatch. This complication may also occur in an underappreciated breast constriction with inadequate internal scoring and release. Repositioning or resizing the implant may be necessary, and a revision of the mastopexy should be considered. A persistent inframammary crease occurs when the pocket is dissected inferiorly to accommodate a large implant or purposefully lower an asymmetric crease or a constricted lower pole. The lower portion of the implant creates a mound below the IMF. Over time, this may improve as pressure from the implant stretches the skin. Correction includes placing smaller implants and plicating the IMF, or creating a neosubpectoral pocket with capsular reinforcement of the fold. If the breast implant position is correct, fat grafting can be used to camouflage the contour depression.

Nipple Sensation and Lactation

Patients should be counseled on the risk of changes in nipple sensation and the potential inability to breast feed following augmentation mastopexy. Large implants pressing laterally on the sensory nerve may increase the risk of nipple numbness, and postoperative edema may create transient changes in sensation. The inability to

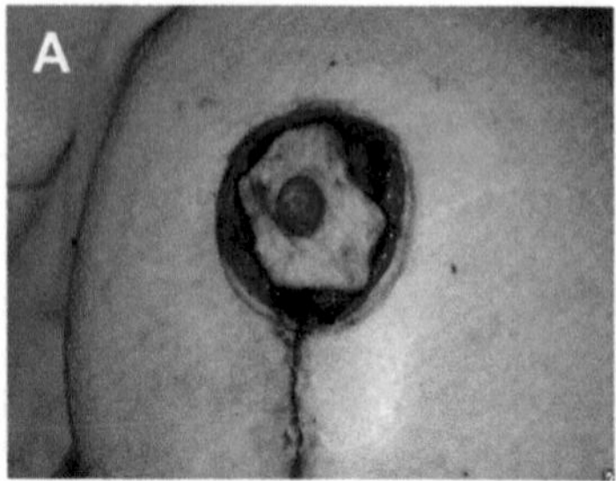

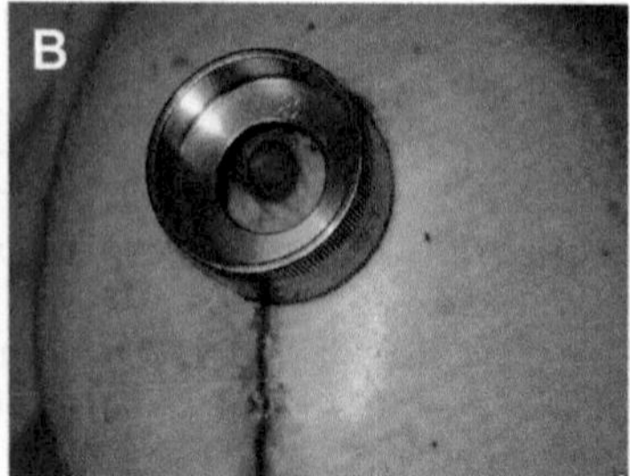

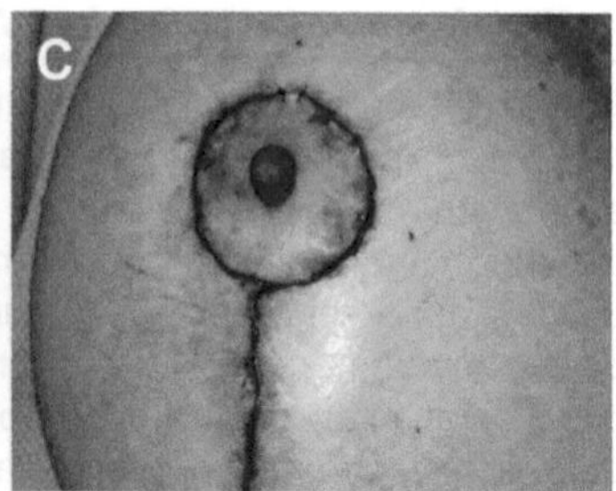

Fig. 8. Correction of asymmetry of the nipple-areolar complex. (*A*) On inset of the nipple-areolar complex, the shape can be evaluated for symmetry and size. (*B*) The nipple marker "cookie cutter" is used to re-mark the areolar shape, paying special attention to meet the vertical incision at right angles and centered. (*C*) Excess edges are trimmed and the inset proceeds.

lactate sufficiently is a possible complication of mastopexy, with or without augmentation, resulting from scar tissue formation and interruption of lactiferous ducts.

Implant-Related Complications

Implant-related complications are due to the inherent nature of breast implants. The implant wall can thin and rupture over time, and there is a small risk of defective implants. Gel fracturing can occur during placement of silicone implants if undue stress is placed on them. It is important to make the incision large enough to place the implants in the pocket without significant trauma. Intraoperative puncturing of the implant with a sharp instrument or retractor should be avoided.

Tissue-Related Complications

Careful tissue handing is important in optimizing scarring. Any excessively traumatized or heated skin edges at the time of the procedure should be excised. Care must be taken to preserve blood flow to the breast tissue and nipple-areolar complex and not to place the tissues or incisions under undue pressure. Consideration of nipple vascularity and conservative tissue undermining is important in decreasing the risk of wound-healing problems or nipple necrosis.

POSTOPERATIVE CARE

Postoperative management includes guidelines for appropriate activity limitations, support garments, and consideration of a bandeau and implant displacement massage when warranted. The authors allow patients to wear an underwire bra and resume full activity after 6 weeks. Scar therapy with silicone gel begins at approximately 3 to 4 weeks following surgery. The authors do not typically use drains during primary augmentation mastopexy, and the patients are discharged to home with a caretaker if they are not to undergo another combined surgery. Patients are encouraged to ambulate on the evening of surgery. Postoperative prophylactic antibiotics are given for a minimum of 24 hours. If textured implants or anatomically shaped implants are used, no massage exercises are recommended. If smooth implants are used, patients are encouraged to do gentle implant mobility exercises starting within the first week of surgery. Bandeaus are not typically used unless the patient exhibits significant upper pole swelling or the implants take longer to settle. Postoperative reassurance for the patient is important, because this implant settling can occur at different rates for each patient. It is reassuring to the surgeon to recall that when the patient was in the operating room the pockets were symmetric and the implants were in good position.

OUTCOMES

The authors recently published a review of 615 consecutive 1-stage mastopexy augmentations[23]: Silicone implants were placed in 79%, and textured implants were used in 92% of cases. The average volume of the implants was 323 mL. Ninety-three percent of implants were placed in a submuscular pocket. Over the period of the study, 16.9% of patients underwent some sort of revision procedure, the most common of which was removal and replacement of the implant with one of a different size. This result demonstrates one of the most difficult aspects of the simultaneous surgery: determining appropriately sized implants that will satisfy the patient in the long term. This and other implant-related complications accounted for 62% of revisions. The placement of saline implants had a statistically significant correlation to higher revision rates because implant deflation was a large contributory factor to implant-related revisions. Tissue-related complications were looked at separately, and poor scarring was the most common indication, with circumareolar mastopexies leading to a statistically higher rate of revision. This finding is consistent with those of other studies.[12,66] The 5 most common complications were poor scarring (5.7%), wound-healing issues (2.9%), implant deflation (2.6%), areolar asymmetry (1.9%), and capsular contracture (1.6%).

For a thorough overview of published outcomes following augmentation mastopexy, the reader is referred to the large meta-analysis by Khavanin and colleagues.[48]

SUMMARY

Primary simultaneous augmentation mastopexy is a challenging and rewarding surgical procedure. Patients differ in the amount of skin laxity, parenchyma distribution, breast dimensions, and nipple position. Patients must be educated about realistic expectations, size limitations, and their native anatomy. Preoperative breast dimensional and soft-tissue analysis must be performed to plan the correct surgery. Precise atraumatic dissection, symmetric muscle release, meticulous hemostasis, and mastopexy closure without excess tension are important factors for good outcomes. Excellent outcomes with low complication rates can be anticipated with proper patient evaluation, education, and operative planning.

DISCLOSURES

M.A. Spring, MD, FACS, Marina Plastic Surgery Associates, Clinical Assistant Professor of Surgery, Keck School of Medicine of USC, is an investigator for Cohera Medical, Inc, and a Physician Advisor to Alphaeon Corporation. E.C. Hartmann, MD, MS, is a Plastic Surgeon and an Aesthetic Surgery Fellow at USC-Marina Plastic Surgery Associates and has no disclosures. W.G. Stevens, MD, FACS, Marina Plastic Surgery Associates, Clinical Professor of Surgery, Keck School of Medicine of USC, is an investigator and speaker for Sientra & Silimed; investigator for Mentor CPG; medical luminary and speaker for SOLTA; medical luminary for Cutera, Merz, Exilis, and Syneron-Candela; speaker for Allergan Academy and Cynosure; consultant for TauTona; medical luminary and speaker for ZELTIQ; Physician Advisor to Alphaeon Corp; editorial board advisor for *Plastic Surgery Practice*; and investigator for Cohera Medical, Inc. No funding was received to assist in the creation of this article.

Editorial Comments by Bradley P. Bengtson, MD

Combined augmentation-mastopexy procedures have been described as the most difficult primary procedure we perform in the breast. It is not surprising then that it carries the highest percentage of complications and litigation rates of the procedures we perform. Drs Spring, Hartmann, and Stevens do a great job of discussing the varying degrees of ptosis and deformities and strategies for their correction. In addition they describe in detail the most common complications and review of outcomes.

REFERENCES

1. Regnault P. The hypoplastic and ptotic breast: a combined operation with prosthetic augmentation. Plast Reconstr Surg 1966;37:31–7.
2. Gonzalez-Ulloa M. Correction of hypertrophy of the breast by exogenous material. Plast Reconstr Surg 1960;25:15–26.
3. Stevens WG, Stoker DA, Freeman ME, et al. Is one-stage breast augmentation with mastopexy safe and effective? A review of 186 primary cases. Aesthet Surg J 2006;26:674–81.
4. Stevens WG, Spring M, Stoker DA, et al. A review of 100 consecutive secondary augmentation/mastopexies. Aesthet Surg J 2007;27:485–92.
5. Stevens WG, Freeman ME, Stoker DA, et al. One-stage mastopexy with breast augmentation: a review of 321 patients. Plast Reconstr Surg 2007;120:1674–9.
6. Hedén P. Mastopexy augmentation with form stable breast implants. Clin Plast Surg 2009;36:91–104.
7. Spear SL, Pelletiere CV, Menon N. One-stage augmentation combined with mastopexy: aesthetic results and patient satisfaction. Aesthetic Plast Surg 2004;28:259–67.
8. Spear S, Boehmler JH 4th, Clemens MW. Augmentation/mastopexy: a 3-year review of a single surgeon's practice. Plast Reconstr Surg 2006;118:136S–51S.
9. Davison SP, Spear SL. Simultaneous breast augmentation with periareolar mastopexy. Semin Plast Surg 2004;18:189–201.
10. Nahai F, Fisher J, Maxwell PG, et al. Augmentation mastopexy: to stage or not. Aesthet Surg J 2007;27:297–305.
11. Swanson E. Prospective comparative clinical evaluation of 784 consecutive cases of breast augmentation and vertical mammaplasty, performed individually and in combination. Plast Reconstr Surg 2013;132:30e–45e.
12. Calobrace MB, Herdt DR, Cothron KJ. Simultaneous augmentation/mastopexy: a retrospective 5-year review of 332 consecutive cases. Plast Reconstr Surg 2013;131:145–56.
13. Tessone A, Millet E, Weissman O, et al. Evading a surgical pitfall: mastopexy—augmentation made simple. Aesthetic Plast Surg 2011;35:1073–8.
14. Parsa AA, Jackowe DJ, Parsa FD. A new algorithm for breast mastopexy/augmentation. Plast Reconstr Surg 2010;125:75e–7e.
15. Don Parsa F, Brickman M, Parsa AA. Augmentation/mastopexy. Plast Reconstr Surg 2005;115:1428–9.
16. Barutcu A, Baytekin C. One-stage augmentation-mastopexy with Wise pattern and inverted-T scar. Aesthetic Plast Surg 2009;33:784–5.
17. Persoff MM. Vertical mastopexy with expansion augmentation. Aesthetic Plast Surg 2003;27:13–9.
18. Persoff MM. Mastopexy with expansion-augmentation. Aesthet Surg J 2003;23:34–9.
19. Karnes J, Morrison W, Salisbury M, et al. Simultaneous breast augmentation and lift. Aesthetic Plast Surg 2000;24:148–54.
20. Nigro DM. Crescent mastopexy and augmentation. Plast Reconstr Surg 1985;76:802–3.
21. Ramirez OM. Reduction mammaplasty with the "owl" incision and no undermining. Plast Reconstr Surg 2002;109:512–24.
22. Loustau HD, Mayer HF, Sarrabayrouse M. The owl technique combined with the inferior pedicle in mastopexy. Aesthetic Plast Surg 2008;32:11–7.
23. Stevens WG, Macias LH, Spring MA. One-stage augmentation mastopexy: a review of 1192 simultaneous breast augmentation and mastopexy procedures in 615 consecutive patients. Aesthet Surg J 2014;34:723–32.
24. Hall-Findlay EJ. Pedicles in vertical breast reduction and mastopexy. Clin Plast Surg 2002;29:379–91.

25. O'Dey D, Prescher A, Pallua N. Vascular reliability of nipple-areolar complex-bearing pedicles: an anatomical microdissection study. Plast Reconstr Surg 2007;119:1167–77.
26. van Deventer PV, Page BJ, Graewe FR. Vascular anatomy of the breast and nipple-areola complex. Plast Reconstr Surg 2008;121:1860–2.
27. Nakajima H, Imanishi N, Aiso S. Arterial anatomy of the nipple-areola complex. Plast Reconstr Surg 1995;96:843–5.
28. Palmer JH, Taylor GI. The vascular territories of the anterior chest wall. Br J Plast Surg 1986;39: 287–99.
29. Gryskiewicz J. Dual-plane breast augmentation for minimal ptosis pseudoptosis (the "in-between" patient). Aesthet Surg J 2012;33:43–65.
30. ASPS Participates in the ABIM Foundation's Choosing Wisely Campaign. 2014. Available at: http://www.plasticsurgery.org/news/past-press-releases/2014-archives/asps-participates-in-the-abim-foundation's-choosing-wisely%C2%AE-campaign.html. Accessed November 20, 2014.
31. Tebbetts JB, Adams WP. Five critical decisions in breast augmentation using five measurements in 5 minutes: the high five decision support process. Plast Reconstr Surg 2005;116:2005–16.
32. Tebbetts JB, Adams WP. Five critical decisions in breast augmentation using five measurements in 5 minutes: the high five decision support process. Plast Reconstr Surg 2006;118:35S–45S.
33. Vegas MR, Martin del Yerro JL. Stiffness, compliance, resilience, and creep deformation: understanding implant-soft tissue dynamics in the augmented breast: fundamentals based on materials science. Aesthetic Plast Surg 2013;37:922–30.
34. Stevens WG, Stoker DA, Fellows DR, et al. Acceleration of textured saline breast implant deflation rate: results and analysis of 645 implants. Aesthet Surg J 2005;25:37–9.
35. Namnoum JD, Largent J, Kaplan HM, et al. Primary breast augmentation clinical trial outcomes stratified by surgical incision, anatomical placement and implant device type. J Plast Reconstr Aesthet Surg 2013;66:1165–72.
36. Puckett CL, Croll GH, Reichel CA, et al. A critical look at capsular contracture in subglandular versus subpectoral mammary augmentation. Aesthetic Plast Surg 1987;11:23.
37. Grace GT, Roberts C, Cohen IK. The role of mammography in detecting breast cancer in augmented breasts. Ann Plast Surg 1990;25:119–23.
38. Leibman AJ, Kruse BD. Imaging of breast cancer after augmentation mammoplasty. Ann Plast Surg 1993;30:111–5.
39. Baran CN, Peker F, Ortak T, et al. Unsatisfactory results of periareolar mastopexy with or without augmentation and reduction mammoplasty: enlarged areola with flattened nipple. Aesthetic Plast Surg 2001;25:286–9.
40. Spear SL, Kassan M, Little JW. Guidelines in concentric mastopexy. Plast Reconstr Surg 1990;85:961–6.
41. Puckett CL, Meyer VH, Reinisch JF. Crescent mastopexy and augmentation. Plast Reconstr Surg 1985; 75:533–43.
42. Snow JW. Crescent mastopexy and augmentation. Plast Reconstr Surg 1986;77:161–2.
43. Marchesi A, Marchesi M, Fasulo FC, et al. Mammaplasties and medicolegal issues: 50 cases of litigation in aesthetic surgery of the breast. Aesthetic Plast Surg 2012;36:1.
44. Mandrekas AD, Zambacos GJ, Anastasopoulos A, et al. Aesthetic reconstruction of the tuberous breast deformity. Plast Reconstr Surg 2003;112:1099–108.
45. DeLuca-Pytell DM, Piazza RC, Holding JC, et al. The incidence of tuberous breast deformity in asymmetric and symmetric mammaplasty patients. Plast Reconstr Surg 2005;116:1894–9.
46. Spear SL, Low M, Ducic I. Revision augmentation mastopexy: indications, operations, and outcomes. Ann Plast Surg 2003;51:540–6.
47. Cardenas-Camarena L, Ramírez-Macías R, International Confederation for Plastic Reconstructive and Aesthetic Surgery, et al. Augmentation/mastopexy: how to select and perform the proper technique. Aesthetic Plast Surg 2006;30:21–33.
48. Khavanin N, Jordan SW, Rambachan A, et al. A systematic review of single stage augmentation mastopexy. Plast Reconstr Surg 2014;134:922–31.
49. Tebbetts JB. Achieving a predictable 24-hour return to normal activities after breast augmentation: part I. Refining practices by using motion and time study principles. Plast Reconstr Surg 2002;109:273–90.
50. Handel N, Cordray T, Gutierrez J, et al. A long-term study of outcomes, complications, and patient satisfaction with breast implants. Plast Reconstr Surg 2006;117:757–67.
51. Adams WP Jr, Rios JL, Smith SJ. Enhancing patient outcomes in aesthetic and reconstructive breast surgery using triple antibiotic breast irrigation: six-year prospective clinical study. Plast Reconstr Surg 2006;117:30–6.
52. Shetty RH, Ottersberg WH. Metals in orthopedic surgery. New York: Marcel Dekker, Inc; 1995.
53. Mladick RA. "No-touch" submuscular saline breast augmentation technique. Aesthetic Plast Surg 1993;17:183–92.
54. Stevens WG, Hirsch EM, Cohen R, et al. A comparison of 500 pre-filled saline breast implants versus 500 standard textured saline breast implants: is there a difference in deflation rates? Plast Reconstr Surg 2006;117:2175–8.
55. Stevens WG, Nahabedian MY, Calobrace MB, et al. Risk factor analysis for capsular contracture: a 5 year Sientra study analysis using round, smooth,

and textured implants for breast augmentation. Plast Reconstr Surg 2013;132:1115–27.

56. Berry MG, Cucchiara V, Davies DM. Breast augmentation: part II—adverse capsular contracture. J Plast Reconstr Aesthet Surg 2010;63:2098–107.
57. Burkhardt BR, Dempsey PD, Schnur PL, et al. Capsular contracture: a prospective study of the effect of local antibacterial agents. Plast Reconstr Surg 1986;77:919–32.
58. Wong CH, Samuel M, Tan BK, et al. Capsular contracture in subglandular breast augmentation with textured versus smooth breast implants: a systematic review. Plast Reconstr Surg 2006;118:1224–36.
59. Barnsley GP, Sigurdson LJ, Barnsley SE. Textured surface breast implants in the prevention of capsular contracture among breast augmentation patients: a meta-analysis of randomized controlled trials. Plast Reconstr Surg 2006;117:2182–90.
60. Dancey A, Nassimizadeh A, Levick P. Capsular contracture—what are the risk factors? A 14 year series of 1400 consecutive augmentations. J Plast Reconstr Aesthet Surg 2008;65:213–8.
61. Collis N, Mirza S, Stanley PR, et al. Reduction of potential contamination of breast implants by the use of 'nipple shields'. Br J Plast Surg 1999;52:445–7.
62. Wixtrom RN, Stutman RL, Burke RM, et al. Risk of breast implant bacterial contamination from endogenous breast flora, prevention with nipple shields, and implications for biofilm formation. Aesthet Surg J 2012;32:956–63.
63. Adams WP Jr, Conner WC, Barton FE, et al. Optimizing breast-pocket irrigation: the post betadine era. Plast Reconstr Surg 2001;107:1596–601.
64. Henriksen TF, Fryzek JP, Holmich LR, et al. Surgical intervention and capsular contracture after breast augmentation: a prospective study of risk factors. Ann Plast Surg 2005;54:343–51.
65. Williams C, Aston S, Rees TD. The effect of hematoma on the thickness of pseudosheaths around silicone implants. Plast Reconstr Surg 1975;56:194–8.
66. Elliott LF. Circumareolar mastopexy with augmentation. Clin Plast Surg 2002;29:337–47.

The Etiologies of Chest Wall and Breast Asymmetry and Improvement in Breast Augmentation

Caroline A. Glicksman, MD[a,b,*], Sarah E. Ferenz[c]

KEYWORDS

- Breast augmentation • Congenital deformities of the chest wall • Highly cohesive breast implants
- Biodimentional planning • 3-dimensional imaging • Shaped breast implants

KEY POINTS

- Patients presenting for correction of breast and chest wall asymmetries may have undergone numerous thoracic procedures in early childhood and some may have suffered profound psychosocial effects.
- Care must be taken to evaluate these patients using objective criteria and biodimentional principles. Long-lasting correction of asymmetry can be obtained when patients are not oversized, and care is taken to avoid visibility, palpability, and malposition problems.
- Complex congenital syndromes often require a more comprehensive preoperative work-up, as well as a detailed history of any previous thoracic or breast procedures.
- Patient education needs to be comprehensive, and patients should be encouraged to have realistic expectations and accept what can and cannot be corrected.
- Shaped highly cohesive breast implants offer plastic surgeons more possibilities and precision by fine-tuning the gel distribution and specific volume required to correct the hypoplastic elements.

OVERVIEW

Today, most children born with mild to severe congenital deformities of the chest survive well into adulthood. Rarely, deep thoracic wall depression leads to displacement or compression of the heart and lungs, and thoracoplasty is indicated. Most affected children survive into adolescence, and the indications for correction of breast and chest wall defects are based on psychological difficulties and issues of self-esteem. As technical skills improved over the last half a century, minimally invasive procedures such as those of Nuss (minimally invasive repair of pectus excavatum) and Ravitch gained popularity, and common chest wall defects are now routinely treated.[1] The spectrum of chest wall abnormalities varies, from complex congenital musculoskeletal deformities to the more common defects like anterior thoracic hypoplasia. The correction of chest wall and breast deformities with breast implants dates back to the early 1970s, and although originally reserved for mild chest wall and breast asymmetry, the availability of shaped highly cohesive breast implants that allow a surgeon to select a specific width, projection, and height independently, may provide a single-stage option to correct more complex deformities.

[a] Glicksman Plastic Surgery, Sea Girt, NJ, USA; [b] Department of Surgery, Jersey Shore University Medical Center, Neptune, NJ, USA; [c] Department of Biology, Cornell University, Ithaca, NY 14853, USA
* Corresponding author. Glicksman Plastic Surgery, Sea Girt, NJ.
E-mail address: docmomcag@aol.com

Clin Plastic Surg 42 (2015) 519–530
http://dx.doi.org/10.1016/j.cps.2015.06.009

EMBRYOLOGY OF CHEST WALL AND BREAST DEVELOPMENT

The development of the musculoskeletal system of the trunk is a multistep process that occurs between the fourth and eighth weeks of development. The paraxial mesoderm divides into 2 subpopulations, the dorsolateral subpopulation (dermomyotome) and the ventromedial subpopulation (sclerotome). Myoblasts within the dermomyotome differentiate into the skeletal musculature, while the sclerotome develops into the vertebrae and ribs. The sternum is derived from somatic mesoderm. The ribs and sternum fuse in the midline in the sixth week of development, and fusion occurs in a cranial–caudal direction completed by the tenth week. Failure to fuse leads to a cleft sternum. The manubrium is formed by primordia between the developing clavicles.[2] The breasts develop during the sixth week of gestation from ectodermal cells along the milk line, which extends from the axilla to the groin. The upper and lower parts of these ridges atrophy, with only the middle or pectoral ridges developing into breast tissue.[3] The exact etiology of chest wall and sternum deformities remains controversial. Causes include overgrowth of costal cartilages, sternal twisting, and a relative weakening of the costal cartilages.[4] The growth and development of the sternum are influenced by both genetic factors and biomechanical factors. Although no specific gene locus has been yet identified for conditions like Poland syndrome and cleft sternum, there is a definite mutation associated with some chest wall and breast deformities. Chest wall and breast deformities can be classified as either monogenic, disruption sequences, isolated chest wall deformities, or acquired chest and breast deformities (**Table 1**).

HISTORICAL MANAGEMENT

Early reconstructive efforts to correct chest wall deformities were primarily performed for improvement in cardiopulmonary function. Aesthetic considerations were usually reserved until patients reached puberty and maximum sternal development. Surgical corrections of chest wall defects were usually delegated to pediatric surgeons, and early invasive procedures have evolved toward more minimally invasive techniques. The 2 most common procedures used today are the Modified Ravitch procedure (transverse sternal osteotomy with subperichondrial costal cartilage resection) and the Nuss procedure (minimally invasive repair of pectus excavatum).[5] With advances in local muscle flaps, contour defects of the chest wall and hypoplastic

Table 1
Etiology of most common chest wall deformities and resultant end organ failure

Origin of Deformity	Anatomic Site	Disorder
Monogenic syndromes	Ventral body wall–rib Sternum Breast Spine	Marfan syndrome Noonan syndrome
Disruption sequences	Thoracic musculature Ventral body wall- rib Breast Spine	Poland syndrome Moebius syndrome
Genetic associations (chromosome aberrations)	Ventral body wall–rib Sternum	PHACE (posterior fossa brain malformations) Cantrell pentalogy Asphyxiating thoracic dystrophy (Jeune syndrome) Cleft sternum
Isolated chest wall deformities	Breast Ventral body wall–rib Sternum Spine	Pectus excavatum Pectus carinatum Thoracic hypoplasia Supranumerary breasts Congenital absence breast Tuberous breast Constricted base breast Gynecomastia
Acquired	Ventral body wall Thoracic musculature Breast	Tetralogy of Fallot

or absent musculature were replaced with local flaps, including the latissimus dorsi flap. Beginning as early as the 1970s, custom-made silicone implants were used requiring the fabrication of a chest wall mold or moulage. It is interesting to note that early silicone rubber chest wall prostheses were firm, having the consistency of muscle tissue. Custom implants were often inserted deep to the serratus, occasionally with a second implant stacked on top to augment the breast. Early custom implants were most often shaped and textured. Several manufacturers supplied custom implants to plastic surgeons until the late 1990s. Inamed (Allergan-Actavis: Irvine, CA, USA and Rockaway, NJ, USA) stopped importing custom implants in 1997, as did Sientra (Santa Barbara, CA, USA) between 2010 and 2011, and Silimed (Rio de Janeiro, Brazil) ceased production of custom silicone implants in 2014. Adjustable saline implants played a significant role in the treatment of chest and breast asymmetry due to the ability to add more volume to the affected hypoplastic chest and breast. Round silicone gel implants have grown in popularity and have largely replaced saline implants, which have high rates of visibility and palpability. The development of shaped highly cohesive gel breast implants has further steered breast augmentation surgeons away from the older volumetric management of asymmetries toward that of shaping the chest and breast with biodimentional planning. Anatomic implants provide not only the increase in volume required to correct the hypoplastic elements, but because surgeons can select the implant by height, base width, and projection, the ability to correct individual chest wall anomalies.[6]

ACQUIRED CHEST WALL DEFORMITIES

Although rare, breast and chest wall asymmetry may be the result of pediatric thoracic surgery. Breast bud injuries can result from chest tube placement as well as thoracotomy procedures. Open thoracotomies can produce significant musculoskeletal morbidity, including atrophy of the serratus anterior muscle and pectoralis due to surgical incisions (**Fig. 1**).[7] Patients may also present to the office after multiple attempts to correct a pectus excavatum or similar sternal deformity, and may have already undergone a breast augmentation with revisions. These cases are certainly more difficult to approach, and patients should be informed that some deformities produced by

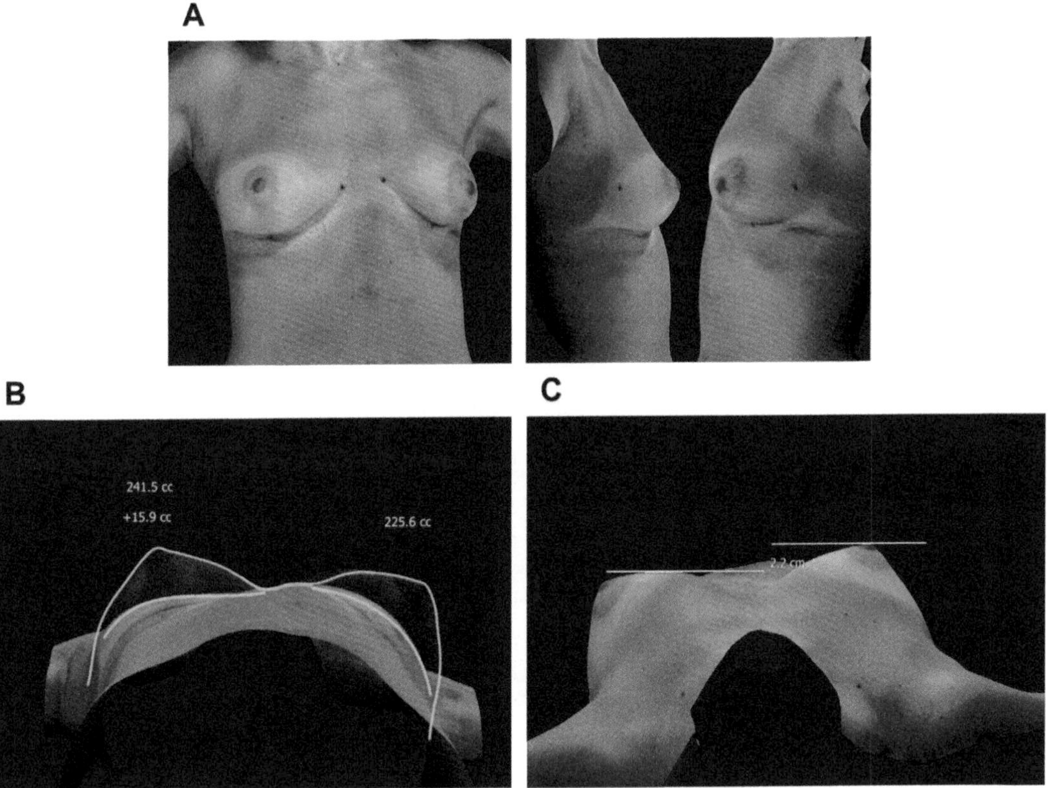

Fig. 1. (*A–C*) 23-year old with history of tetralogy of Fallot. Vectra 3-dimensional image demonstrates degree of chest wall deformity in a patient who underwent multiple cardiac surgeries within the first 5 years of life.

detachment of muscles, scarring, or thinning of overlying soft tissues may be uncorrectable (**Fig. 2**).

PSYCHOSOCIAL IMPLICATIONS

For young women with isolated chest and breast deformities, concerns about body image often drive them into a plastic surgeon's office. For those patients with genetic mutations that affect multiple organ systems, their physicians and family often underestimate the significance of their deformity. Most children affected with chest wall deformities begin to recognize that they are different from other children around the age of 4 to 6 years. Teasing and peer ridicule continue into adolescence. Clothing often hides breast deformities, but self-esteem issues worsen through the teenage years.[8] The psychological and social impact of breast asymmetry has been well documented. Poor body image and impaired psychosocial functioning increase with age in patients who have not had surgery.[9] Just as a young woman is establishing an independent identity, going off to college, or beginning sexual relationships, she must also deal with the distress associated with her deformity. Her physical condition can deeply upset her ability to do all of those things. The effect on quality of life, self-esteem, and psychological well-being advocates early intervention for these patients.

PATIENT ASSESSMENT AND PREOPERATIVE PLANNING

Chest wall and breast asymmetries can vary, from significant unilateral defects involving the sternum, ribs, muscle, and breast, to very subtle asymmetries that are difficult to detect and quantify.[10] Technological advances available today increase a plastic surgeon's ability to evaluate patients with chest and breast asymmetry. For patients with more complex monogenic and chromosomal aberrations, chest computed tomography (CT) may be useful for thoracic surgeons and plastic surgeons to establish a proper preoperative plan. Computerized algorithms have been developed to facilitate quicker and more accurate diagnosis of the defects.[11] CT images may include axial images and 3-dimensional CT reconstruction. If available, these studies can be valuable in the preoperative planning for breast augmentation (**Fig. 3**).

For several years, the option of in-office 3-dimensional imaging has provided plastic surgeons the ability to generate reproducible and clinically valid data for studying breast volume, chest contour, and asymmetries.[12] In-office 3-dimensional imaging can be integrated into the preoperative consultation, improving physician–patient communication and the management of patient expectations. Simulations can illustrate possible outcomes using selected implants and also demonstrate what may be a correctable or uncorrectable deformity. Simulations can also streamline the implant selection process, reducing the number of implants ordered and possibly the need for multiple sizers (**Fig. 4**).

CORRECTION OF CHEST WALL AND BREAST ASYMMETRIES WITH SHAPED HIGHLY COHESIVE GEL IMPLANTS

Shaped highly cohesive breast implants provide a greater degree of individualization and choices for

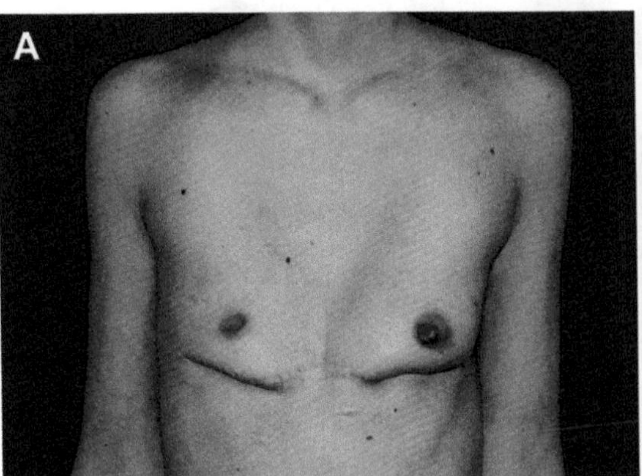

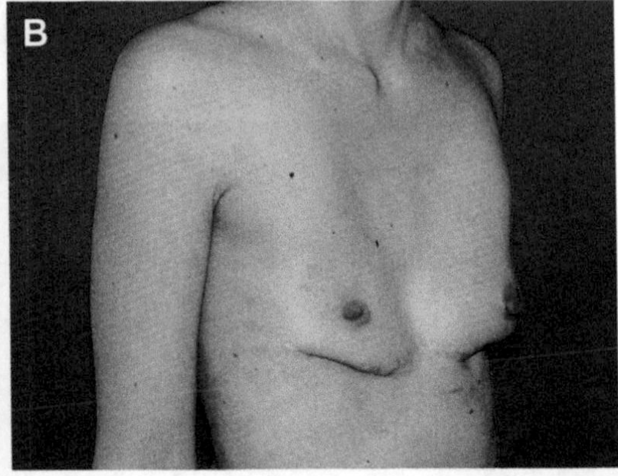

Fig. 2. (*A, B*) 31-year-old with Marfan syndrome. Minimally invasive pectus repair at age 10 years, revision at 18 years, and 2 scoliosis surgeries. First breast augmentation at age 18 with subglandular saline implants. Developed inferior malposition and synmastia. Revision with pocket change to submuscular saline at age 20 followed by another revision for recurrent malposition. Third revision with bilateral inferior capsulorrhaphy age 21. She subsequently developed recurrent synmastia and malposition and presents 10 years after explantation.

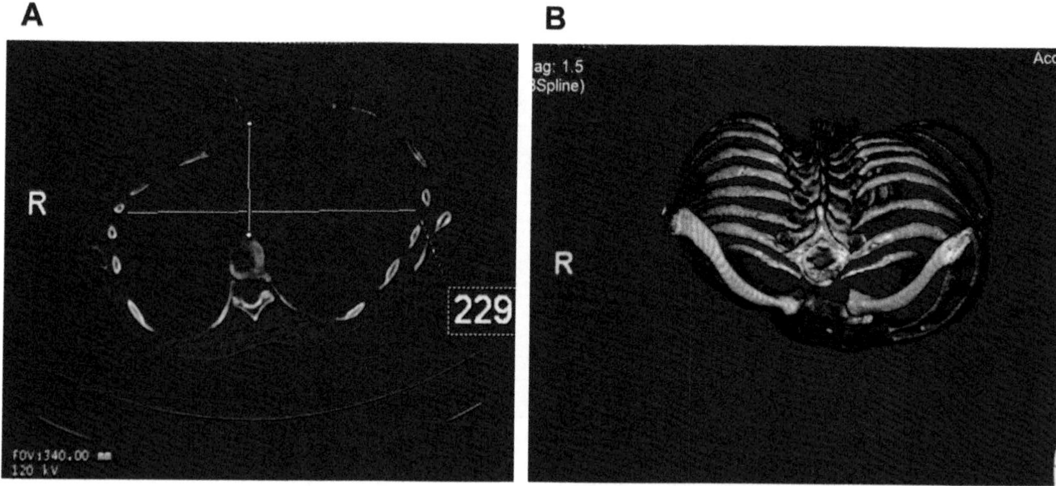

Fig. 3. (*A, B*) 22-year old with Marfan syndrome. Preoperative CT scan demonstrates severe chest wall deformity and presence of 2 asymmetric round gel implants. 3-dimensional CT reconstruction demonstrates significant chest wall asymmetry.

each patient. The ability to select an implant based on the base width, height, and projection as independent variables makes these implants especially valuable in the correction of chest wall and breast deformities. Detailed preoperative evaluation of thoracic and glandular asymmetries with objective measurements will provide the surgeon and patient with a small range of possible implant choices. Additional considerations include the assessment of the patient's soft tissue coverage, each breast type (tight, average, or loose-fatty), and patient desires. All of these parameters will contribute to the final implant selection.

Tissue-Based Planning

Tissue-based planning in breast augmentation has been well described and is critical when using shaped highly cohesive gel breast implants to correct chest wall and breast deformities.[13] Implant selection begins with determining the base width. This may be a bit more challenging in patients with chest wall deformities and asymmetry; however, the principles should be respected to avoid implant palpability and visibility. Soft tissue coverage is critical with all implants, as even the most highly cohesive implants available on the US market may be visible and palpable if oversized. The tissue type of the breast helps to define the projection of the device and may vary between breasts. Implant projection should be determined considering the need to correct asymmetry in both volume and shape, while respecting the breast fill, skin elasticity, and stretch. The sternal notch-to-nipple distance will help determine the height of the selected device. Here too, the desire to correct chest wall deformities needs to be balanced with the shape of the chest, which may vary between the right and left sides. The key measurements used in the selection of a shaped breast implant should be determined individually for each breast (**Fig. 5**). the authors attempt to correct the smaller breast or hypoplastic chest deformity to its optimal fill, and select a slightly smaller implant for the larger breast or chest wall. Oversizing a breast implant to correct a chest wall deformity or breast asymmetry will not produce a long-term stable outcome and may contribute to higher revision rates.

Techniques for Correction

It is recommended to use an inframmamary incision for the placement of a highly cohesive gel implant.[14] The planned incision should be well hidden in the new inframmary fold (IMF), which often needs to be adjusted. Lowering of the fold may help to achieve an optimal ratio between the base width (BW) and volume of the selected implant, and the new nipple-to-fold distance on stretch. The existing nipple-to-fold distance in patients with a chest wall deformity or breast asymmetry will likely differ between the 2 breasts. Ideally, although the location of the IMF on the chest may differ between the 2 sides, the final nipple-to-fold distance should not. Lowering 1 IMF beyond the recommended nipple-to-fold to BW ratio in an attempt to match the contralateral breast may result in an implant becoming inferiorly displaced over time, creating an upward pointing nipple-areolar complex (**Figs. 6** and **7**).

Whenever possible, the authors plan on placing the shaped implants in the dual-plane subpectoral pocket. This provides for optimal soft tissue

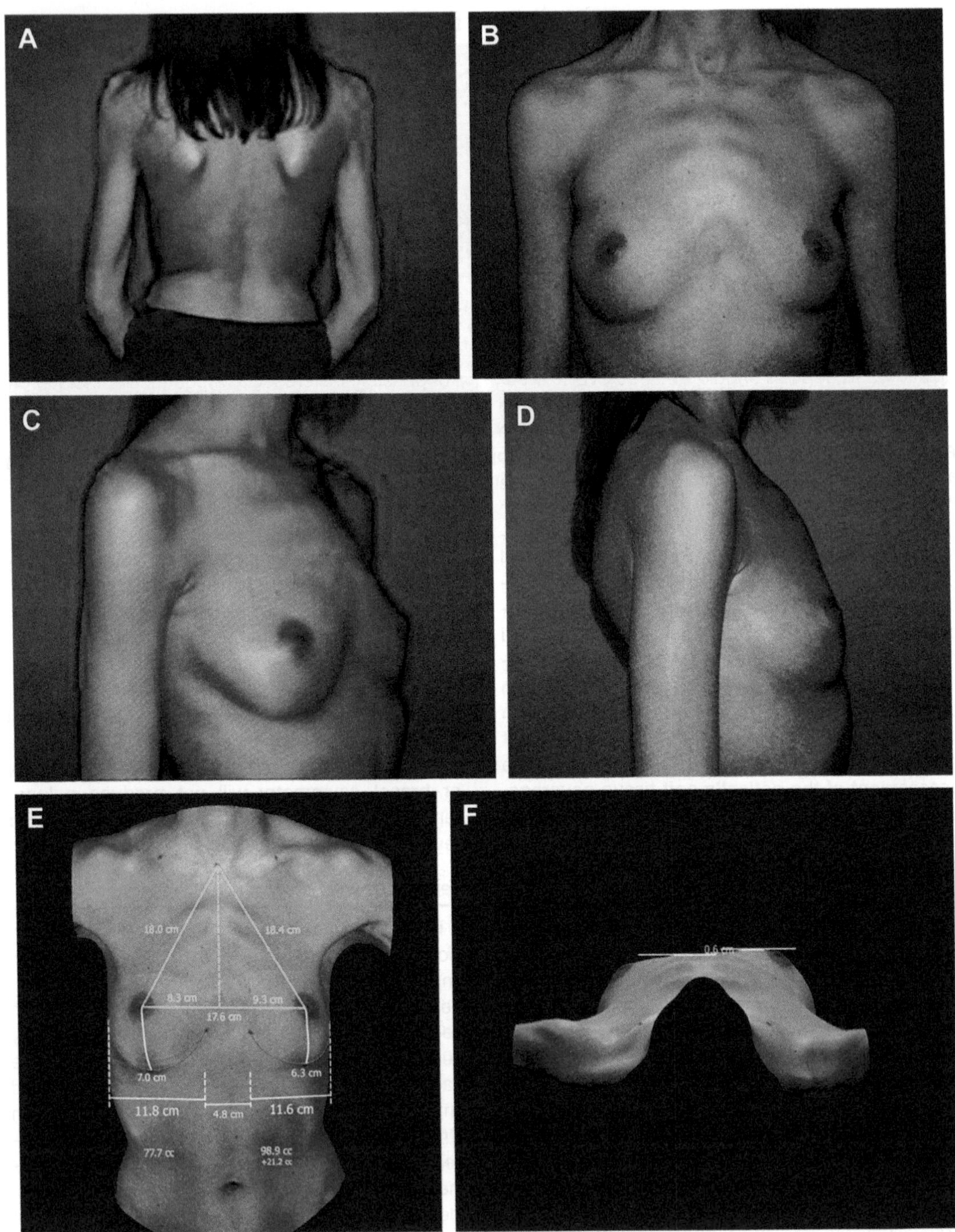

Fig. 4. (*A–D*) Standard photography documents the degree of chest wall and breast deformity in 30-year-old patient with Nail-Patella syndrome. (*E, F*) Preoperative 3-dimensional simulation can provide more detailed information on degree of breast asymmetry and location of chest wall defects.

coverage, especially in patients with hypoplastic breast tissue. A minimum incision length should be planned so as not to damage the implant during insertion. It has been well documented that pocket dissection and preparation for the implant should be dry and produce a hand-in-glove fit with the selected device. Intraoperative sizers can be avoided in most straightforward

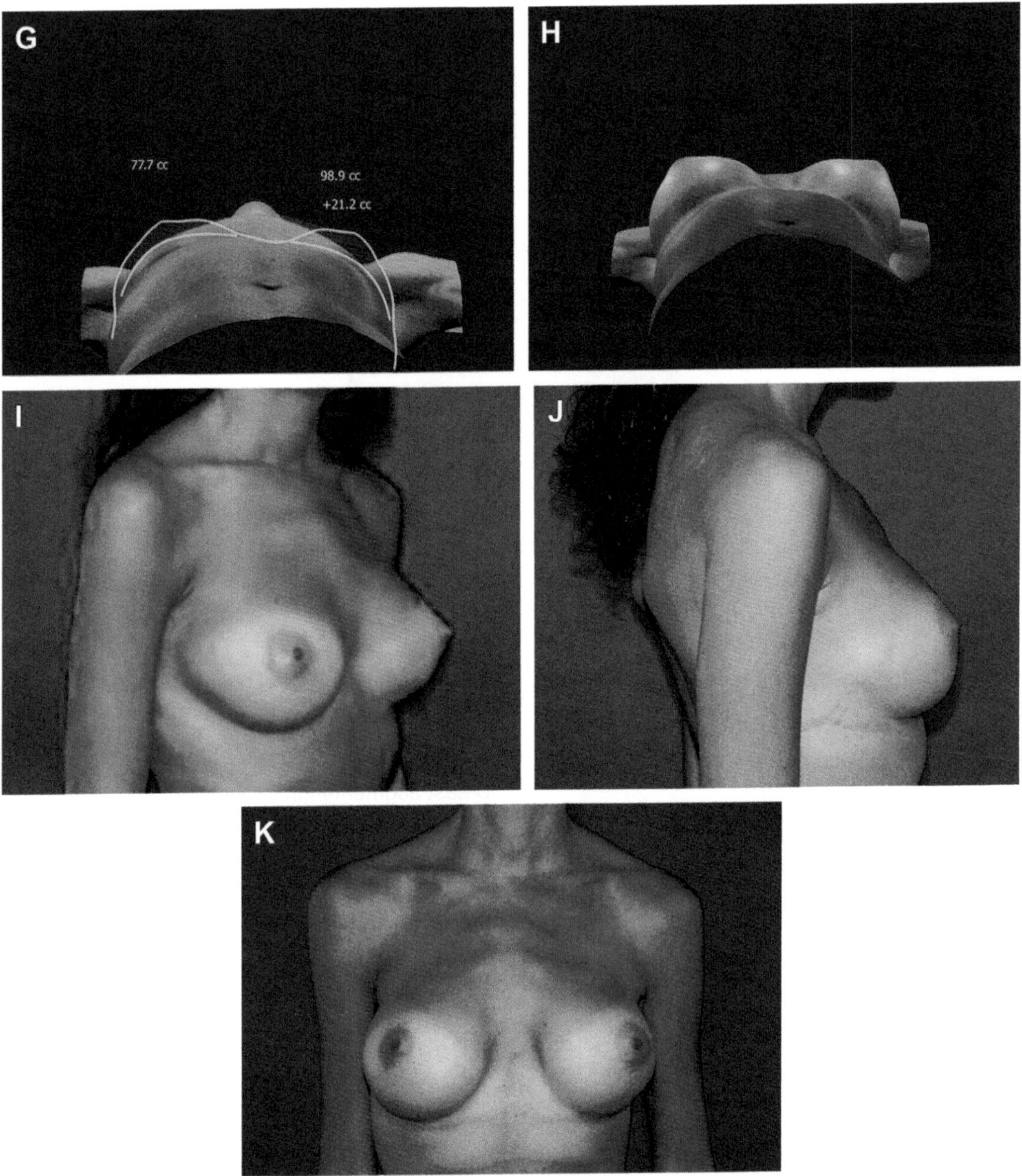

Fig. 4. (*continued*). (*G, H*) Preoperative and 1-year postoperative 3-dimensional simulation of the chest wall reveals improvement in projection of hypoplastic elements and symmetry. (*I–K*) Breast augmentation with style 410 FM270 right, FX315 left. Although there is not exact symmetry, the 3-year results remain stable.

breast augmentation cases; however, they may be useful in complex chest and breast asymmetries, especially in revision procedures. If used, care should be taken to limit the introduction of sizers to a bare minimum while using techniques to avoid contamination of the pocket. Finally, if the IMF has been adjusted, a sturdy suture repair that includes deep sutures from the chest wall to the fascia, followed by deep dermal sutures and skin, will help prevent inferior malposition and keep the incision well hidden in the new fold (**Fig. 8**).

ISOLATED BREAST ASYMMETRIES

By far, the most common deformities that a plastic surgeon will encounter are isolated breast asymmetries. These differences can be in volume alone, but more likely will also include

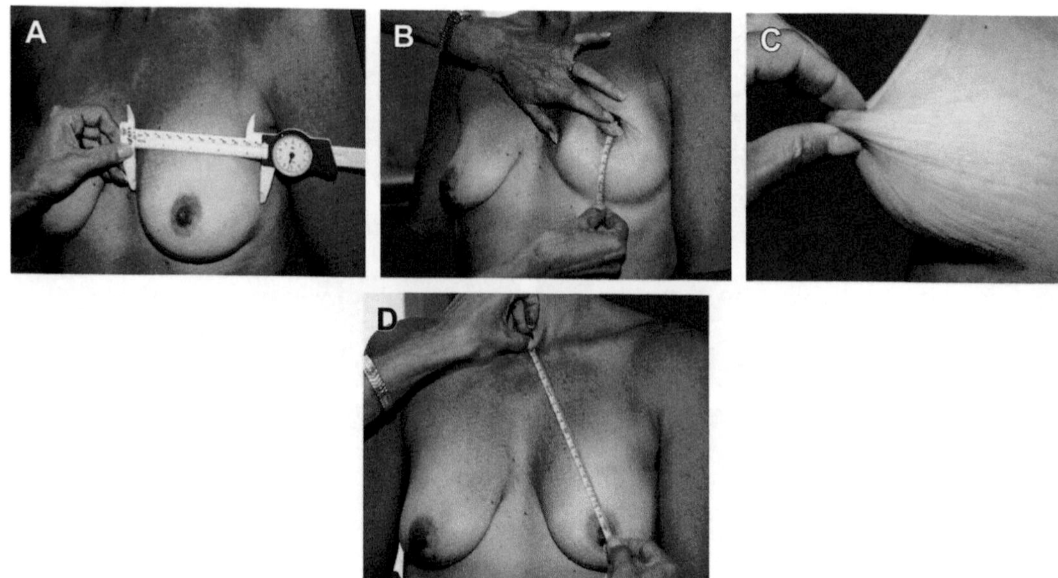

Fig. 5. (*A–D*) Tissue-based planning. (*A*) Base width—BW. (*B*) Nipple-to fold distance—N:IMF. (*C*) Breast type: skin stretch and elasticity. (*D*) Sternal notch-to-nipple distance-SN:N.

asymmetries in shape and parenchymal fill. The true beauty of the anatomic highly cohesive breast implant is its ability to produce shape while simultaneously adding volume, and the capacity to control the distribution of the gel.

During the initial consultation, the patient may initiate the discussion on breast asymmetry, but quite often it is only during the preoperative planning that the conversation about using 2 different implant styles or shapes begins. Some patients with breast asymmetries may not be aware of the extent of their asymmetry, while others are acutely aware of their dissimilar breasts. It is wise to document all objective measurements, 2-dimensional photographs, and computer scored measurements preoperatively and to thoroughly discuss these findings with the patient during the implant selection process. The availability of a full range of implant sizes and styles in the United States will finally allow surgeons the ability to fine-tune breast augmentation for women with asymmetries (**Figs. 9** and **10**).

CORRECTION OF BREAST AND CHEST WALL ASYMMETRY WITH IMPLANTS AND FAT

Fat transfer is becoming a more common procedure in the treatment of chest wall and breast deformities. When used in conjunction with shaped highly cohesive gel implants, autologous fat may be able to provide additional soft tissue coverage and contour improvements that implants alone may not be able

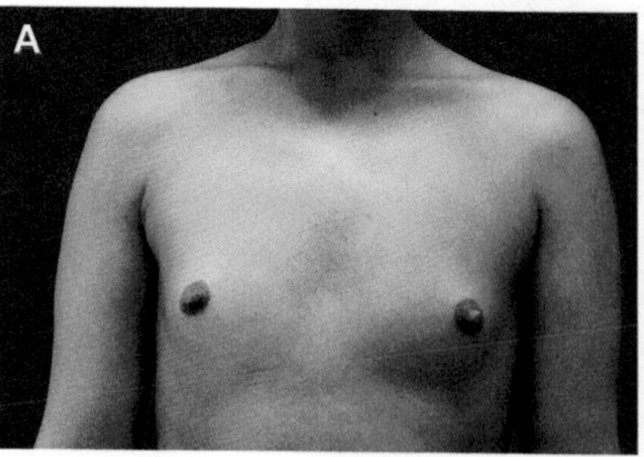

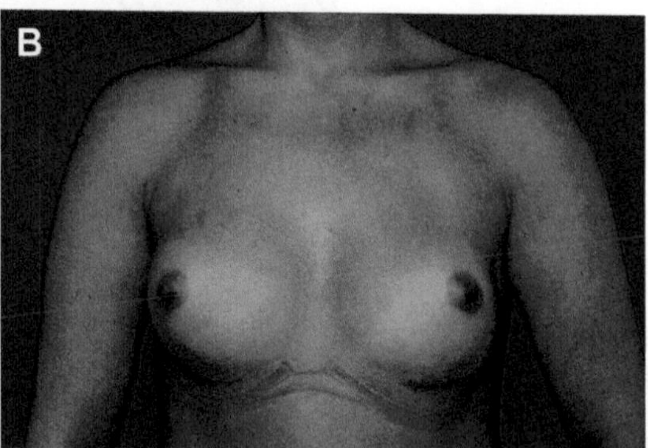

Fig. 6. (*A, B*) This patient underwent correction of her asymmetry with a style 410 MM320 on the left and an MF335 on the right. The nipple-to-fold distance was lowered on the right to match the lowered left. This resulted in both folds being placed too low and upward pointing nipples at 3 years.

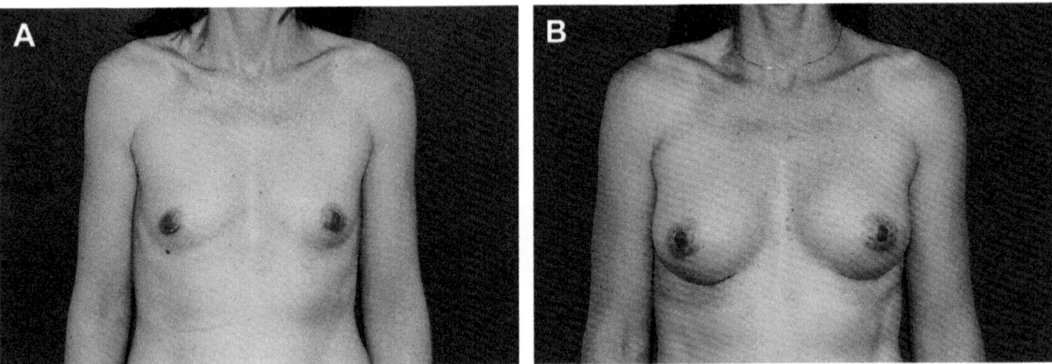

Fig. 7. (*A, B*) This patient underwent correction of her mild asymmetry with an MM280 on the left and an MF295 on the right. The nipple-to-fold distance was set at 7.8 cm on the left and 8.0 cm on the right. The location of the IMF may be different on each side, but the nipples will point forward not upward. 3-year result.

to achieve. Autologous fat transplantation to improve contour defects in breast reconstruction was described in 2005.[15] Chest wall deformities like pectus excavatum have been treated with lipomodeling as either an adjunct to minimally invasive procedures or alone in milder cases, with reported high satisfaction rates.[16] Composite breast augmentation can be defined as the simultaneous

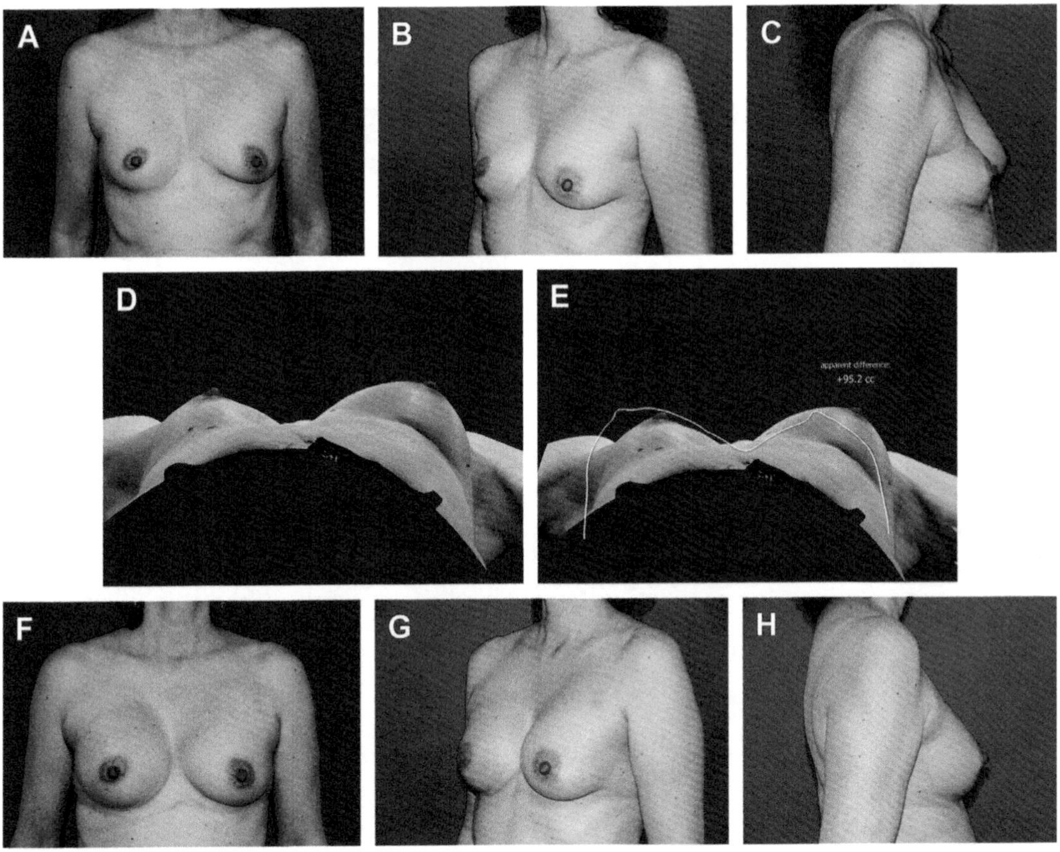

Fig. 8. (*A–E*) The preoperative photographs and 3-dimensional chest wall views, including a reflection view, can provide a better evaluation of the existing unilateral thoracic hypoplasia. (*F–H*) Style 410 FM270 right, ML125 left. Patient underwent a single lipofilling session at 2 years, with stable results at 3 years.

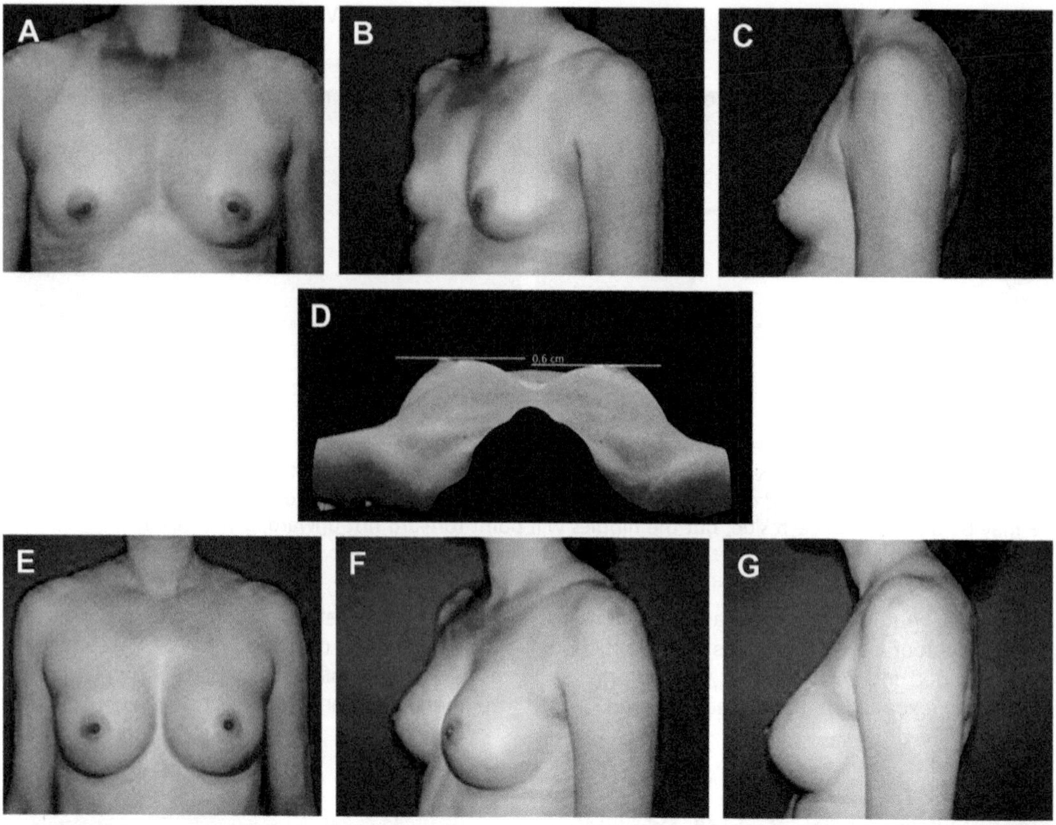

Fig. 9. (*A–D*) Preoperative 3-dimensional assessment reveals a .6 cm difference in projection between the left and right breasts. (*E–G*) Breast augmentation for asymmetry with style 410 MM280 left, MF295 right. Results at 3 years.

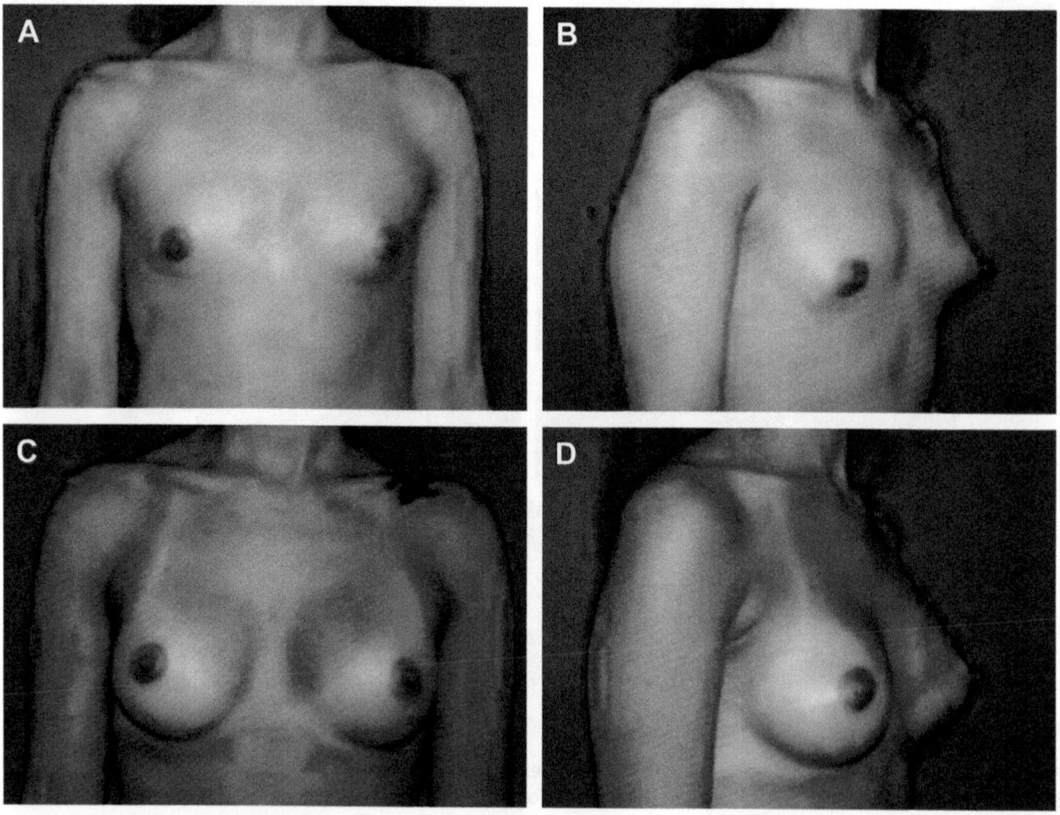

Fig. 10. (*A, B*) Preoperative views and (*C, D*) 5-year results in a patient with breast asymmetry and constricted base breast right. Right: 410 style MF255, left: 410 style MM245.

use of breast implants with autologous fat.[17] Some of the complications associated with large-volume transfer, such as calcifications and cysts, can be potentially be reduced when lower volumes of fat are required for fine-tuning the desired volume or shape. Fat transfer does not have to be performed at the time of augmentation and may be staged to further correct residual asymmetries or changes that occur with aging and time. With improvements and modifications in harvesting, processing, and injection techniques, there has been a documented increase in the survival rate of transferred fat. For younger patients with a very low body mass index (BMI), the benefits of harvesting fat must be weighed against the potential risks of additional donor site deformities and the possibility that harvesting sufficient fat may not be feasible. Fat grafting used in conjunction with shaped highly cohesive gel implants does offer further options for patients with moderate-to-severe chest wall deformities and breast asymmetry.

SUMMARY

Patients presenting for correction of breast and chest wall asymmetries may have undergone numerous thoracic procedures in early childhood, and some may have suffered profound psychosocial effects for years. Care must be taken to evaluate these patients using objective criteria and biodimentional principles. More complex congenital syndromes will require a more comprehensive preoperative work-up as well as a detailed history of any previous thoracic or breast procedures. Even the most mild of breast asymmetries needs to be carefully documented using measurements, photography, and 3-dimensional simulations when available. Patient education needs to be comprehensive, and patients need to understand that absolute correction of underlying chest wall and breast asymmetry may not be possible. Shaped highly cohesive breast implants offer plastic surgeons more possibilities and precision by fine-tuning the gel distribution and specific volume required to correct the hypoplastic elements. Preoperative planning and implant selection can be more interactive, with patient involvement in the decision-making process. Patients need to be willing to accept what can and cannot be corrected, and have realistic expectations. Long-lasting correction of asymmetry can be obtained when patients are not oversized, and care is taken to avoid visibility, palpability, and malposition problems. Finally, fat grafting for residual small defects is becoming a useful adjunct to the use of shaped implants alone.

Editorial Comments by Bradley P. Bengtson, MD

Some form of breast and chest wall asymmetry or deformity can be identified in essentially every breast augmentation patient. As one of my favorite mentors taught me: "Breasts are sisters not twins!". The preoperative assessment of the patient's chest wall and breasts are even more critical in these patients. 3-D imaging and simulation is extremely helpful in both planning and implant selection as well as setting patients expectations and establishing acceptable outcomes. In addition, shaped implants can provide a huge number of options with four different projection and three height options along with a large number of implant widths. In addition fat grafting or transfer is often important in achieving the best outcome in these patients thickening the soft tissues over thin asymmetric areas of the chest or over devices.

REFERENCES

1. Nuss D, Croitoru DP, Kelly RE. Congenital chest wall deformities. In: Ascraft KW, Holcomb GW III, Murphy JP, editors. Pediatric surgery. 4th edition. Philadelphia: Elsevier Saunders; 2005. p. 245–63.
2. Engum S. Chest wall deformities embryology, sternal clefts, ectopia cordis, and Cantrell's pentalogy. Semin Pediatr Surg 2008;17(3):154–60.
3. van Aalst J, Phillips JD, Sadove AM. Pediatric chest wall and breast deformities. Plast Reconstr Surg 2009;124(1):38e–49e.
4. Mathes S, Seyfer A, Miranda E. Congenital anomalies of the chest wall. In: Hentz VR, editor. Plastic surgery. vol. 6. 2nd edition. Philadelphia: W. B. Saunders; 2005. p. 1–80.
5. Bianco F, Elliot S, Sandler A. Management of congenital chest wall deformities. Semin Plast Surg 2011;25(1):107–16.
6. Spear S, Goldstein J, Pelletiere C. Augmentation mammoplasty in women with thoracic hypoplasia. In: Spear SL, editor. Surgery of the breast principles and art. 3rd edition. Chapter 120. Philadelphia: Lippincott Williams & Wilkins; 2011. p. 1410–15.
7. Sadove AM, van Aalst J. Congenital and pediatric breast anomalies: a review of 20 year's experience. Plast Reconstr Surg 2005;115(4):1039–50.
8. Kelly RE Jr, Cash TF, Shamberger RC, et al. Surgical repair of pectus excavatum markedly improves body image and perceived ability for physical activity: multicenter study. Pediatrics 2008;122(6):1218–22.
9. Nuzzi LC, Cerrato FE, Webb ML, et al. Psychological impact of breast asymmetry on adolescents: a prospective cohort study. Plast Reconstr Surg 2014;134(6):1116–23.

Surgical Strategies in the Correction of the Tuberous Breast

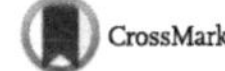

Mitchell H. Brown, MD, MEd, FRCSC[a,*],
Ron B. Somogyi, MD, MSc, FRCSC[b]

KEYWORDS

• Tuberous breast • Congenital breast • Constricted breast • Breast asymmetry

KEY POINTS

- The tuberous breast is a congenital abnormality of breast development that incorporates a constricted base of the breast and 1 or more of the following: high inframammary fold, areola hypertrophy, pseudoherniation of tissue through the areola, ptosis, hypoplasia, and breast asymmetry.
- Advanced forms of tuberous breast are readily apparent clinically; however, the diagnosis of more minor forms of tuberous breast requires careful examination and a high index of suspicion.
- The principles of treatment of the tuberous breast include:

a. Release of the constricted base through expansion, scoring, or internal flaps.
b. Lowering of the inframammary fold and restoring a normal nipple to inframammary fold distance.
c. Correction of herniated breast tissue.
d. Reduction of the size of the areola.
e. Augmenting the breast volume, when necessary.
f. Correction of underlying breast asymmetry.

INTRODUCTION

Breast anomalies characterized by an abnormality or asymmetry of the breast base have been called many names including tuberous breasts, tubular breasts, herniated nipple areolar complex (NAC), Snoopy deformity, lower pole hypoplasia, and constricted breasts.[1–5] These terms all represent varying degrees of the same deformity, with a multitude of different techniques described for their correction. No matter the name, it is broadly characterized by a deficiency in the vertical and horizontal dimensions of the breast, frequent underdevelopment of the breast, asymmetry, and herniation of breast tissue into the areola accompanied by expansion of the areola. Since its first description in 1976 by Rees and Aston,[1] this deformity, now most commonly referred to as the tuberous breast, has been the subject of several classification systems and a host of surgical management options.

It has been said that no other condition of the breast presents the same type of surgical challenge as the tuberous breast deformity.[6] Understanding its features and implementing a methodical approach to its surgical management is paramount, as the psychological and emotional effect these deformities can have on women are significant.[7]

Disclosures: Dr M.H. Brown is a shareholder in Strathspey Crown. Dr R.B. Somogyi has no financial disclosures.
[a] Department of Surgery, University of Toronto, 790 Bay Street, Suite 410, Toronto, Ontario M5G 1N8, Canada;
[b] North York General Hospital, 790 Bay Street, Suite 410, Toronto, Ontario M5G 1N8, Canada
* Corresponding author.
E-mail address: drbrown@torontoplasticsurgery.com

Clin Plastic Surg 42 (2015) 531–549
http://dx.doi.org/10.1016/j.cps.2015.06.004

Despite several large reported series, the prevalence of tuberous breast deformity is not firmly established. DeLuca-Pytell and colleagues[8] reported a prevalence of 73% in a retrospective analysis of 375 patients presenting for mammoplasty. Zambacos and Mandrekas[9] suggested that the actual percentage of tuberous breast is unknown but is actually much lower (6%–7%) than the one reported in the study by DeLuca-Pytell and colleagues.[8] Although some investigators consider this to be a problem of the female breast only,[7] several recent studies have described similar features in the male breast.[10] Asymmetry in tuberous breast deformity is almost always present[7]

A high index of suspicion is important in recognizing all forms of a tuberous breast. The unique anatomic features require specific surgical decisions and techniques in comparison with a standard breast augmentation. Failure to recognize this will predispose the patient to an unsatisfactory outcome and increase the likelihood of problems such as implant malposition, implant edge visibility and palpability, persistence of the old inframammary fold (IMF), and secondary soft-tissue deformities.

ANATOMY AND HISTOPATHOLOGY

The clinical features of the tuberous breast are illustrated in **Fig. 1**, and include a reduced breast base diameter, a high and constricted IMF, breast hypoplasia, ptosis, areola hypertrophy, herniation of tissue into the areola, and variable asymmetry of the breast.

The etiology of this deformity is unclear. Glaesmer (1930) suggested a phylogenetic relapse and Pers (1968) postulated that there is a failure of tissue differentiation in a limited zone of the fetal thorax.[3] These theories were effective in explaining deformities consistent with amastia and Poland syndrome, but more recent theories point to a simpler explanation that highlights the abnormal superficial fascia or weakness of the periareolar supporting tissues in the tuberous breast.

In earlier description and classification of tuberous breast deformity, Grolleau hypothesized in 1999 that the tuberous form is the result of stronger than normal adherence between the dermis and underlying muscle in the lower quadrants of the breast, which the developing breast cannot release. This adherence restricts peripheral expansion of the breast, causing it to develop in a forward direction and giving the breast its tubular appearance. In cases where the connective and muscular structure of the areola is weak, the gland herniates into the areola. These theories have been more recently expanded with Mandrekas' description of the ring theory[1] and Costagliola's discussion of the role of the weakened peri-NAC skin and fascia in predisposing to herniation of tissue into the areola.[6]

Together, these theories describe the breast as contained within a superficial fascial envelope, continuous with Camper fascia in the abdomen. The superficial layer covers the breast parenchyma, and the deep layer lies on the pectoralis fascia and forms the posterior boundary. A constricting ring at the level of the areola caused by a thickening of the superficial fascia, the joining of the 2 fascial layers at a higher level, or a thickening of the suspensory ligaments in this area inhibits normal development of the breasts. This constriction, combined with the absence of the superficial layer of the fascial envelope under the areola, allows for preferential development of the growing breast in a vertical direction with herniation through the weakened peri-NAC skin, resulting in the tuberous shape with areolar widening.

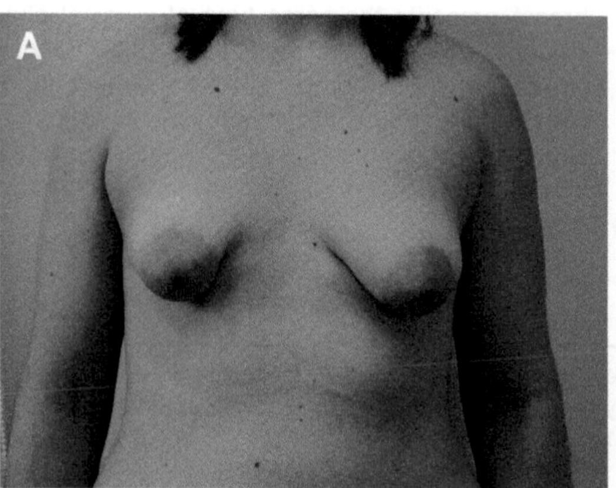

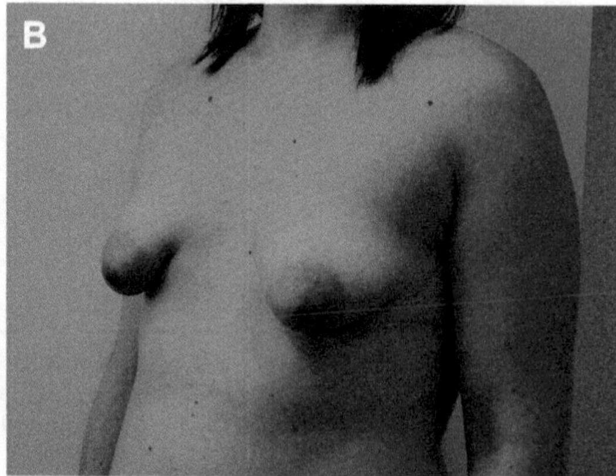

Fig. 1. (*A*, *B*) Clinical features of the tuberous breast: constricted base, high IMF, areola hypertrophy, herniation of tissue into areola, hypoplasia, asymmetry.

CLASSIFICATION

In 1996, Von Heimberg reviewed preoperative photos of 40 patients (68 breasts) with varying degrees of the tuberous breast deformity to describe a classification of 4 types (**Fig. 2**):

Type I: Hypoplasia of the lower medial quadrant
Type II: Hypoplasia of the lower medial and lateral quadrants with sufficient skin in the subareolar region
Type III: Hypoplasia of the lower medial and lateral quadrants with skin deficiency in the subareolar region
Type IV: Severe breast constriction with minimal breast base

Grolleau later examined 37 patients with breast base deformity, and modified the Von Heimberg classification to describe only 3 groups, as no objective or clinical difference could be seen between Von Heimberg types II and III. This study graded constricted breast base as Type I (lower medial quadrant deficiency), Type II (deficiency in both lower quadrants), and Type III (deficiency of all 4 quadrants). Of his patients, 54% had type I, 26% had type II, and 18% had type III. Seventy percent had volume asymmetry of greater than 100 g. Virtually all type III were hypoplastic and required an implant to restore adequate volume; 74% of type II and 100% of type I had sufficient volume to make an implant unnecessary. This classification also noted areolar herniation to be more frequent in type III breasts but did not include this feature in the classification.

More recently, a paradigm shift in the classification of tuberous breast deformity has been suggested based on the degree of areolar herniation. Pacifico and Kang[11] described an objective classification using the Northwood Index (NI), a ratio between the amount of forward projection of the areola divided by the areolar diameter. Fifty-five breasts were examined (20 tuberous) from photos, and NI was found to be 0.19 in normal breasts and 0.54 in tuberous breasts (on average). Tuberous breasts were then further divided into mild, moderate, and severe based on NI. Any NI higher than 0.4 was considered tuberous.[11]

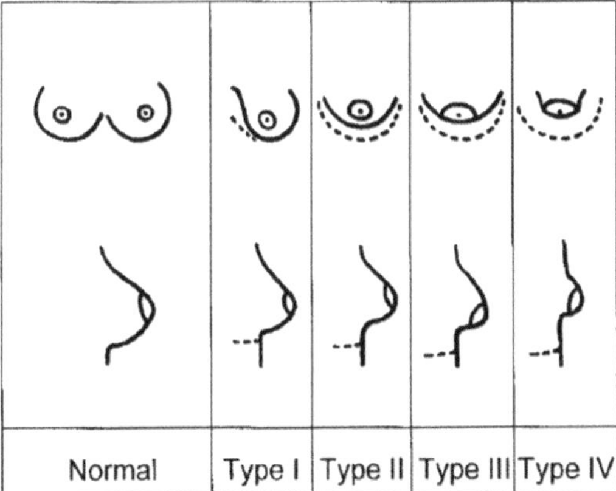

Fig. 2. Von Heimberg classification of the tuberous breast. The higher the type of deformity, the higher the severity. Type I, hypoplasia of the lower medial quadrant; Type II, hypoplasia of the lower medial and lateral quadrants, sufficient skin in the subareolar region; Type III, hypoplasia of the lower medial and lateral quadrants, deficiency of skin in the subareolar region; Type IV, severe breast constriction, minimal breast base. (*From* von Heimburg D. Refined version of the tuberous breast classification. Plast Reconstr Surg 2000;105(6):2269–70.)

TREATMENT GOALS AND PLANNED OUTCOMES

Principles of Treatment

A cornerstone of any successful aesthetic procedure is having a defined process for patient education and management of expectations. This tenet holds particularly true for patients with a tuberous breast. These patients dwell on the boundary between aesthetic and reconstructive surgery. Most patients appreciate that their breasts have an unusual shape or appearance, and in many cases desire an increase in volume. Patients frequently comment that they knew something was not quite right about their breasts but just did not know what it was. Often, however, patients do not have a full appreciation of the degree of anatomic abnormality, and the difficulties that will be faced by the surgeon to restore a near normal appearance to the breast. Without proper education, many patients expect outcomes similar to those seen with routine primary breast augmentation.

Surgical management of the tuberous breast is ultimately determined by the severity of presentation, and requires both the surgeon and patient to address each aspect of the deformity. The principles of treatment should include the following:

1. Release of the constricted base in both a vertical and horizontal plane
2. Restore a normal nipple to IMF distance through a combination of mastopexy and lowering of the IMF
3. Obliterate the old IMF to avoid a double-bubble appearance
4. Reduction of herniated tissue
5. Correction of areola hypertrophy
6. Restoration of breast volume
7. Correction of breast asymmetry

In addition, the decision must be made whether to address the multiple elements of this deformity in 1 or 2 stages. Whenever possible, correction is offered in a single stage; however, in cases of type IV deformity or severe herniation of tissues into the areola, a 2-stage approach is suggested (**Fig. 3**).

Photographs can be helpful in the process of managing expectations. Patients should be aware that in comparison with a primary augmentation, they are more likely to have residual asymmetry, require additional scars, have implant edge visibility or palpability, and may have persistence of an old inframammary scar. The complexity of these patients will result in an increased incidence of secondary surgery compared with the population undergoing primary breast augmentation. Ensuring that patients have a full understanding and acceptance of these issues before their initial treatment is a necessary component of patient selection and preparation.

Minor degrees of tuberous deformity are often seen in women presenting with concerns of ptosis, hypertrophy, or asymmetry. A high index of suspicion is necessary to appreciate the constrictive component of the presentation.

Patients with ptosis and adequate volume can be treated using mastopexy and breast-reduction techniques. Care should be taken to adjust and customize the skin patterns of excision to account for areas of tissue deficiency. For example, in a type I deformity with medial deficiency, it is important to excise skin laterally and maintain skin in the deficient medial quadrant. Tissue excision is also guided by the type of deformity, and internal breast flaps may be helpful to redistribute tissue to areas of apparent deficiency (**Fig. 4**).

It is also necessary to appreciate the difference between the tubular breast deformity and the tuberous breast deformity.[12] Despite the similarity in pathogenesis, tubular and tuberous breasts are distinct deformities that present with different clinical features. The tuberous breast is characterized by reduction of both vertical and horizontal diameters, alteration of areola shape and size, and moderate to severe hypoplasia of the skin and glandular tissue. By contrast, a tubular breast presents with a long vertical diameter of the upper quadrants, extending downward far beyond the IMF, and a normal or relatively reduced horizontal diameter. Volume is either normal or increased. In general, tubular breasts can be corrected with mastopexy/reduction patterns of glandular resection and reshaping, whereas tuberous breasts require more release, reshaping of lower quadrants

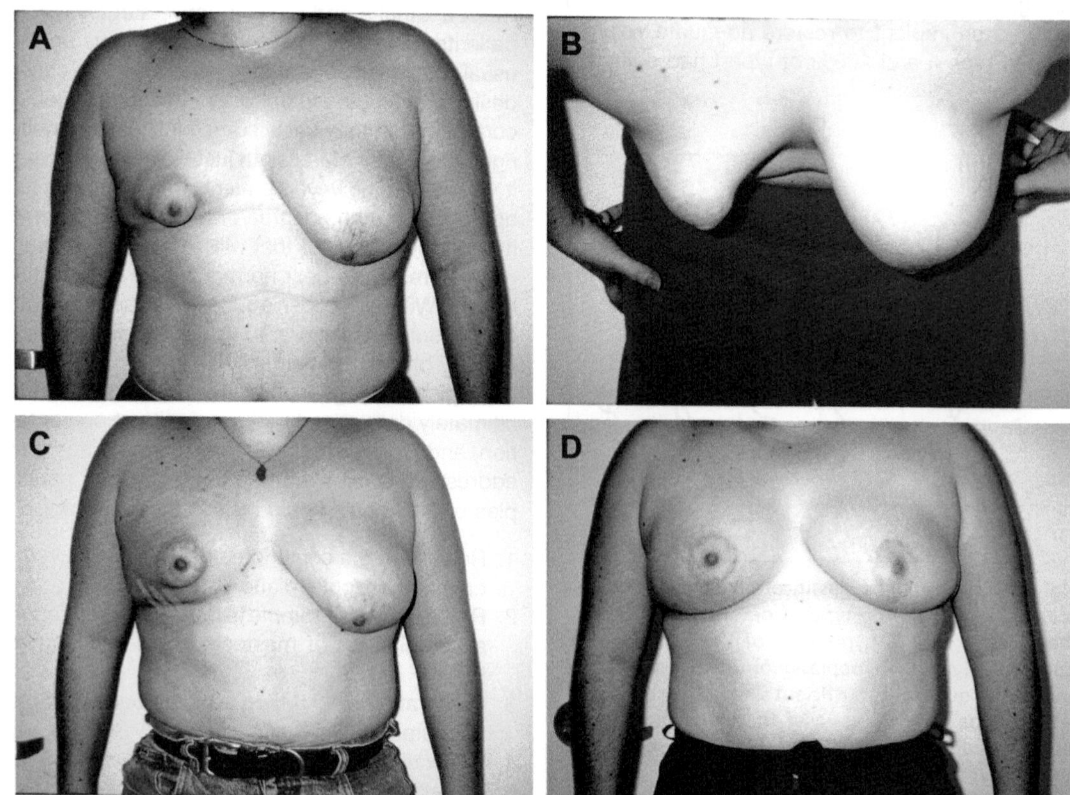

Fig. 3. Type IV deformity on the right and type I deformity on the left. (*A, B*) Preoperative view; (*C*) expander in place; (*D*) implant and areola reduction with balancing lift and reduction.

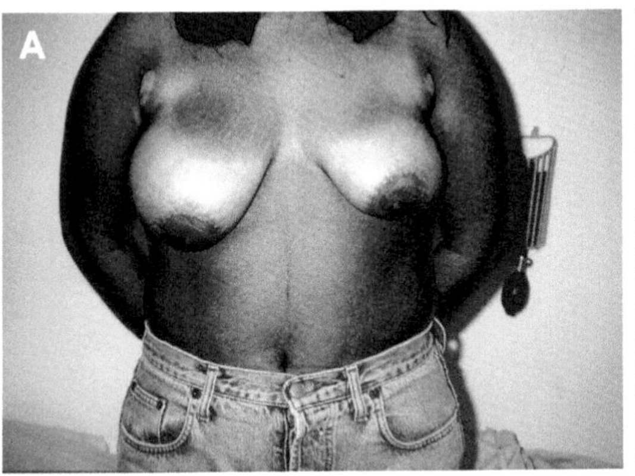

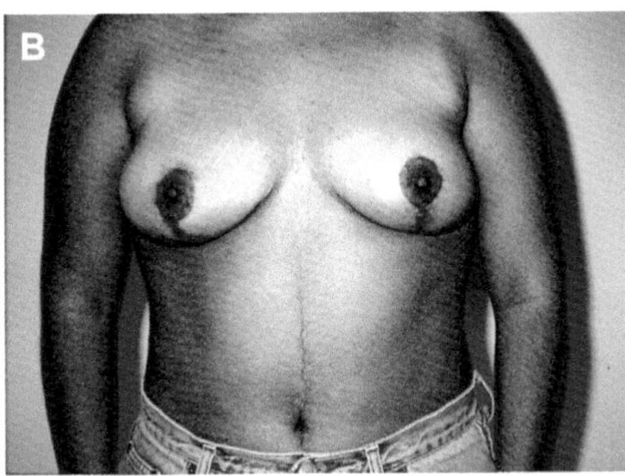

Fig. 4. Bilateral mastopexy with asymmetric resection of lateral tissue only because of a deficient medial quadrant in a type I deformity. (*A*) Preoperative. (*B*) 3 months postoperative.

with glandular flaps, autologous fat, or the use of an implant.

The Constricted Base

Successful correction of the tuberous breast must include adequate expansion of the constricted base of the breast. Since the first descriptions of the tuberous deformity, most investigators have highlighted techniques to release, resurface, or camouflage the constricted base (**Fig. 5**). Adequate release can often be achieved through implant pocket dissection with radial scoring as required. In severe cases, 2-stage release with the use of tissue expansion may be indicated. More recently, fat has been considered for filling a tight lower pole in conjunction with preoperative external expansion (see later discussion). Although Rees and Aston[1] were first to discuss radial scoring, they did not actually transect the constricting ring. Dinner and Dowden[13] considered that the skin itself was constricting, and advocated full-thickness skin and glandular incisions with transposition of local skin and subcutaneous tissue flaps.

More recently, internal glandular reshaping has allowed for correction of the constricted base without significant external scars or contour irregularities. Internal flaps fashioned from subareolar parenchyma, based anteriorly on the subareolar tissue or posteriorly on the chest wall, can be folded down to reconstitute the constricted lower pole.[14–17] The unfolded subareolar gland flap was recently described in 42 breasts (26 patients).[7] This modified Puckett technique, which included lengthening of the subareolar flap with 2 L-shaped releasing incisions, allowed further unfolding, elongation, and homogeneity of the flap to allow it to reach the new IMF and provide full coverage of a prosthesis.

Mandrekas and Zambacos[5] used a modified inferior pole flap in 41 breasts over 10 years. These investigators used a periareolar donut excision and inferior pole exteriorized through the periareolar incision that was then transected vertically at 6 o'clock, releasing the constriction ring and forming 2 pillars that could be redraped and sutured if necessary to reform the lower pole of the breast. Implants were used if additional volume was required. Reported complications included bruising and swelling, hematoma, capsular contracture (secondary to hematoma), and asymmetry. No reoperations were required with a minimum follow-up of 18 months.[5]

Volume Correction

In most cases, it will be necessary to increase volume either to establish a normal breast shape or to satisfy patient expectations. Volume can be increased with either autogenous or alloplastic techniques. The use of flaps for the correction of a tuberous breast has been described (see earlier discussion), although microfat injection is becoming a common method for the use of autogenous tissue.

Fat can be used to increase breast volume, with the added benefit of being able to control distribution of volume throughout the breast. Most often, fat will be added to the lower pole of the breast. When combined with techniques such as needle band release (also known as rigottomies), fat can be used to restore contour in the inferior pole and lower the IMF. External tissue expansion using a BRAVA device is a useful adjunct to fat injection and is thought to assist in retention of the fat graft through expansion of the recipient site, increasing the graft to capacity ratio and improving recipient site vascularity (**Fig. 6**).

Fig. 7 shows a 27-year-old woman with bilateral lower pole constriction. She was treated with 2 sessions of fat injection, 2 months apart.

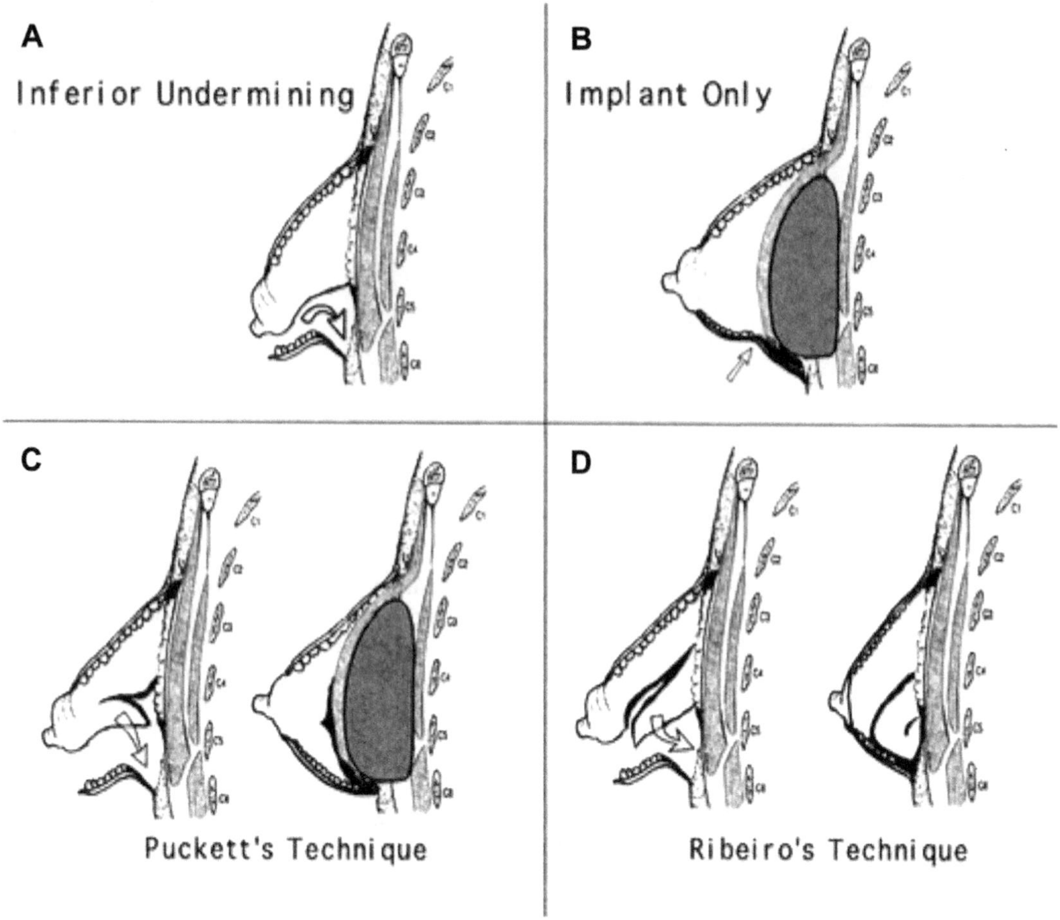

A
Inferior Undermining

B
Implant Only

C
Puckett's Technique

D
Ribeiro's Technique

Fig. 5. Techniques for releasing the constricted base; (*A*) subcutaneous dissection and scoring, (*B*) implant pocket dissection, (*C*) areola-based flap, (*D*) chest wall–based flap. (*From* Grolleau JL, Lanfrey E, Lavigne B, et al. Breast base anomalies: treatment strategy for tuberous breasts, minor deformities, and asymmetry. Plast Reconstr Surg 1999;104(7):2040–8; with permission.)

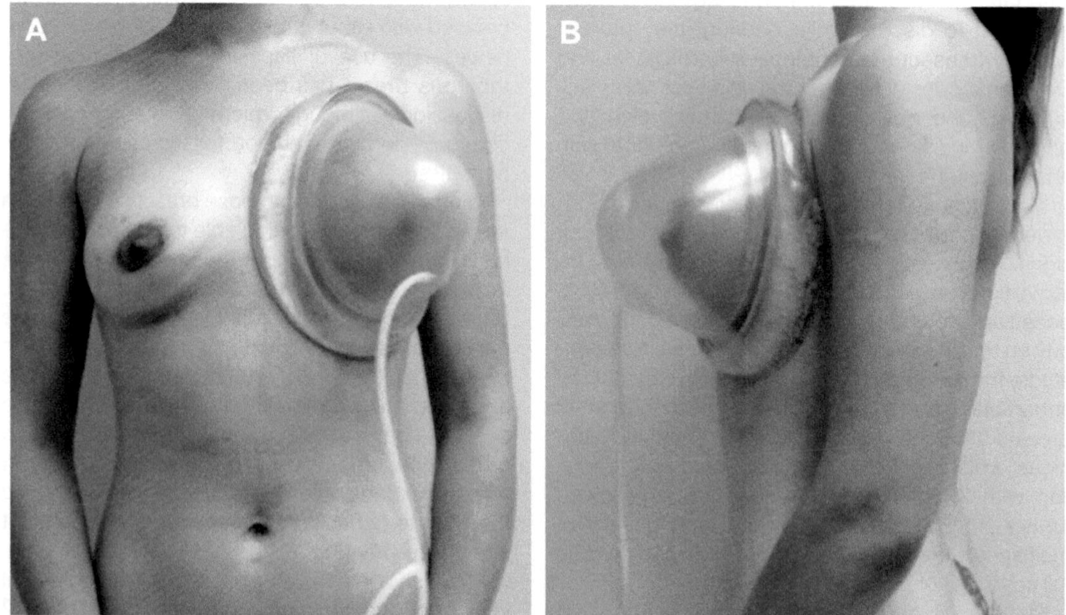

Fig. 6. (*A, B*) BRAVA external expansion as preparation for fat injection of the breast.

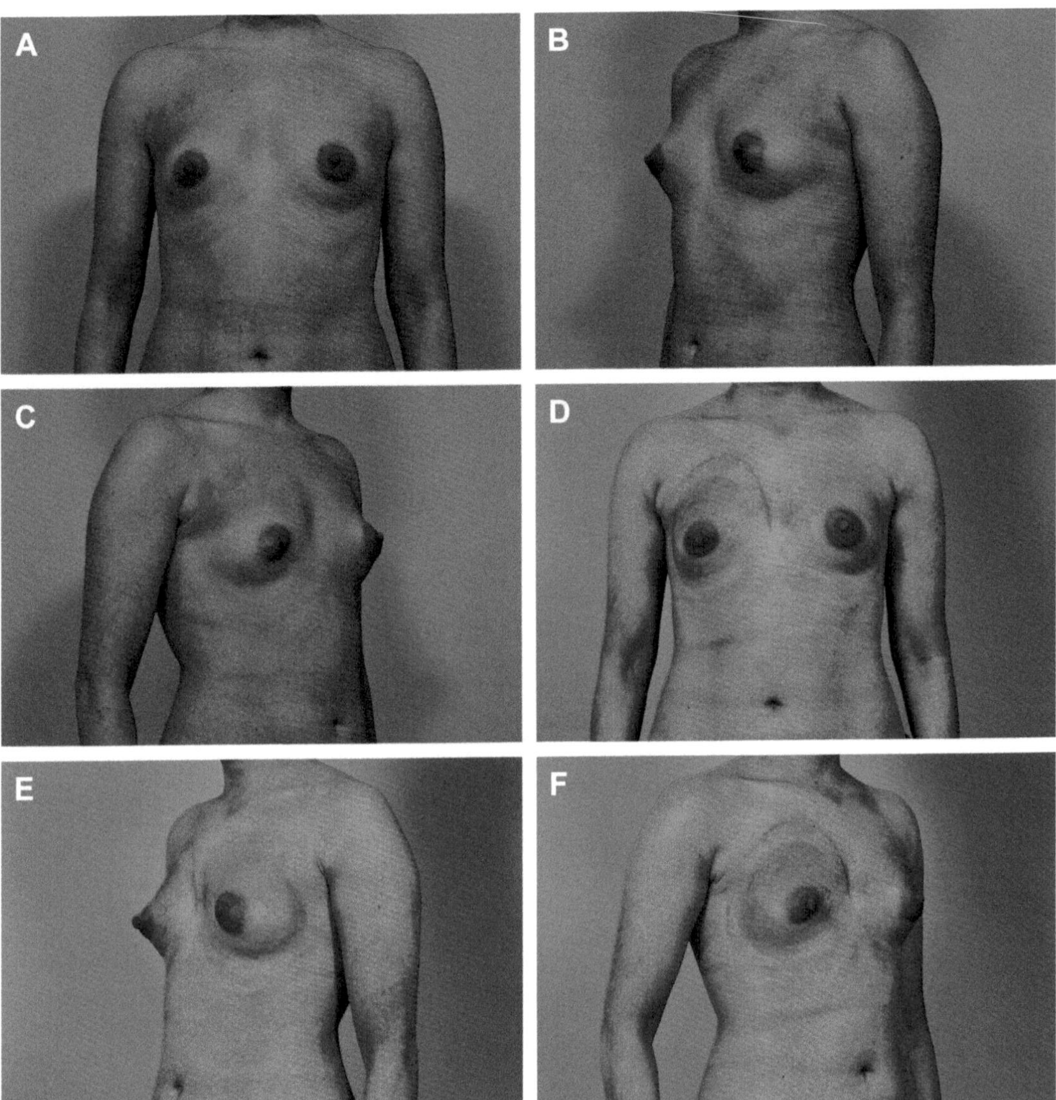

Fig. 7. Bilateral tuberous breast treated with external expansion and 2 sessions of fat injection. (*A–C*) Preoperative views; (*D–F*) following external expansion.

Approximately 600 mL of fat was injected in the first stage and 300 mL in the second stage. BRAVA expansion was applied for 6 hours per day, 3 weeks before each procedure.

BREAST IMPLANTS AND THE TUBEROUS BREAST

Most tuberous breasts are hypoplastic and require some form of augmentation; this is most often performed with an implant. The use of an implant requires a methodical approach with regard to both the surgical technique (incision location, pocket selection, adjunctive procedures such as fat grafting or 2-stage reconstruction with a tissue expander) and implant selection (shape, texture, adjustable).

Saline-filled implants are not preferred because of the lack of soft-tissue coverage, especially laterally and at the IMF. Both round and anatomic cohesive gel implants have a role in the correction of the tuberous breast, and selection is often based on both surgeon and patient preference. When correction is unilateral, an implant should be selected to best match the shape of the opposite breast.

The senior author has a strong preference for the use of form-stable anatomic gel implants when correcting the tuberous breast.[18] These implants are able to maintain their shape in all

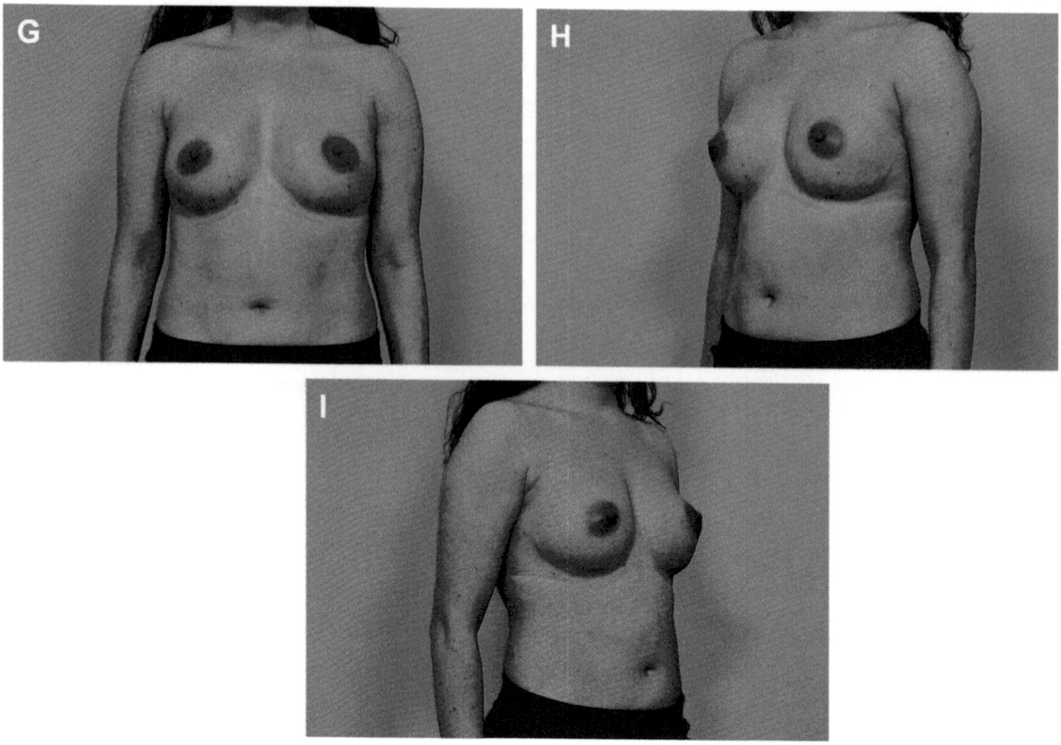

Fig. 7. (*continued*). (*G–I*) After 2 sessions of fat grafting. (*Courtesy of* Dr Lou Bucky, Philadelphia, PA.)

positions, and resist deformation. Compared with traditional round implants, anatomic implants are designed to resemble more closely the shape and dimensions of a normal breast, which can be particularly useful in a breast that is tuberous with an abnormal shape and a tight skin envelope (**Fig. 8**).

Selection of the implant is based on dimensional planning processes that include an objective measurement of breast height, width, and tissue compliance, and an assessment of the degree of tissue deficiency in the lower pole of the breast.[19–21] Full-projection or extra-projection implants are particularly helpful to augment the lower pole deficiency and maintain expansion of the released constricted base without producing unnatural fullness of the upper pole. Many unique characteristics make an anatomic cohesive gel implant an excellent choice for treatment of the tuberous breast. For patients with an asymmetric deformity, the matrix of implants available allow for selection of different implants based on specific measures of width, height, and projection. Given the constricted nature of the breast base,

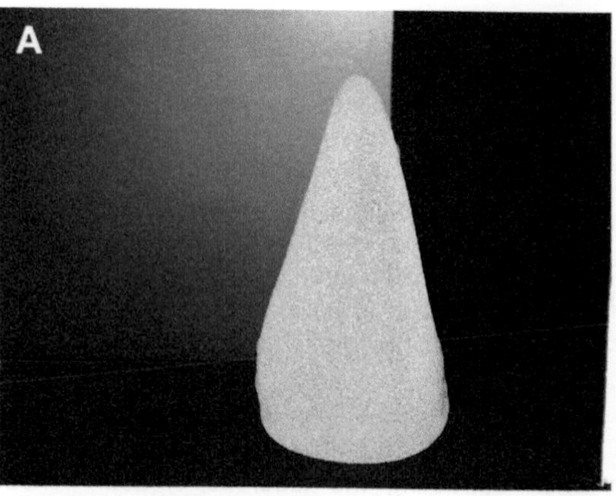

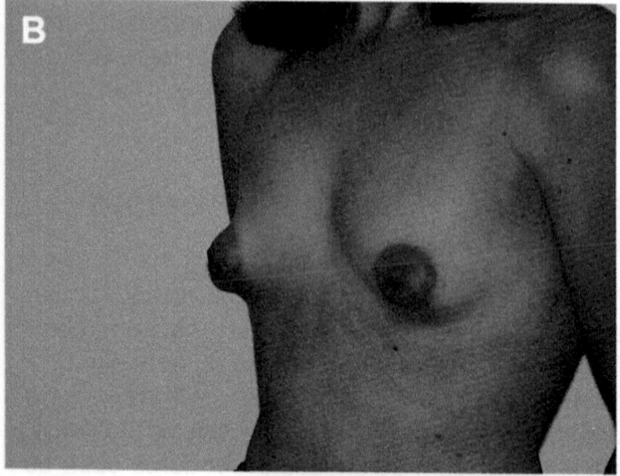

Fig. 8. Form-stable anatomic implant (*A*), ideally shaped for the correction of a tuberous breast (*B*).

a subglandular pocket is often preferred. This pocket allows the implant to exert direct force on the breast base and maximize the stretch of the tissues. Placement of an implant in a subglandular position with minimal overlying tissue may result in palpability and rippling of the implant edge. Form-stable implants should minimize the likelihood of this occurring in comparison with less cohesive devices.

The typical tuberous breast requires volume replacement in the lower pole, elevation of the NAC, and avoidance of excessive fullness in the upper pole. An anatomically shaped device is an ideal choice for dealing with these issues. The degree of nipple elevation that can be achieved with full-projection or extra-projection devices can be dramatic, and in some circumstances allows the surgeon to avoid a simultaneous mastopexy.

The senior author has previously described his experience in more than 50 tuberous breast cases using a single-stage approach with anatomic implants. Most implants were placed in a dual-plane pocket with muscle coverage in the upper pole and subglandular placement in the lower pole. This approach allowed for a natural contour superiorly while maximizing stretch on the constricted lower tissues. Complication rates were low, and no patients required conversion to a 2-stage expander procedure.[18]

Incision Selection

The surgical approach and exposure is selected to minimize visible scarring on the breast, allow adequate exposure for pocket dissection and glandular repositioning, remove redundant skin when necessary, and correct any existing areola deformity. In cases where there is minimal areola hypertrophy or herniation of soft tissues, an IMF approach may be selected. The resultant scar will be well hidden under the breast, avoiding a scar around the small areola. This approach requires precise presurgical planning to determine the exact position of the new IMF (see later discussion). **Fig. 9** shows a woman with a type III tuberous breast, severe hypoplasia, and a small areola diameter. She has been corrected in a single stage through an IMF incision with a medium-height, moderate-projection 320-g implant placed in a subpectoral pocket. The scar is well hidden in the new IMF. Note the persistence of the old IMF on the left breast 4 years after surgery.

Most commonly, the incision for implant insertion is placed around the areola in conjunction with a circumareolar approach to manage areola hypertrophy (**Fig. 10**).

Dissection can proceed directly through the breast tissue to the muscle (breast splitting approach), or alternatively can follow an inferior subcutaneous plane down to the IMF (unroofing approach). Once the constricted base has been released, the implant inserted, and the herniated tissue reduced, the areola diameter is controlled with the use of a wagon-wheel Gore-Tex suture[22,23] (**Fig. 11**). When performing a mastopexy or areola reduction, it is important not to commit to the skin excision until after the implant is inserted. Although the large size of the areola

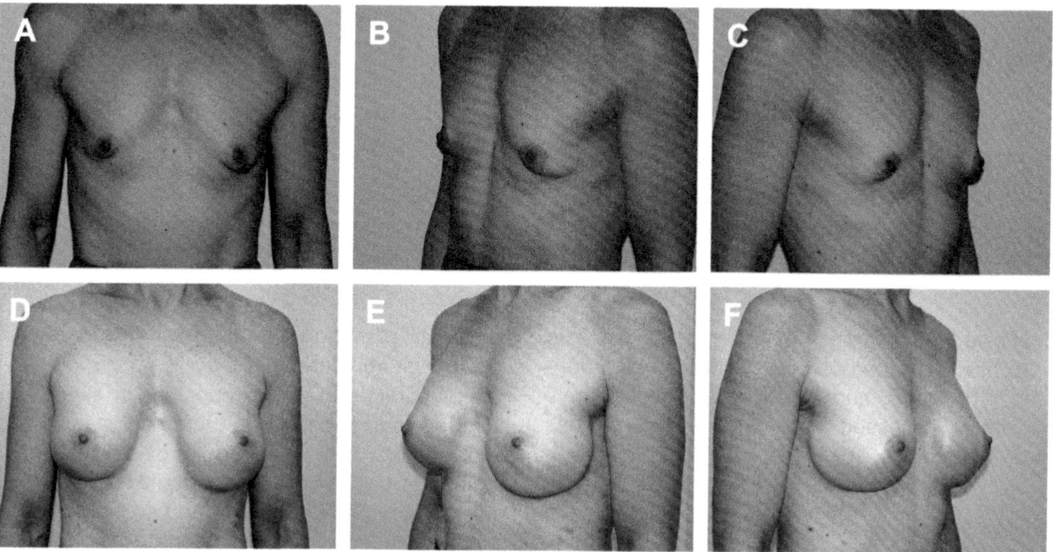

Fig. 9. Bilateral type III deformity with a small areola and no herniation of tissue. (*A–C*) Preoperative views; (*D–F*) 4 years after correction with shaped MM 320-g implants through an IMF incision.

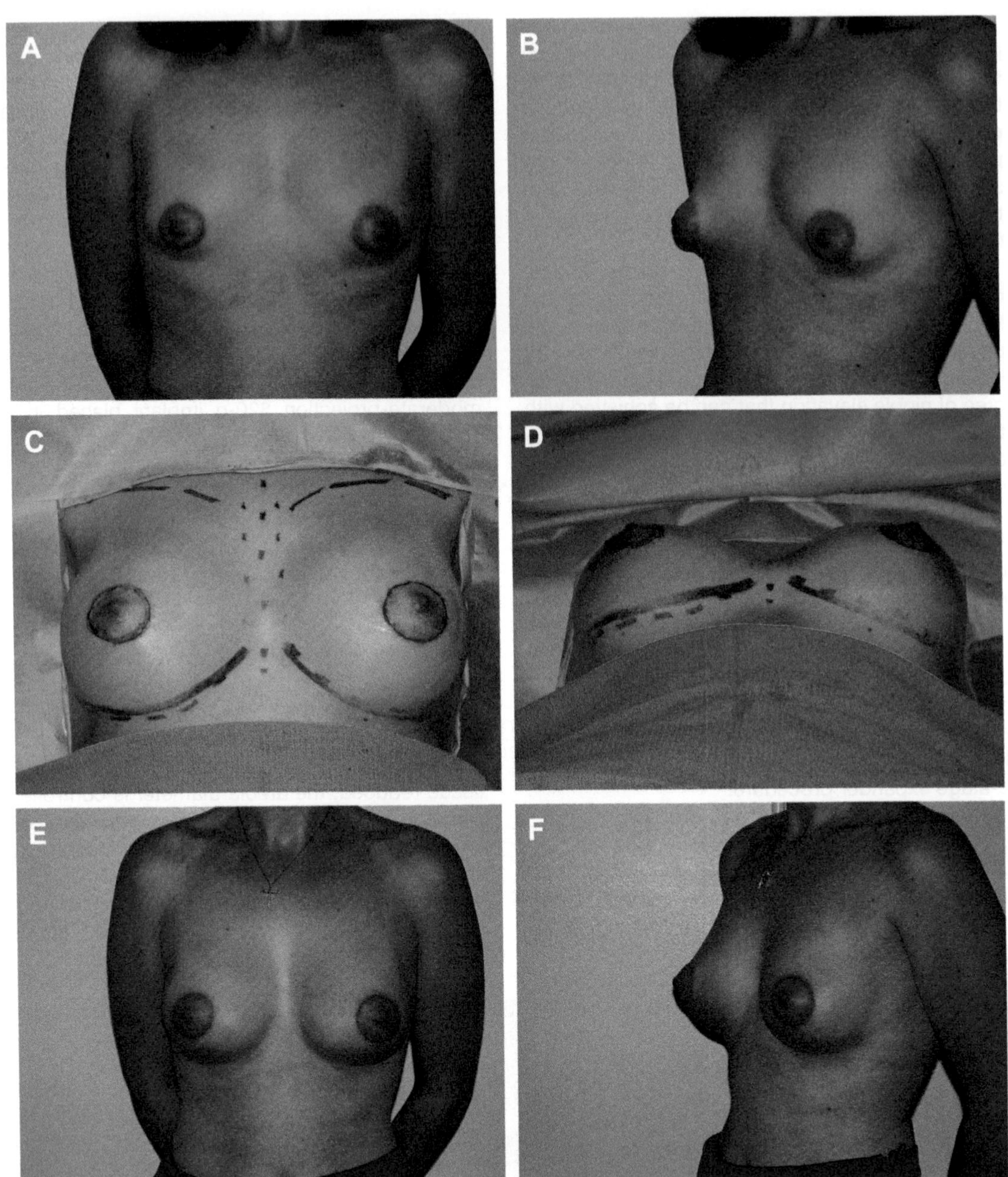

Fig. 10. Type III deformity treated with circumareolar reduction and a shaped MF 295-g implant in a subglandular pocket. (*A, B*) Preoperative views; (*C, D*) on-table result; (*E, F*) 6 weeks postoperatively.

may give the impression that there is excess skin to excise, the tuberous breast always has a deficiency of tissue, and areola reduction can only be safely assessed once breast volume has been restored.

Pocket Selection

Ideal pocket selection will allow for maximum expansion of the constricted base of the breast while still providing adequate soft-tissue cover of the breast implant.

For patients in whom constriction exists both inferiorly and superiorly in the breast, a subglandular pocket is preferred, providing there is adequate tissue in the upper pole. Occasionally, fat injection can be used to add soft-tissue cover where needed. Some surgeons advocate for a subfascial dissection, suggesting that the fascia provides stability for the implant and adds some

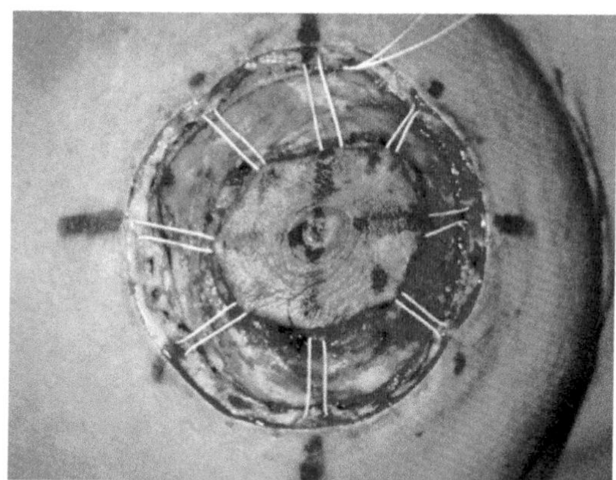

Fig. 11. Wagon-wheel approach to controlling areola diameter.

degree of soft-tissue support.[24] The senior author has not found that the minor addition of tissue cover justifies the added element of separating the fascia from its underlying muscle.

Pocket dissection is performed under direct vision using electrocautery. Dissection is accomplished in as atraumatic a manner as possible to minimize accumulation of blood and fluid in the pocket. This aspect is especially relevant with the use of anatomically shaped devices to minimize the risk of implant rotation or malposition. **Fig. 12** shows a young woman with circumferential constriction. A small shaped implant was inserted in a subglandular pocket through a circumareolar incision. The patient is seen initially at 1 year, and then 10 years after surgery with an implant exchange to a 600-mL device in the same subglandular space.

In cases with insufficient tissue in the upper pole (<2-cm pinch) a dual-plane procedure is performed, with a subpectoral dissection in the upper pole and a subglandular dissection in the lower pole. This approach maximizes the direct stretching effects of the implant on the constricted lower pole tissues while adequate coverage in the upper part of the breast is maintained. When performing a dual-plane dissection, the pectoral muscle is divided inferiorly to the level of the sternum. No medial release of the muscle is performed. The dual plane is then created by slowly releasing the superior cut edge of the muscle from the overlying gland. Only a few millimeters of release is necessary. Excessive release will result in superior migration of the muscle with resultant window shading and animation deformity. **Fig. 13** shows a woman with lower pole constriction and a normal breast contour superior to the areola. She is an ideal candidate for a dual-plane approach to fill the lower pole and maintain maximum soft-tissue cover in the upper pole.

Preoperative Markings and Determining the New Inframammary Fold

Preoperative markings are performed before surgery with the patient standing. The sternal notch, the midline, and the breast meridian for each breast are marked. When areola lifting or reduction is indicated, the estimated position of the new nipple is marked along the breast meridian, measured from the sternal notch to ensure symmetry. This marking will serve as an initial estimate only, as the final nipple position is determined intraoperatively once the implant has been inserted. When using a shaped implant, it is important to plan the pocket dissection to closely match the dimensions of the implant. Markings are placed to define the extent of dissection medially, laterally, inferiorly, and superiorly. Pocket dissection must follow these markings precisely.

The medial and lateral markings are generally planned as equidistant from the breast meridian. **Fig. 14** shows the preoperative markings for a subpectoral implant of medium height, full projection, and 295 g. The base width of the implant is 12.5 cm, so medial and lateral markings are each roughly 6 cm from the meridian.

The inferior markings will define the new level of the IMF. In primary breast augmentation, it is the senior author's preference to avoid lowering the IMF whenever possible. The IMF is a defined anatomic structure, and release of the entire IMF predisposes to inferior implant malposition or deformities of the lower pole contour. In most patients with a tuberous breast, this luxury is not possible and the IMF must be lowered. Determining the new position of the IMF can be difficult. Malucci and Branford[25] identified certain relationships that are common in breasts perceived by many as beautiful, one of which is that 55% of the breast volume should be below the nipple and 45% of the volume above the nipple. In our example, the implant height is 11.1 cm. Applying this rule, approximately 6 cm of vertical height should be from the final nipple position to the new IMF ($11.1 \times 0.55 = 6.1$). The patient is asked to place her hands on top of her head; this approximates the new nipple position following implant insertion (see **Fig. 14**). A line is then dropped inferiorly from this point, a distance of 6 cm, and the new IMF is marked. The superior markings are then measured from the new IMF, a distance equal to the height of the implant.

Skin Excision

Of the many techniques described to correct the constricted base, reduction of the areola diameter

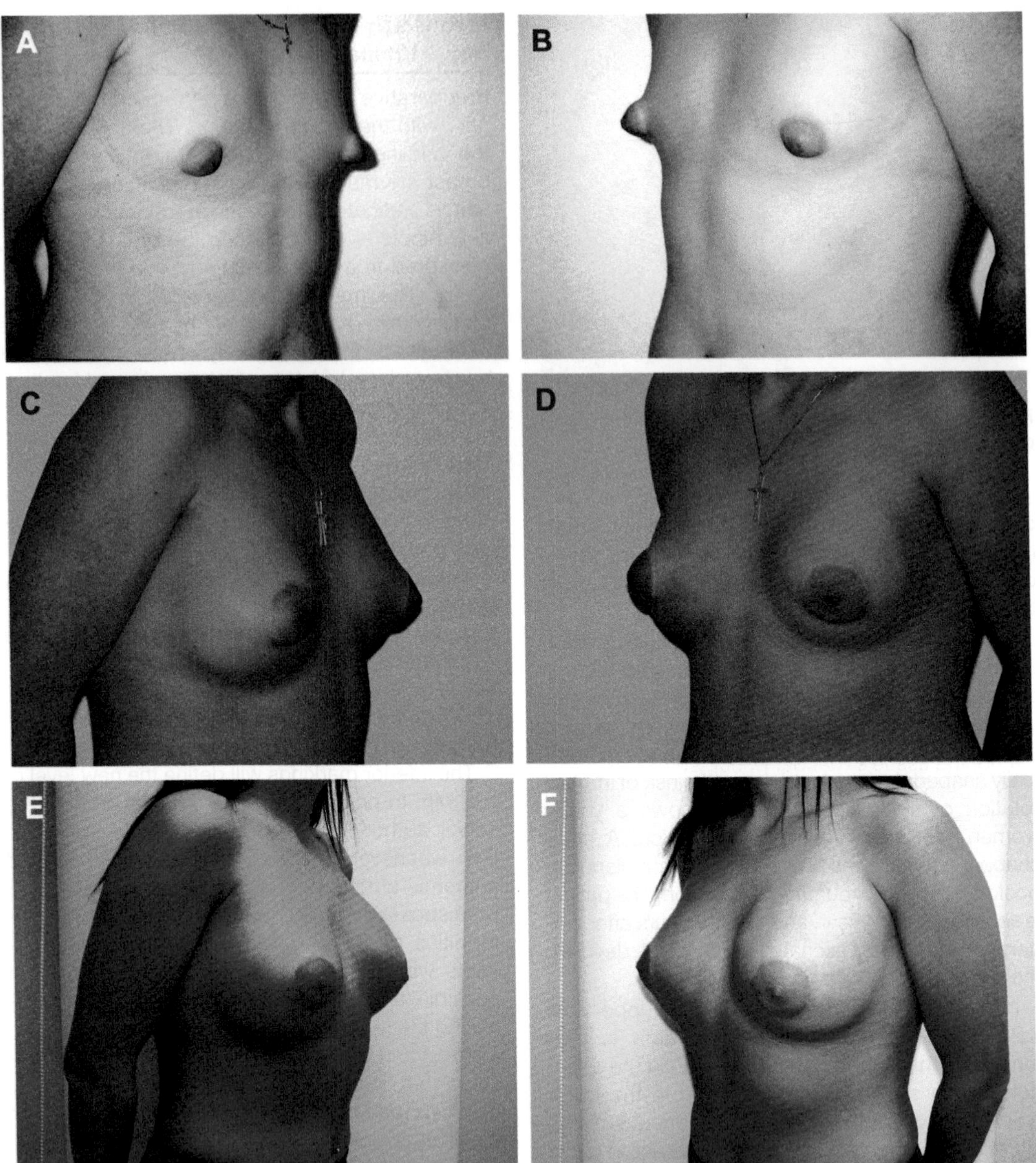

Fig. 12. Type IV deformity treated in a single stage with implants placed in subglandular pocket. (*A, B*) Preoperative views, (*C, D*) results at 1 year; (*E, F*) results at 10 years following weight gain and exchange to larger implant. Note maintenance of adequate soft-tissue cover.

via a Benelli circumareolar excision is common to most surgical approaches. Skin excision is planned based on the degree of ptosis, the size of the areola, and the location of tissue deficiency. A circumareolar component is generally required to excise redundant areola skin and provide access for suturing to control the areola diameter. Inclusion of a vertical or horizontal component of skin excision is often necessary, although care must be taken to avoid overresection of skin. Compared with a standard mastopexy, tuberous breasts have a deficiency of tissue, and the surgeon must ensure that reshaping is performed with minimal skin removal. This aspect is particularly important when the surgical correction includes the insertion of a breast implant.

Patient Positioning and Rapid Recovery Process

All procedures are performed under general anesthesia. The patients are placed supine with the

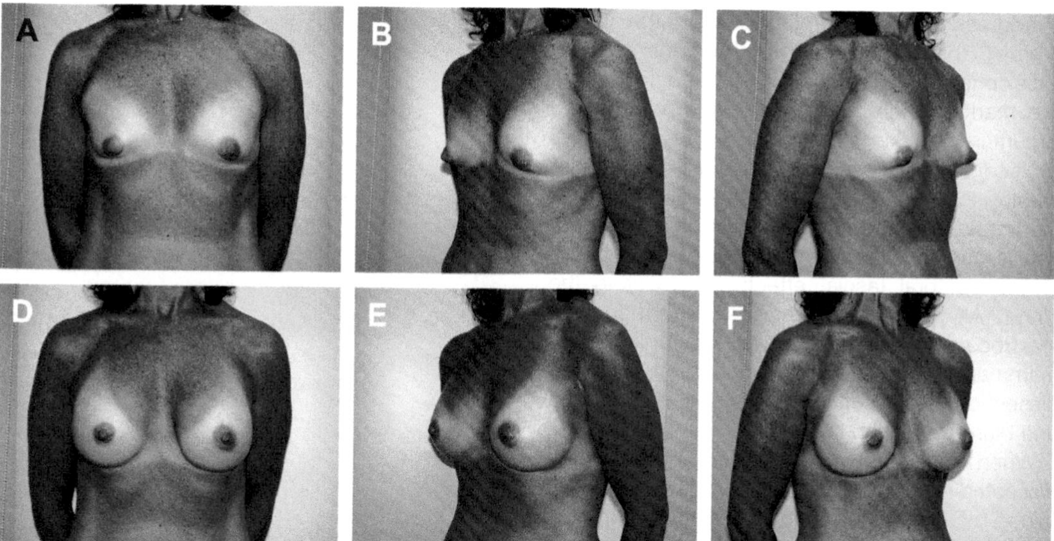

Fig. 13. Bilateral type II deformity treated with dual-plane pocket. (*A–C*) Preoperative views; (*D–F*) 1 year postoperatively after using shaped MF 255-g implant.

arms extended to 90°. The patient is supported on arm boards that will stabilize the arms when she is placed in a sitting position. A pillow is placed under the knees and a warming blanket is applied to the lower body.

The rapid recovery process is a series of steps designed to maximize recovery with minimal morbidity. The process begins with education of the patient regarding what to expect during surgery and how to prepare for the first few days after surgery. Patients receive an anti-inflammatory and acetaminophen 1 hour before surgery. A single intravenous dose of antibiotics is given on induction. All patients receive intraoperative decadron, muscle relaxation, and minimal narcotics. The muscle paralysis is carefully timed to wear off once the subpectoral dissection is completed; this makes it easier to retract the muscle and, when combined with precise nonblunt dissection, minimizes postoperative muscle pain. As blood is a strong inflammatory mediator, care is taken to dissect the pocket with prospective hemostasis and avoid damage to the subchondral vessels of the anterior ribs. Following surgery, patients remain on a regular anti-inflammatory and acetaminophen for 5 days. Narcotics are prescribed only as needed.

Procedural Approach

In most circumstances, an areola incision is required to manage the hypertrophy of the areola

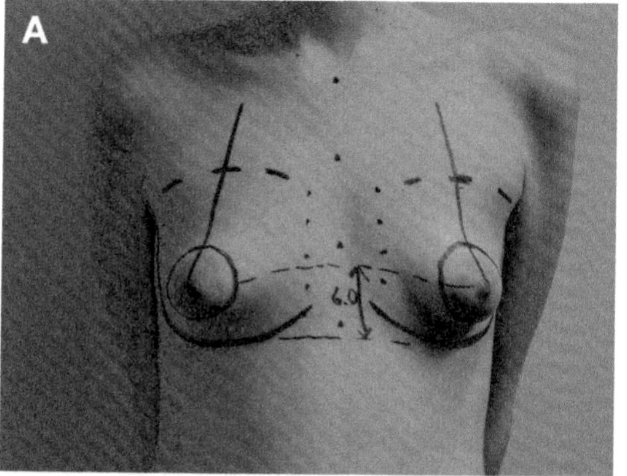

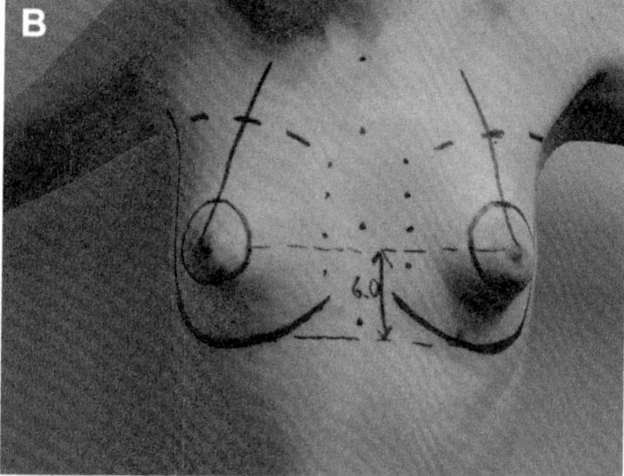

Fig. 14. (*A*) Preoperative markings. (*B*) Determining the level of the new IMF.

or address the herniation of tissue into the areola. A small Opsite is placed over the nipple to minimize contamination of the surgical field. Preoperative markings will have been made for planned circumareolar skin excision; however, no skin is excised until the implant is inserted. An inferior areola incision is made along the lower 40% of the areola circumference. In most cases, dissection is carried directly through the breast tissue to the pectoral fascia, effectively bisecting the gland. All pocket dissection is performed with electrocautery and under direct vision. A lighted mammary retractor is used to assist with the dissection. Prospective hemostasis is achieved and blunt dissection is avoided.

When indicated, subglandular pockets are dissected precisely according to the predetermined markings. This action is particularly important when using a shaped implant to produce a tight-fitting pocket that will minimize the risk of implant rotation. When placing the implant in a dual plane, the pectoral muscle is approached on its lateral border. The pocket is dissected and the muscle is divided horizontally at the level of the lower border of the areola. Dissection is then carried inferiorly to the level of the planned IMF, superficial to the cut edge of the muscle. This maneuver creates a subpectoral pocket superior to the areola and a subglandular pocket inferior to the areola. Aggressive radial scoring is then performed with electrocautery until the skin and gland has been adequately released. It is often necessary to take the scoring directly to the dermis, and care must be taken not to damage the skin or produce an uneven contour (**Fig. 15**).

If pocket dissection and radial scoring do not produce enough release of the constricted base, a tissue expander is inserted. Otherwise, the surgery proceeds with placement of the final implant.

Although the senior author prefers to avoid sizers in primary breast augmentation, the use of sizers in patients with tuberous breasts can be helpful. Sizers will demonstrate the degree of soft-tissue release and allow for an assessment of the accuracy in positioning the new IMF. Sizers will also assist in determining the implant volume that will best fill the tight lower pole and maintain a natural contour in the upper pole. The patient is assessed in both supine and upright positions.

The implant pocket is irrigated with an antibacterial solution and inspected again for hemostasis. Drains are not routinely used. Gloves are changed, the implant is bathed in the antibacterial solution, and the implant is inserted using an insertion funnel.

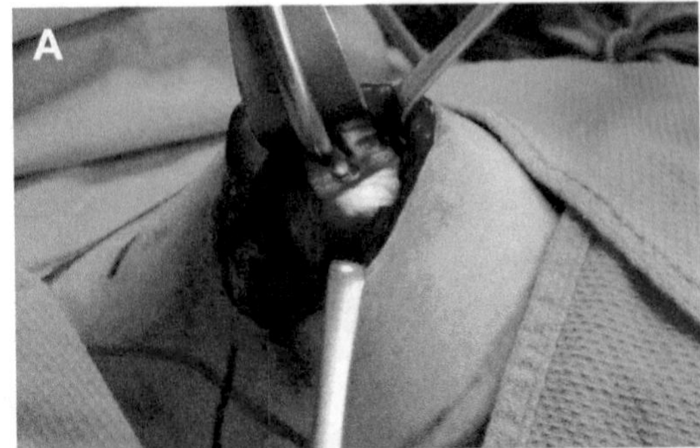

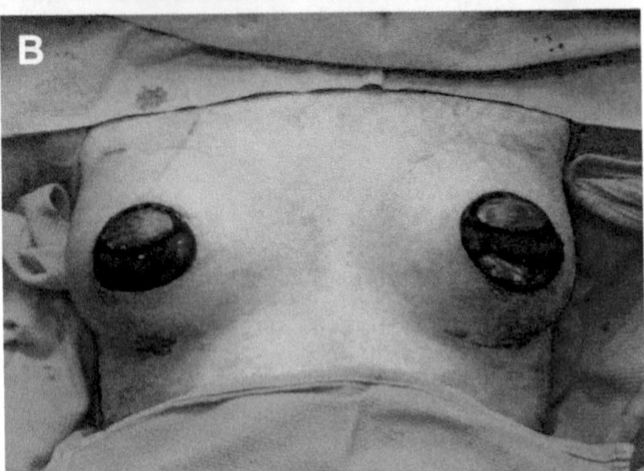

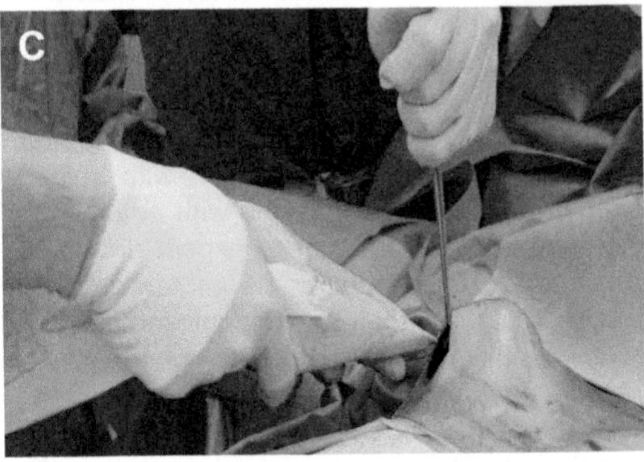

Fig. 15. Surgical technique. (*A*) Areola approach and scoring to release the base; (*B*) patient upright with sizers to determine degree of skin resection; (*C*) minimal touch technique with insertion funnel.

The funnel minimizes contact between the implant and the skin and soft tissues; this is particularly helpful when using textured surface devices. Once the implant is in place, the extent of circumareolar skin excision can be planned. Excision is performed with the patient upright to ensure symmetry of the eventual nipple position.

Closure of the areola begins with superficial subcutaneous undermining around the outer border of the areola. The diameter is controlled with a wagon-wheel suture. Although any nonabsorbable monofilament suture can be used, the senior author prefers Gore-Tex because of its

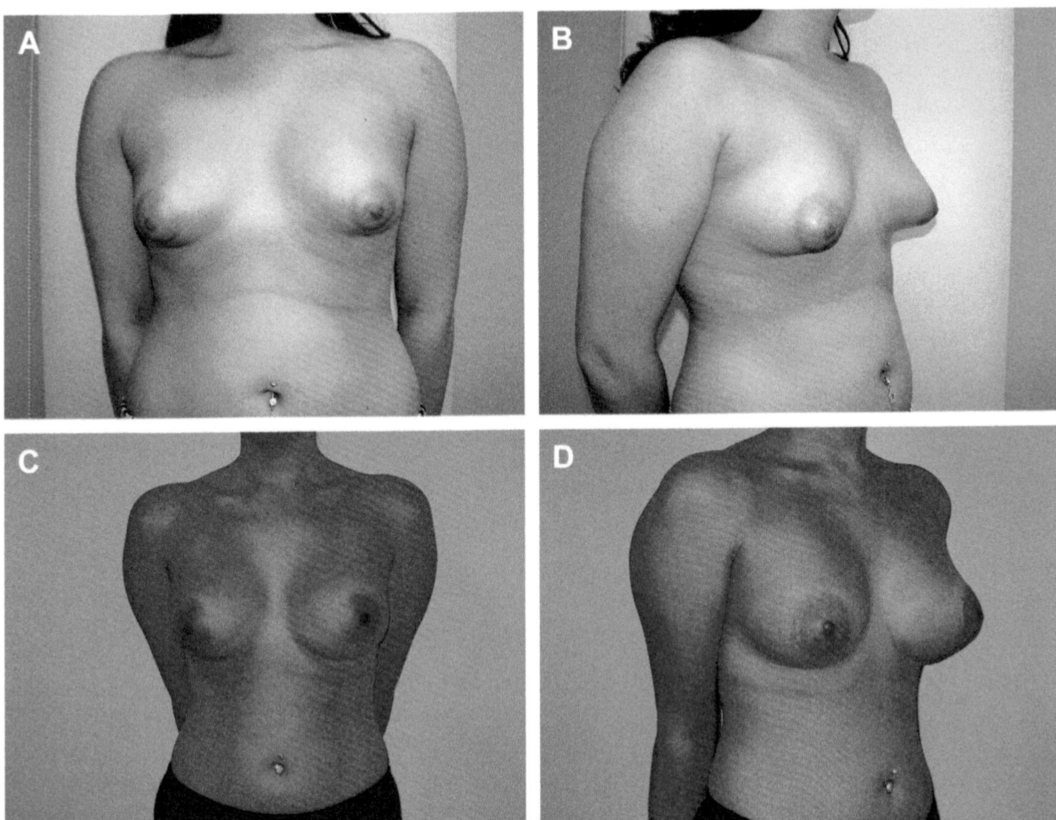

Fig. 16. Case 1. Preoperative (*A, B*) and 18-month postoperative (*C, D*) views.

soft feel and ability to easily glide through tissue. It is important to avoid the temptation of overtightening the areola, as this may compromise the blood supply. Final closure is performed with subcuticular absorbable suture.

A minimal dressing is applied that includes a waterproof Opsite bandage. Patients are placed in a comfortable sports bra and allowed to shower after 48 hours. Anti-inflammatory and acetaminophen therapy is continued for 5 days, and patients generally return to normal activity within 1 week.

POTENTIAL COMPLICATIONS AND MANAGEMENT

Complications in managing a tuberous breast deformity are similar to those encountered in patients undergoing mastopexy, implant insertion, or fat grafting. However, there are unique complications related specifically to the tuberous breast.

Persistence of the IMF may be seen in type III or IV deformities. Even though the implant has been placed where intended, the need to lower a tight IMF may produce a double-bubble contour. Often this will subside with time as the lower pole stretches under the pressure of the breast implant. Persistent old IMFs have traditionally been corrected with reoperation to release the band, glandular rearrangement, or tissue expansion. More recently, fat grafting has been a useful adjunct in this regard.[17,26,27] Fat injection can obliterate the persistent fold, especially when combined with aggressive needle band release.

If the residual fold is significant, consideration is given to further surgical release and possible insertion of a tissue expander.

Because of the hypoplastic nature of most tuberous breasts, implant dimensions are frequently larger than the amount of tissue available to adequately cover the device. This situation may result in visibility, palpability, and rippling of the implant edge. The use of a form-stable device assists in minimizing rippling, and placement of the implant in a partially submuscular plane will add cover in the upper pole. Further correction can be achieved with fat injection, which is an ideal option for covering or camouflaging implant edges.

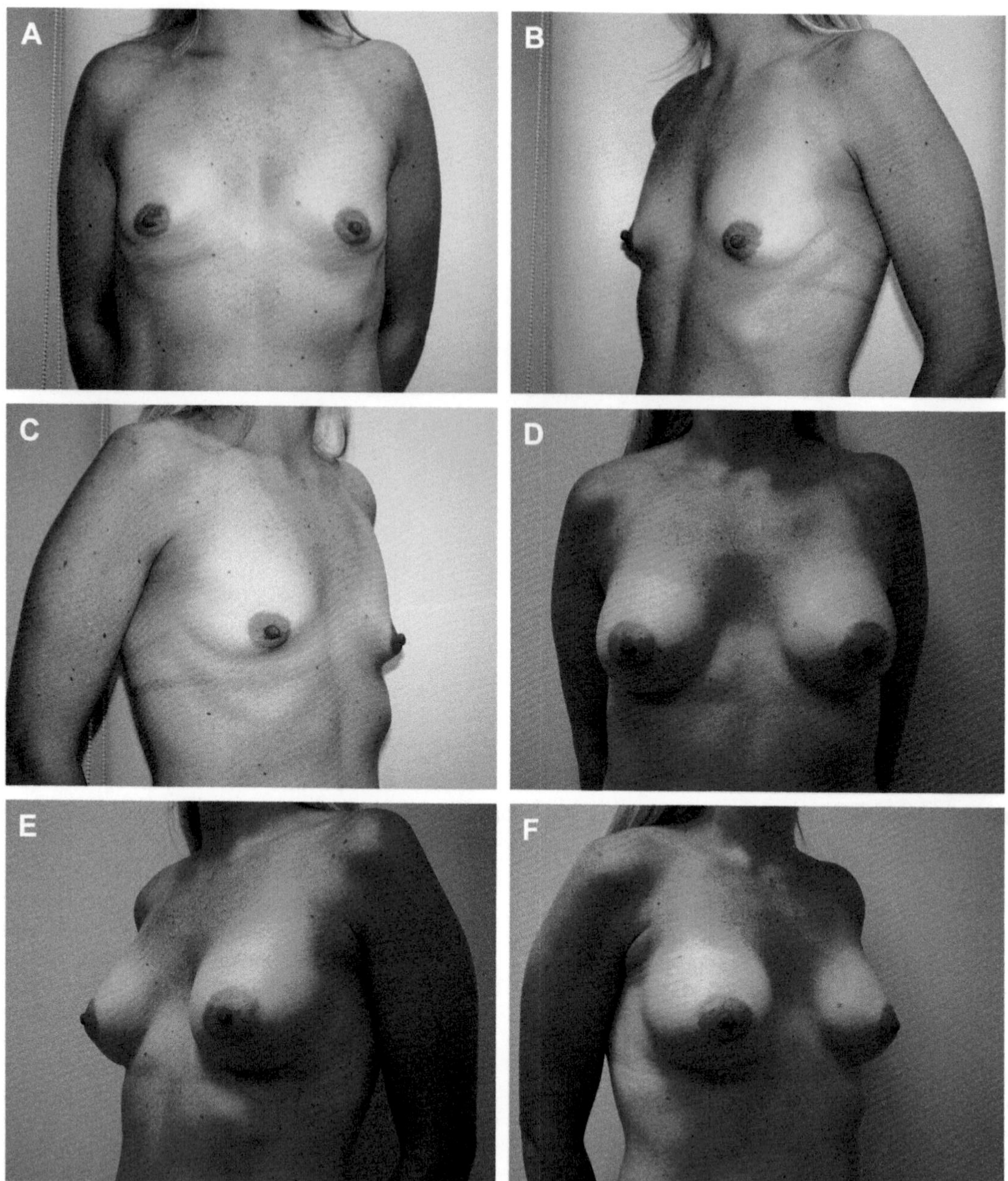

Fig. 17. Case 2. Preoperative (*A–C*) and 6-month postoperative (*D–F*) views.

A common concern following surgery is a large areola, despite areola reduction and support with a Gore-Tex suture. The need to increase breast volume in a tight skin envelope works against the forces required to decrease areola diameter. Excessive areola reduction will result in widened scars and possible delayed healing. Patients must be educated to understand the limitations of skin excision. With time, the soft-tissue envelope will stretch and become more compliant. Occasionally, subsequent pregnancy or weight loss will assist with increasing compliance of the soft tissues. Once this has occurred, further areola reduction can be offered.

Asymmetry is another concern sometimes raised by patients. Education of the patient preoperatively is important. All patients have some degree of breast asymmetry, and this is magnified in most patients with tuberous breasts. Although

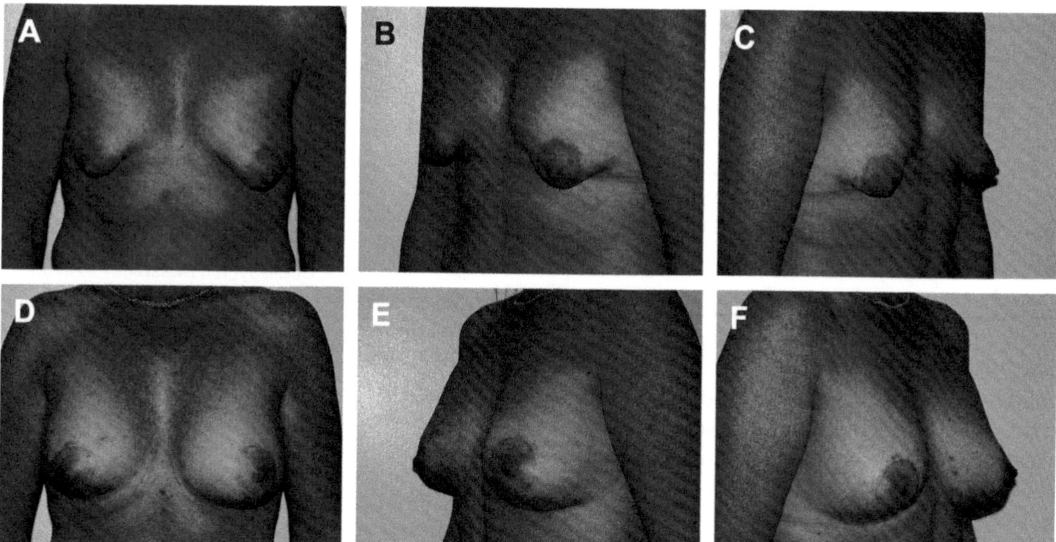

Fig. 18. Case 3. Preoperative (*A–C*) and 6-month postoperative (*D–F*) views.

correction may involve the use of different implants or different soft-tissue procedures, it is certain that some degree of asymmetry will persist. If significant, options for managing asymmetry include adjustment of implant size or shape, adjustment of the nipple position, or modification of the soft tissues with targeted fat injection.

OUTCOMES

Case 1

A 21-year-old woman with asymmetric type III tuberous breasts. Note the asymmetry of the IMFs. She was treated in a single stage with circumareolar lift, resection of 25 g of tissue from the right breast, and insertion of medium-height, full-projection, 335-g implants. Implants were placed subpectorally; after pocket dissection, aggressive radial scoring was performed to release the constricted lower base. The patient is shown in **Fig. 16**, before and 18 months after surgery.

Case 2

A 36-year-old woman with type III tuberous breasts involving constriction medially and

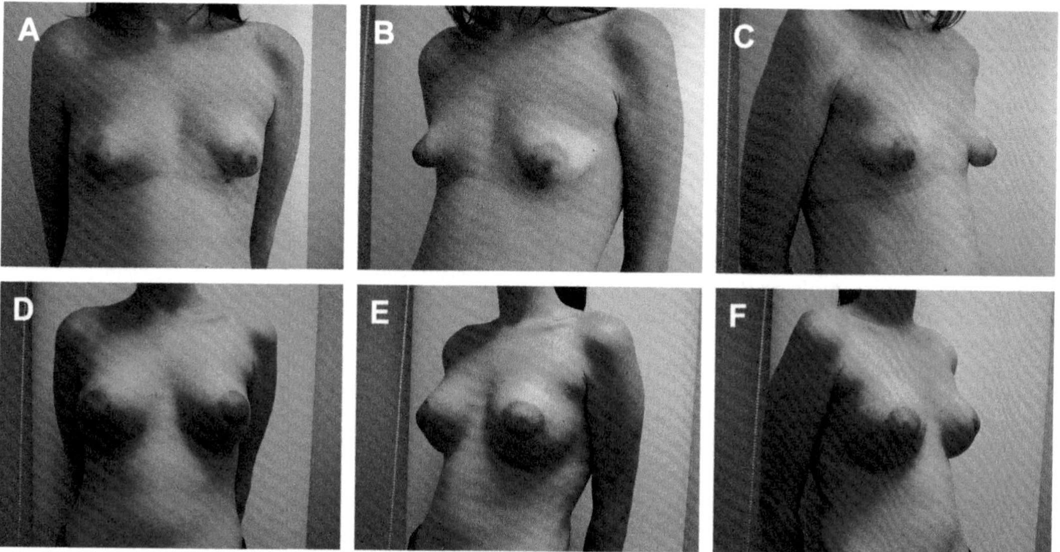

Fig. 19. Case 4. Preoperative (*A–C*) and 6-month postoperative (*D–F*) views.

laterally, with short nipple to IMF distance and deficient infra-areolar tissue. She was treated in a single stage with an inframammary incision, subpectoral pocket, and insertion of medium-height, full-projection, 295-g implants. It was necessary to drop the IMF 2.5 cm on the right and 1.5 cm on the left. The patient is shown in **Fig. 17**, before and 6 months after surgery.

Case 3

A 26-year-old woman with type IV tuberous deformity, asymmetry, and elevated IMF. She was treated with circumareolar lift and creation of a subglandular pocket. The lower pole was released with bisection of the gland and aggressive radial scoring of the lower pole. The patient had been prepared for insertion of a tissue expander; however, after preparing the pocket, it was decided that the surgery could be completed in a single stage with the insertion of full-height, full-projection, 375-g implants. She is shown in **Fig. 18**, before and 6 months after surgery.

Case 4

A 24-year-old woman with asymmetric type III deformity and a high IMF. Her surgical markings are shown in **Fig. 14**, which demonstrate planning for lowering the IMF. She was treated in a single stage with dual-plane dissection, lower pole radial scoring, circumareolar lift, and insertion of form-stable shaped medium-height, full-projection, 295-g implants. She is shown in **Fig. 19**, before and 6 months after surgery.

Editorial Comments by Bradley P. Bengtson, MD

Along with mastopexy operations, proper surgical correction of patients with Tuberous or Constricted breasts are among the most difficult plastic surgeons are asked to address in plastic surgery. In addition, inadequate recognition or improper treatment of the tuberous breast in the primary operation creates a large number of uncorrectable or difficult to correct secondary deformities. My friend and colleague Dr Brown has done an excellent job reviewing, categorizing and methodically addressing the specific, critical components of the Tuberous deformity and strategies for correction. Both Highly Cohesive implants helpful in shaping the breast, adequate scoring of the breast parenchyma, and often mastopexies are essential in achieving a successful result in these challenging patients.

REFERENCES

1. Rees T, Aston S. The tuberous breast. Clin Plast Surg 1976;3:339.
2. Grolleau J, Lanfrey E. Breast base anomalies: treatment strategy for tuberous breasts, minor deformities, and asymmetry. Plast Reconstr Surg 1999;104(7): 2040–8. Available at: http://journals.lww.com/plasreconsurg/Abstract/1999/12000/Breast_Base_Anomalies__Treatment_Strategy_for.14.aspx. Accessed September 9, 2014.
3. Von Heimburg D, Exner K, Kruft S, et al. The tuberous breast deformity: classification and treatment. Br J Plast Surg 1996;49(6):339–45. Available at: http://www.ncbi.nlm.nih.gov/pubmed/8881778.
4. Teimourian B, Adham MN. Surgical correction of the tuberous breast. Ann Plast Surg 1983;10:190–3.
5. Mandrekas AD, Zambacos GJ. Aesthetic reconstruction of the tuberous breast deformity: a 10-year experience. Aesthet Surg J 2010;30(5):680–92.
6. Spear SL, Willey S, Robb G, et al, editors. Surgery of the breast. 3rd edition. Philadelphia: Wolters Kluwer Health/Lippincott Williams and Wilkins; 2010.
7. Oroz-Torres J, Pelay-Ruata M-J, Escolán-Gonzalvo N, et al. Correction of tuberous breasts using the unfolded subareolar gland flap. Aesthetic Plast Surg 2014;38(4):692–703.
8. DeLuca-Pytell DM, Piazza RC, Holding JC, et al. The incidence of tuberous breast deformity in asymmetric and symmetric mammaplasty patients. Plast Reconstr Surg 2005;116(7):1894–9.
9. Zambacos GJ, Mandrekas AD. The incidence of tuberous breast deformity in asymmetric and symmetric mammaplasty patients. Plast Reconstr Surg 2006;118(7):1667.
10. Klinger M, Caviggioli F, Villani F, et al. Gynecomastia and tuberous breast: assessment and surgical approach. Aesthetic Plast Surg 2009;33(5):786–7.
11. Pacifico MD, Kang NV. The tuberous breast revisited. J Plast Reconstr Aesthet Surg 2007;60: 455–64.
12. Persichetti P, Cagli B, Tenna S, et al. Decision making in the treatment of tuberous and tubular breasts: volume adjustment as a crucial stage in the surgical strategy. Aesthetic Plast Surg 2005;29(6):482–8.
13. Dinner MI, Dowden RV. The tubular/tuberous breast syndrome. Ann Plast Surg 1987;19:414–20.
14. Ribeiro L, Accorsi A, Argencio V. Tuberous breasts: a periareolar approach. Aesthet Surg J 2005;25(4): 398–402.
15. Choupina M, Malheiro E, Pinho C, et al. Tuberous breast: a surgical challenge. Aesthetic Plast Surg 2002;26(1):50–3.
16. Puckett CL, Concannon MJ. Augmenting the narrow-based breast: the unfurling technique to prevent the double-bubble deformity. Aesthetic Plast Surg 1990;14:15–9.

17. Serra-Renom JM, Muñoz-Olmo J, Serra-Mestre JM. Treatment of grade 3 tuberous breasts with Puckett's technique (Modified) and fat grafting to correct the constricting ring. Aesthetic Plast Surg 2011;35: 773–81.
18. Panchapakesan V, Brown MH. Management of tuberous breast deformity with anatomic cohesive silicone gel breast implants. Aesthetic Plast Surg 2009;33(1):49–53.
19. Hedén P, Bronz G, Elberg JJ, et al. Long-term safety and effectiveness of style 410 highly cohesive silicone breast implants. Aesthetic Plast Surg 2009; 33(3):430–6 [discussion: 437–8].
20. Somogyi RB, Brown MH, Street B. Outcomes in primary breast augmentation: a single surgeon's review of 1539 consecutive cases. Plast Reconstr Surg 2015;135(1):87–97.
21. Tebbetts JB. A system for breast implant selection based on patient tissue characteristics and implant-soft tissue dynamics. Plast Reconstr Surg 2002;109:1396–409 [discussion: 1410–5]. Available at: http://content.wkhealth.com/linkback/openurl?sid=WKPTLP:landingpage&an=00006534-200204010-00030.
22. Bassot J. Comment obtenir dans Les Plasties periareolairies avec ou sans cicatrices verticales, un effet de pince transversale, sous areolaire efficace qui assure une forme harmonieuse, evite l'elargissement de l'areol et une cicatrice verticale trop longe. La Rev Cherurgie Esthet Lang Fr 1999.
23. Hammond DC, Khuthaila DK, Kim J. The interlocking Gore-Tex suture for control of areolar diameter and shape. Plast Reconstr Surg 2007; 119(3):804–9.
24. Graf R, Bernardes A, Rippel R, et al. Subfascial breast implant: a new procedure. Plast Reconstr Surg 2003;111(2):904–8.
25. Mallucci P, Branford OA. Concepts in aesthetic breast dimensions: analysis of the ideal breast. J Plast Reconstr Aesthet Surg 2012;65:8–16.
26. Serra-Renom JM, Muñoz-Olmo J, Serra-Mestre JM. Endoscopically assisted aesthetic augmentation of tuberous breasts and fat grafting to correct the double bubble. Aesthetic Plast Surg 2012;36(5):1114–9.
27. Delay E, Sinna R, Ho Quoc C. Tuberous breast correction by fat grafting. Aesthet Surg J 2013; 33(4):522–8.

The Subfascial Approach to Primary and Secondary Breast Augmentation with Autologous Fat Grafting and Form-Stable Implants

João Carlos Sampaio Goes, MD, PhD[a,b,*],
Alexandre Mendonça Munhoz, MD, PhD[c,d],
Rolf Gemperli, MD, PhD[a,e]

KEYWORDS

• Breast augmentation • Silicone implant • Form-stable implants • Fat grafting • Subfascial
• Outcome • Complications

KEY POINTS

- The latest generations of silicone implants and the introduction of surgical techniques such as the subfascial approach have improved esthetic outcomes following breast augmentation.
- The advantages of the subfascial pocket are soft tissue coverage and avoidance of the limitations of the submuscular position. In the upper breast pole, this technique is useful in minimizing the appearance of the edges of the implant and provides an adequate supporting system.
- Autologous fat grafting has been performed more frequently. Based on various clinical studies, fat grafting may be considered to treat breast defects secondary to oncological diseases and esthetic deformities.
- Most candidates for primary and secondary breast augmentation can be successfully treated with this present technique. Ideal primary candidates are those with significant hypomastia/amastia with less soft tissue to adequately cover the implant. Ideal secondary candidates are those with partial/total soft tissue deficiency with visible implant contours and rippling, and patients with stretched breast tissue and irregularities of the implant surface.

Funding Sources/Financial Disclosures: This work was not supported by any external funding. Dr J.C. Sampaio Goés and A.M. Munhoz are consultants to Allergan Corporation. Dr R. Gemperli is consultant to Ethicon and Johnson & Johnson Corporations.
Contributor's Statement: J.C. Sampaio Goés is principal investigator of this study. A.M. Munhoz and R. Gemperli are coinvestigators. The principal investigator made significant contributions to the conception and design of this study. A.M. Munhoz and R. Gemperli made substantial contributions to the acquisition, analysis, and interpretation of data. A.M. Munhoz drafted the article. All authors revised the article for intellectual content, gave final approval of the version to be published, and have sufficiently participated in the work to take public responsibility for appropriate portions of the content.
[a] Department of Plastic Surgery, Hospital Albert Einstein, Avenida Albert Einsten, 627/701 - Morumbi, São Paulo - SP 05652-900, Brazil; [b] Breast Surgery and Plastic Surgery Department, Instituto Brasileiro do Controle do Câncer, Av. Alcântara Machado, 2576 - Móoca, São Paulo - SP 03102-002, Brazil; [c] Department of Plastic Surgery, Hospital Sírio-Libanês, Rua Dona Adma Jafet, 115 - Bela Vista, São Paulo - SP 01308-050, Brazil; [d] Breast Plastic Surgery, Department of Plastic Surgery, University of São Paulo School of Medicine and Instituto do Câncer do Estado de São Paulo, Avenida Doutor Arnaldo, 251 - Cerqueira César, São Paulo - SP 01255-000, Brazil; [e] Department of Plastic Surgery, University of São Paulo School of Medicine, São Paulo, Brazil
* Corresponding author. Rua Campos Bicudo, 98-cj-111-Jardim Europa, São Paulo - SP 04536-010, Brazil.
E-mail address: clinica@sampaiogoes.com

Clin Plastic Surg 42 (2015) 551–564
http://dx.doi.org/10.1016/j.cps.2015.06.017
0094-1298/15/$ – see front matter

INTRODUCTION

Breast augmentation is a well-known procedure and continues to be one of the most frequently performed esthetic surgeries worldwide.[1,2] The development of modern silicone implants as well as new surgical techniques has led to widespread acceptance of breast augmentation in recent years.[3–6]

Although breast augmentation has a high rate of patient satisfaction, some patients may present unsatisfactory results and will require surgical revision.[5–7] In the authors' experience, many of these reoperations are required for soft tissue–related problems, such as implant visibility and rippling, and not necessary for implant failure. In fact, although providing satisfactory postoperative recovery, subglandular implant placement may sometimes result in visibility of the implant edge and limited soft tissue coverage.[7–10] With the introduction of subpectoral implant placement, reduced implant visibility and a lower incidence of capsular contracture were observed in some series. However, undesirable superior displacement of the implant and implant animation are frequently observed in some groups of patients.[9–11]

Recently, a new implant position uses the subfascial plane, which is gaining popularity because of the more satisfactory postoperative recovery it yields compared with submuscular techniques.[12–22] It has been the authors' experience, as with other investigators, that a satisfactory outcome and good results following subfascial breast augmentation can be achieved in selected patients.[12–22]

As observed with the subfascial approach, there has been a resurgence in the use of autologous fat grafting for breast surgery for a variety of indications over the past 10 years.[23–36] In fact, autologous fat grafting has been performed more frequently since 2008, when new clinical recommendations were released.[37,38] Based on various clinical studies, the American Society of Plastic Surgeons (ASPS) concluded that fat grafting may be considered for treatment of breast defects associated with oncological diseases and esthetic deformities.[37] Although refinement in fat-grafting procedures has improved reproducibility, it has been the authors' impression that a standardized technique remains to be described.

Given that form-stable breast implants and the subfascial technique are effective and predictable procedures for esthetic breast surgery, a variety of poor outcomes in breast augmentation may result from the limited ability of the overlying soft tissue to adequately cover the silicone implant.[35] Consequently, the relevance of autologous fat grafting as an associated technique to improve the results of breast augmentation may be investigated. In addition, it is reasonable to emphasize that if autologous fat grafting and implant-based breast augmentation are equally reproducible, and involve similar risk and surgical time, it is possible to combine both techniques in one surgical procedure.

The objective of this article is to provide an overview of the subfascial approach to primary and secondary breast augmentation with form-stable implants associated with autologous fat grafting. Although breast augmentation is a well-studied procedure, previous reports concerning the subfascial technique are limited, especially related to the most recent generations of form-stable breast implants.[13,14,16,17,21] In addition, there are few detailed clinical reports that specifically address the operative planning, outcomes, and complications following simultaneous autologous fat grafting.[35] Therefore, in this article a detailed description of the authors' method, including the preoperative evaluation and intraoperative care is provided, for patients undergoing primary and secondary breast augmentation associated with lipofilling. The surgical technique, advantages, and limitations are also discussed. When combined with clinical expertise, this evidence will help the plastic surgeon provide patients with predictable and safer esthetic outcomes.

THE SUBFASCIAL APPROACH

Introduced in the 1990s, the subfascial approach is especially interesting for surgeons who have been seeking alternative planes with less morbidity.[12–14] In fact, placing the silicone implant next to the glandular tissue may result in a disappointing outcome in terms of.[13–22] A visible implant edge is especially apparent in underweight patients with severe hypomastia and less soft tissue coverage, where a transition can be seen at the borders of the silicone implant.[12–14,16] From an anatomic point of view, the pectoral fascia is a distinct, identifiable layer and is suitably strong, as is apparent during intraoperative manipulation[13,14] (**Fig. 1**A, B). Although the fascia may be thin in the lower pole, it is not thin in the upper sector corresponding to the underlying muscles such as pectoralis muscle. According to Ventura and Marcello,[20] this anatomic aspect is helpful for creating a foundation to support the implant at the lower edge, preventing inferior displacement and palpation of the implant border. In a study of 1000 cases of subfascial breast augmentations, Tijerina and colleagues[22] observed that the upper displacement of the implant can be limited because the pectoral fascia force the implant downward. In the upper thorax, the pectoral fascia is useful in minimizing the visibility of the

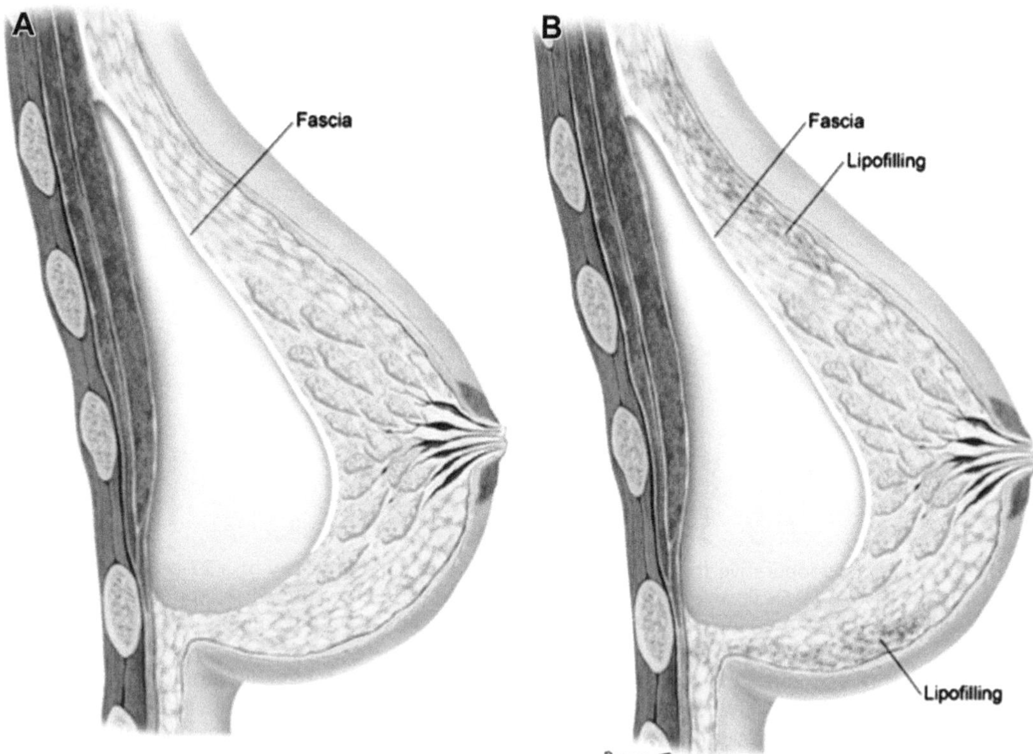

Fig. 1. (*A, B*) Breast and pectoral fascia anatomy following subfascial form-stable breast augmentation. The anterior wall of the implant pocket consists of pectoral fascia, breast parenchyma, subcutaneous tissue, and skin. The stronger support system that results from placing the implant under the fascia tends to keep the implant's upper third from altering its shape and position (*A*). Breast and pectoral fascia anatomy following subfascial form-stable breast augmentation associated with autologous fat grafting (*B*).

edges of the implant and provides coverage over an anatomic implant (**Box 1**).

Despite the controversy concerning the suboptimal soft tissue coverage provided by the subfascial approach and the limitation involved with the thickness of the pectoral fascia,[39] some studies have demonstrated a satisfactory outcome in selected patients.[13,14,16–19,21,22] In the authors' previous clinical long-term study using the subfascial approach, they emphasized the importance of the pocket plane in the dynamics between the implant and the soft tissues.[14,16] In fact, it has been their impression that besides the positive aspects of the supplementary soft tissue coverage, the subfascial approach provides more rapid postoperative recovery than the total submuscular pocket and avoids breast animation when the pectoral muscle is contracted (**Fig. 2**).

Box 1
Advantages of subfascial approach for breast augmentation

- Improved upper pole contour
- Avoids implant edge visibility
- Helps keep the implant in place
- Avoids muscular dynamics over the implant

FORM-STABLE IMPLANTS

Silicone breast implant technology has advanced over the last 3 decades with the introduction of new textures and high-cohesive anatomic implants.[40–51] These implants resemble the natural shape of the breast, granting them wide acceptance by both patients and surgeons.

In the authors' clinical experience,[14,48] form-stable implants are available with 3 different types of gels: soft cohesive (MemoryShape, Contour Profile Gel-CPG; Mentor Corporation, Santa Barbara, CA, USA), highly cohesive (Style 410; Allergan, Inc, Irvine, CA, USA), and dual-gel soft touch (Style 510; Allergan, Inc). The Style 410 implant and the Contour Profile Gel CPG implant have been available in Brazil since the 1990s and 2000, respectively, to women seeking breast

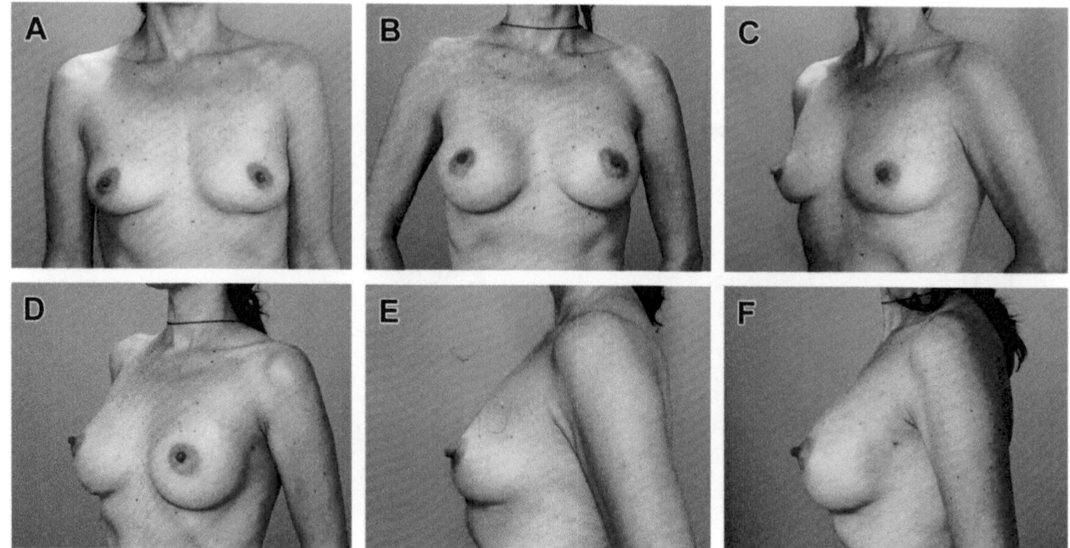

Fig. 2. (*A–F*) (Case 1) Preoperative frontal view, left oblique view, and left view of a 27-year-old patient with hypoplastic breasts (*A, C, E*). Postoperative (2 years) frontal view, left oblique view, and left view following bilateral implant with Allergan Style 510 MX (290 g), showing a very good outcome (*B, D, F*).

augmentation and reconstruction.[48] The Style 410 implant is a form-stable, highly cohesive, silicone gel-filled breast implant designed with a low-diffusion silicone elastomer shell (Intrasheil barrier technology).[44–46,48,49] These implants also use a Biocell surface texture available in various sizes in Europe and Brazil since 1994, in Canada since 2006, and in the United States since 2012. Biocell texturing on the implant shell promotes tissue adherence to reduce implant rotation and capsular contracture. Both Style 410 and 510 implants are available in a wide range of shapes to permit the selection of an implant appropriate to each patient's anatomy. The CPG MemoryShape is a textured contoured implant filled with cohesive silicone gel, intended for use in esthetic and reconstructive breast surgery and available in a wide range of shapes.[47] The differences between the CPG implant and 410 are slightly increased crosslinking of the gel, and more textured outer surface.[48]

In the authors' clinical experience, they have observed a significant benefit in placing the Style 410 implant in the subfascial pocket. Recently, they have been using this same position with the Style 510 implant with satisfactory outcomes.[48] In fact, the newest dual-gel Style 510 implants have a concave posterior that conforms and adheres better to the chest wall, and the edging of the Style 510 implant makes this device easier to control during insertion (**Box 2**). In addition, this biodimensional, anatomically shaped implant preserves the teardrop configuration, maintaining projection and, consequently, breast shape. In fact, Nipshagen and colleagues,[52] using a 3-dimensional MRI for in vitro and in vivo shape evaluation of subpectoral round and shaped silicone gel-filled implants, observed that Style 510 implants preserved projection, probably because of the high-density silicone core.

Another important aspect is related to satisfactory outcomes in terms of implant visibility and wrinkling. In a study of 163 patients, Hedén and colleagues[45] demonstrated a high satisfaction rate with the Style 410 shaped, form-stable gel implant and a low rate of wrinkling. Similarly, Lista and colleagues,[50] in a sample of 440 patients who underwent primary subglandular breast augmentation with the Style 410 implant, concluded that this property helped decrease wrinkling and rippling, which was observed in only one patient (0.2%).

Despite the advantages of these form-stable implants, the use of highly cohesive, textured, anatomically shaped implants has its drawbacks

Box 2
Last generation of form-stable silicone implants (510 style)—implant aspects to avoid displacement/rotation

- Texturized with large pores (capsule adherence)
- Thin implant edge (better implant adaptation)
- Concave base (better implant stability)
- Form stable with dual gel consistence

(**Box 3**). Schots and colleagues,[53] in a sample of 73 cases of augmentation mammaplasty using the Style 510 implants, observed unilateral malrotation in 8.2% of patients after a mean period of 10 months; 7 patients underwent reoperation. Lista and colleagues,[50] in a retrospective review, observed a 16.6% rate of complications, with 10.7% of patients requiring reoperation. The most common complication was malrotation (5.2% of patients), and this was predominantly managed nonoperatively.

In order to avoid this complication and to ensure implant stability, it is crucial to evaluate the exact dimensions of the implant's height and width, which helps to create an adequate pocket and avoid implant rotation (**Box 4**). If an implant has insufficient volume compared with the dimension of the available pocket, rotation will occur more frequently. If necessary, the skin may be adjusted with vertical or periareolar resections in order to achieve an appropriate match between the implant and pocket volume. It has been the authors' impression that the Style 410 or 510 implant can achieve excellent results without the customary submuscular placement often used with older-style round implants.[48]

Box 4
Surgical technique to avoid form-stable implant rotation

- Subfascial plane
- Superior edge contention with muscular-fascia system
- Precise implant pocket and skin adjustment
- In reoperations, partial/total capsulectomy
- Vacuum drain and postoperative immobilization
- No physical activities and massage

AUTOLOGOUS FAT GRAFTING

Autologous fat grafting is extensively used in reconstructive and esthetic surgery to repair volume and contour defects with technical variations on fat harvesting, preparation, and reinjection.[54–58] According to the International Society of Aesthetic Plastic Surgery in 2009, fat grafting represented almost 6% of the nonsurgical procedures within the realm of esthetic surgery, with more than 514,000 procedures performed worldwide.[56,59]

Over the past 10 years, there has been a reintroduction in the use of autologous fat grafting for breast surgery. In fact, there are numerous clinical studies that corroborate esthetic outcome and patient satisfaction.[26–36,54,56–58] First introduced by Bircoll[23,24] in the 1980s for esthetic breast surgery, autologous fat grafting had the major advantage of autologous tissue transplantation in terms of natural and long-term results, even when secondary and tertiary surgical sessions were necessary. However, at that time, the American Society of Plastic and Reconstructive Surgery (ASPRS) Ad Hoc Committee on New Procedures concluded that the potential scarring and calcifications could interfere with diagnosis of breast cancer.[38,60] According to the available data, the ASPRS committee demonstrated that fat grafting could result in the formation of nodule formation and calcifications, potentially affecting breast cancer screening.[60]

Box 3
Form-stable implants rotation/displacement causes

- Lack of a capsule adherence
- Large surgical pocket
- Lateral and superior muscular mobilization
- Seroma, hematoma
- Double capsule
- Postoperative massage

In 2008, the ASPS established a new committee, the Fat Grafting Task Force, which concluded that fat grafting may be considered for breast augmentation and correction of defects associated with oncological conditions.[37] In their report, the Task Force emphasized that no evidence was found in the previous studies that suggested interference with early diagnosis of breast cancer.[37] Therefore, fat grafting can be considered a surgical tool for breast shaping because of its relative ease of use and low morbidity.[54,56–58]

Although various surgical procedures have been described for improving survival of fat grafts, including washing,[36,61,62] centrifugation,[27,63–65] decantation,[61] and not washing,[66] there is still controversy about their esthetic outcome, complications, and long-term results.[36,54,56–58]

Coleman and Saboeiro[27] introduced the structural fat grafting technique and emphasized the importance of removing nonviable aspirate components, such as oil and blood cells by centrifugation.[65] Following the initial description, Coleman's technique has been popularized; it also emphasizes an atraumatic method of fat harvesting, centrifugation, and, especially, a small amount of fat injection in order to provide maximal contact between fat and the recipient tissue. This technique has gained clinical application and has become crucial to many procedures described in numerous further studies.[54,56–58] In fact, it has been the authors' experience that grafted fat that is too large for injection may present central necrosis due to a lack of adequate blood perfusion and secondary neoangiogenesis. Thus, minimizing the amount of fat grafted during injection will maximize the surface area of contact between the fat and recipient tissue.[27,36,65]

Contrary to the centrifugation principles, Khater and colleagues[67] concluded in a clinical and experimental study that in noncentrifuged adipose tissue, more active preadipocytes were maintained, which could possibly lead to enhanced survival of injected fat.[36] Similarly, Rohrich and colleagues[68] performed a quantitative analysis of the role of centrifugation and harvest site and found that the fat survival rate after centrifugation was no better than after filtration. Ramon and colleagues[69] compared fat prepared either via centrifugation or via cotton towel drying in a mouse model and observed no differences in fat weight or volume.

Recently, some investigators have described a satisfactory outcome for grafting fat to the breast in order to improve contour deformities.[26,28–30,32,35] Spear and colleagues[26] observed satisfactory outcomes after fat injections to the breast in 37 patients, recommending autologous fat grafting in and around reconstructed breasts as a safe procedure. However, the effectiveness of fat grafting associated with silicone breast augmentation has not been determined and justified by a significant clinical series in the literature.

Zheng and colleagues[29] studied 66 patients who underwent autologous fat grafting for breast augmentation, following them for up to 5 years. In this series, overall esthetic improvement was observed in about 80% of patients, as evaluated by independent plastic surgeons or judged by patients themselves. Auclair and colleagues,[35] in a series of 197 patients treated over a 3-year period, described a new concept for composite breast augmentation surgery that combines silicone breast implants with natural overlying fat grafting. According to the investigators, the technique was indicated when the overlying soft tissue was insufficient to adequately cover the underlying silicone, in both breast implant revision and primary breast augmentation. Through quantitative 3-dimensional imaging of the grafted fat in the subcutaneous space, the investigators concluded that breast augmentation with simultaneous implants and fat represents a versatile approach and achieves a synergistic outcome. In this sample, 57% of the injected graft volume persisted at 1 year, and cysts, masses, and fat necrosis were not observed.

Despite the benefits and satisfactory results described, there is a lack of controlled, prospective clinical studies evaluating the technical aspects related to autogenous fat grafting such as fat harvesting and processing methods, injection techniques, as well as donor site areas and outcomes of fat intake. In fact, harvested fat contains different types of cells, including mature fat cells, fibroblasts, adipose-derived stem cells, and endothelial cells, and the percentages of these cell populations may differ between patients. Similarly, there is no consensus concerning the viability of cell types between the various fat harvesting and preparation techniques. These limitations were clearly observed in the earlier systematic reviews described above.[54,56–58]

From the authors' point of view, and despite the good results observed in their sample, the long-term complications of fat grafting for esthetic breast surgery have still not been reported and determined in a large series. Existing data concerning fat grafting for esthetic breast surgery are restricted to case series and retrospective reviews.[56–58] Some studies demonstrate that fat grafting may result in varying degrees of nodule formation and calcifications, which could potentially interfere with breast cancer screening. Nonetheless, recent clinical studies have demonstrated that fat-grafting results have improved, with a decreased incidence of local complications and less fat necrosis after autologous fat transplantation.[30,57]

SURGICAL PLANNING/TECHNIQUE

Patient Selection

Primary augmentation

In general, most candidates for breast augmentation can be successfully treated with autologous fat grafting. Ideal candidates are slim and have significant hypomastia/amastia. In the authors' experience, rippling was observed most frequently in patients classified as underweight. According to Codner and colleagues[70] in a series of 812 patients, thinner patients frequently had less soft tissue to adequately cover the implant. In the authors' sample, most of the patients were thin with a body mass index (BMI) less than 20. Despite this limitation in terms of fat volume, it was possible to find adequate volumes of fat in the hip and flank region. In addition, the technique is indicated for patients with less upper pole coverage (eg, pinch test result of <2 cm). It has been the authors' impression that in patients with a pinch test result greater than 2 to 3 cm, associated fat grafting is not necessary and is considered a relative contraindication to the present technique and an indication for conventional subfascial breast augmentation (**Box 5**).

Secondary augmentation

Most candidates for secondary breast augmentation can be successfully treated with the present technique. This group of patients frequently present with partial or total soft tissue deficiency with visible implant contours and rippling. In patients with thinned, stretched breast tissue, distortion and irregularities of the implant surface become noticeable. It has been the authors' impression that this aspect is frequently present in thin patients. In some cases, large implant pockets can also contribute to this result, and correction of this factor is important to achieve a good result. Therefore, implant replacement and subcutaneous placement of autologous fat graft where needed (frequently the upper pole or the superomedial area) provide additional soft tissue that reinforces thin tissue, thus masking surface irregularities. In the authors' experience with revision, surgery using subfascial form-stable implants associated with fat grafting was performed for one or more of the following primary indications: (1) local soft tissue deficiency/irregularities; (2) implant contour palpability; (3) implant contour visibility; (4) rippling. Some patients had multiple indications for the use of the present technique during their revision procedure. In addition, the same primary augmentation principles were used (**Box 6**).

Box 6
Subfascial form-stable and autologous fat grafting—patient selection: secondary augmentation

- Partial or total soft tissue deficiency
- Thin patients (BMI <20)
- Pinch test result of less than 2 cm
- Visible implant contours
- Rippling
- Stretched breast tissue
- Implant contour palpability

Preoperative Evaluation/Implant Selection

Incision choice should be based on a thorough discussion with the patient regarding factors such as individual preference and the advantages and limitations of each approach. The inframammary approach offers well-known advantages, such as simple access (ensuring accurate dissection and hemostasis), nondisruption of the breast parenchyma, and the ability to use virtually any type/size of implant. The incision is usually 4 cm long and should be located slightly lateral to the nipple-areola complex (NAC)'s inferior projection on the inframammary fold and approximately 0.5 cm above the anticipated new fold. In patients desiring an areolar approach, the incision location depends on whether a change in the position of the areola is anticipated. Usually, the incision should be placed in the lower half of the areola when its position is considered satisfactory.

Implant size is selected considering factors such as height and weight, thoracic wall, the presence of breast ptosis, and thickness of the subcutaneous tissue in the upper and the lower pole. Usually, volume is determined by both the patient's desired postoperative size and the physical examination to determine the patient's breast width and dimensions. In the authors' practice, sizers may be inserted to determine intraoperative size dimensions. Before surgery, the following skin markings are planned with the patient in a sitting position: current inframammary sulcus, anterior axillary line, the limits of the pocket, and the future inframammary fold. Limits of the dissection are defined depending on the anatomy of the breast and size of the implant. Breast width is measured from the medial to the lateral aspect of the breast mound. Before surgery, the anterior axillary line and the thoracic medial line are planned with the patient in the standing position. The existing inframammary fold is marked and is used as a landmark to highlight any asymmetry. The new inframammary fold is marked at a new position approximately 0.5 to 2.5 cm below, based on the desired breast volume, any existing asymmetry, and the implant base diameter. Slight pressure is applied to the top of the gland to mark the inferior limit of the pocket. The same maneuver is performed to mark the medial limit of the pocket. The superior limit of the pocket depends on the

Box 5
Subfascial form-stable and autologous fat grafting—patient selection: primary augmentation

- Severe hypomastia/amastia
- Thin patients (BMI <20)
- Less upper pole coverage
- Pinch test result of less than 2 cm

height of the implant. Preoperatively, areas of soft tissue deficiency are marked out on the patient.

Surgical Technique

Subfascial dissection

The operative procedure begins with the patient under general anesthesia. With the patient's arms abducted at 90°, an incision is made and the superficial fascia of the pectoralis muscle is identified and opened. In the areolar approach, dissection after the incision is performed parallel to the skin, for approximately 4 cm. The breast parenchyma is then incised in a radial direction (perpendicular to the skin incision) and vertically until the fascial layer is reached. Dissection of the implant pocket is then performed in the well-defined subfascial plane using electrocautery. When planning the position of the inframammary fold, it should be lowered so that the horizontal midaxis of the implant is centered on the nipple, and the amount of lowering correlates with the implant diameter. The attachments from the fascia to the skin at the level of the fold must be disrupted in order to avoid deformities, such as high-riding implants and "double-bubble" contours in the lower breast. Undermining should not be extended laterally beyond the lateral border of the breast because of the innervation of the NAC, and to avoid implant displacement after surgery. The fascia is raised by cauterization of the perforators. With the aid of customized retractors, subfascial dissection is continued on the pectoralis muscle beneath the fascia moving toward the upper, lateral, and medial breast pole. The glandular tissue is lifted away from the chest, consequently elevating the gland and muscular fascia, facilitating the passage between them and the retractors. Medially, dissection then proceeds approximately 1–2 cm lateral to the sternal border depending on the preoperative markings. Laterally, dissection should be limited to the anterior axillary line in order to avoid lateral displacement of the implant. The boundaries of the pocket and the new inframammary fold are checked and enlarged if necessary. In order to avoid injury to the lateral cutaneous nerves and the lymphatic channels, the lateral aspect of the pocket dissection should be minimized.[16,71] Before implant insertion and following meticulous hemostasis, the implant is bathed in Cephalothin solution and is inserted into the subfascial pocket, and the patient is positioned upright to assess implant position and breast shape. Layered wound closure is performed using absorbable sutures (in the subcutaneous and subdermal planes) and Monocryl subcuticular running sutures. Suction drains are inserted, usually through the axilla, and are maintained until output decreases to less than than 30 mL/day on each side.

Autologous fat grafting

Areas for liposuction are previously marked with the patients in the upright position and included the abdomen, flanks, inner thigh, trochanteric

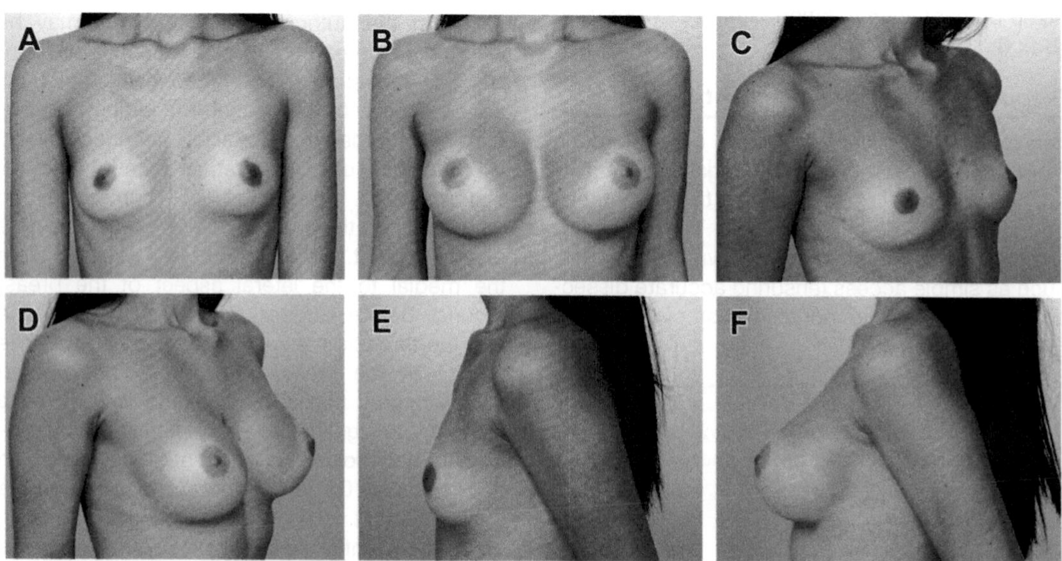

Fig. 3. (*A–F*) (Case 2) Preoperative frontal view, right oblique view, and right view of a 23-year-old patient with hypoplastic breasts (*A, C, E*). Postoperative (1 year) frontal view, right oblique view, and right view following bilateral implant with Allergan Style 510 MX (335 g) associated with autologous fat grafting, showing a very good outcome (*B, D, F*).

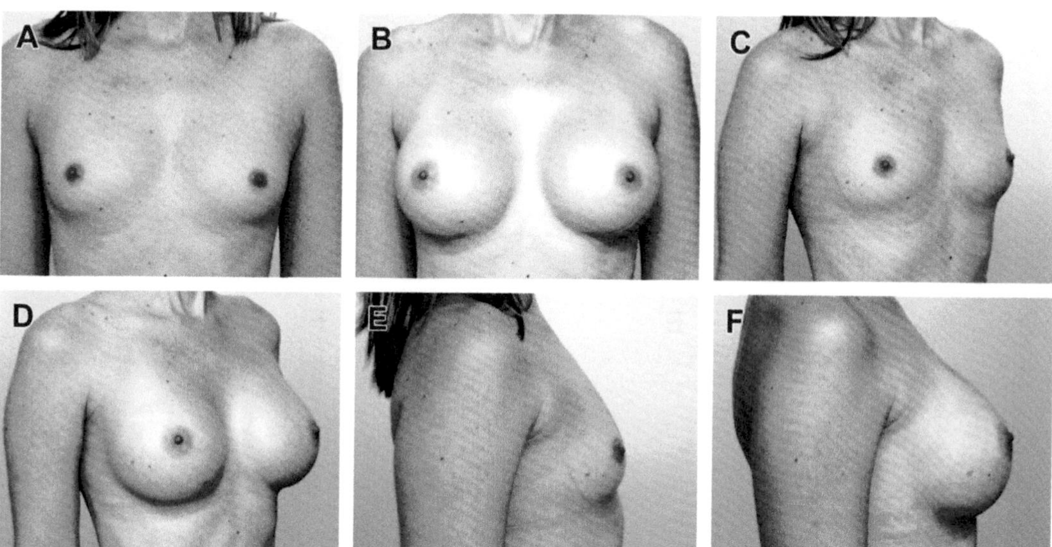

Fig. 4. (*A–F*) (Case 3) Preoperative frontal view, right oblique view, and right view of a 29-year-old patient with hypoplastic breasts (*A*, *C*, *E*). Postoperative (2 years) frontal view, right oblique view, and right view following bilateral implant with Allergan Style 510 MX (220 g) associated with autologous fat grafting, showing a very good outcome (*B*, *D*, *F*).

region, and medial aspect of knees, depending on the patient's fat distribution. Usually the lateral thigh/flank area serves as the donor site for most patients. The authors use a modified Coleman technique for fat graft harvest. Following injection of local anesthesia (40–100 mL/area of 1% lidocaine and 1:100,000 epinephrine), fat is harvested using a blunt 2-mm cannula with several 0.8-mm holes (Byron Medical, Inc, Tucson, AZ, USA). Usually, fat is washed and condensed by a vacuum system. The aspiration is a closed system until the fat is collected and injected in the syringes. Purified fat is transferred into 10-mL syringes in preparation for injection through blunt cannulas. Usually, 1 to 2 small incisions are performed associated with the breast incision in each breast.

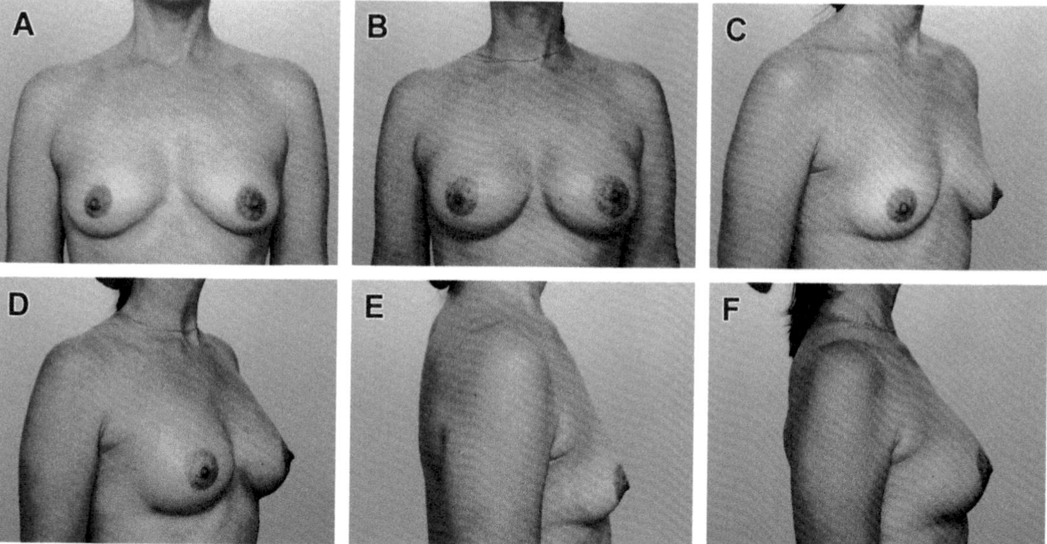

Fig. 5. (*A–F*) (Case 4) Preoperative frontal view, right oblique view, and right view of a 22-year-old patient with hypoplastic breasts (*A*, *C*, *E*). Postoperative (1 year) frontal view, right oblique view, and right view following bilateral implant with Allergan Style 510 MX (290 g) associated with autologous fat grafting, showing a very good outcome (*B*, *D*, *F*).

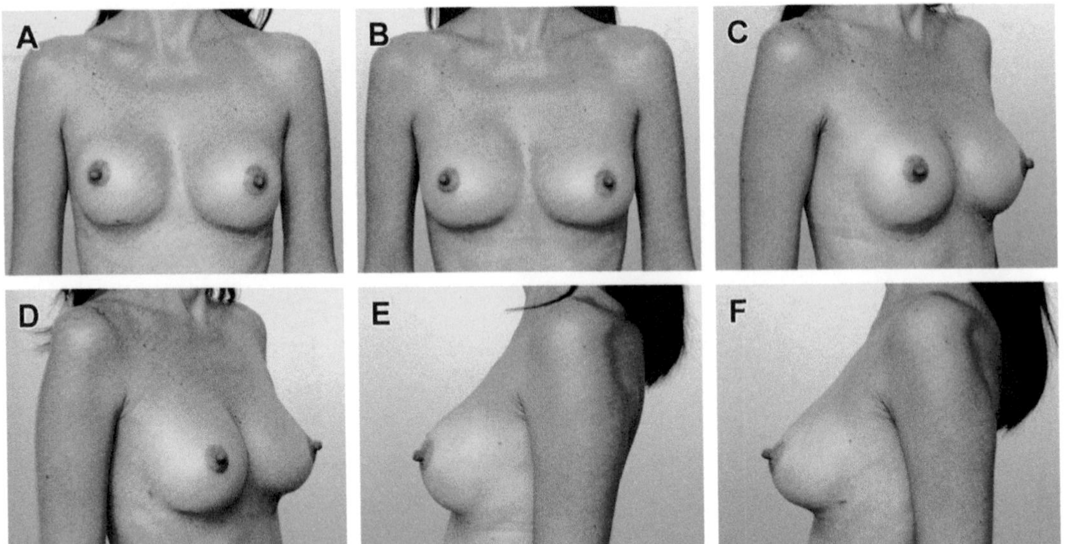

Fig. 6. (*A–F*) (Case 5) Preoperative frontal view, right oblique view, and right view of a 31-year-old patient with previous subglandular breast augmentation and right breast capsular contracture (*A, C, E*). Postoperative (1 year) frontal view, right oblique view, and right view following bilateral implant with Allergan Style 510 MX (290 g) associated with autologous fat grafting, showing a very good outcome (*B, D, F*).

Through a periareolar incision or inframammary incisions, the fat grafts are injected into the subcutaneous tissue of the medial, superior, lateral, and inferior aspect of the breast. The technique for injecting fat grafts into the breast relies on preoperative topographic markings, where small amounts of fat are infiltrated by means of multiple passes along several planes. The fat is placed in multiple planes from deep to subcutaneous tissue. At this point, care must be taken to avoid penetrating the implant capsule or causing harm to the silicone implant. For this purpose, it must be stressed that blunt cannulas in the subdermal region must be used gently. In some cases, a blunt cannula is used before, depending on the degree of cicatricial adherence observed. Following the

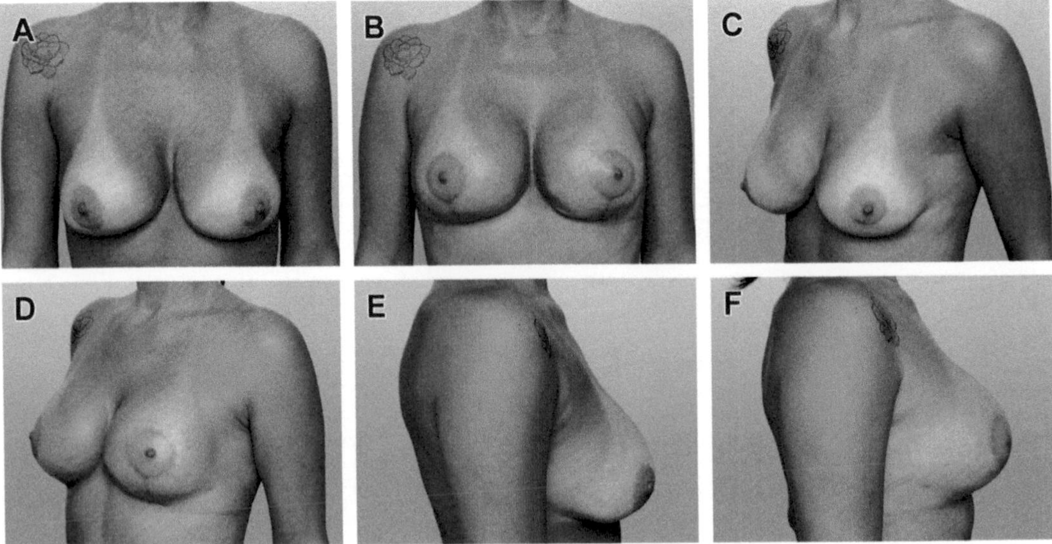

Fig. 7. (*A–F*) (Case 6) Preoperative frontal view, left oblique view, and left view of a 39-year-old patient with previous subglandular breast augmentation and ptosis (*A, C, E*). Postoperative (1 year) frontal view, left oblique view, and left view following bilateral implant of Allergan Style 510 MX (360 g) associated with autologous fat grafting, showing a very good outcome (*B, D, F*).

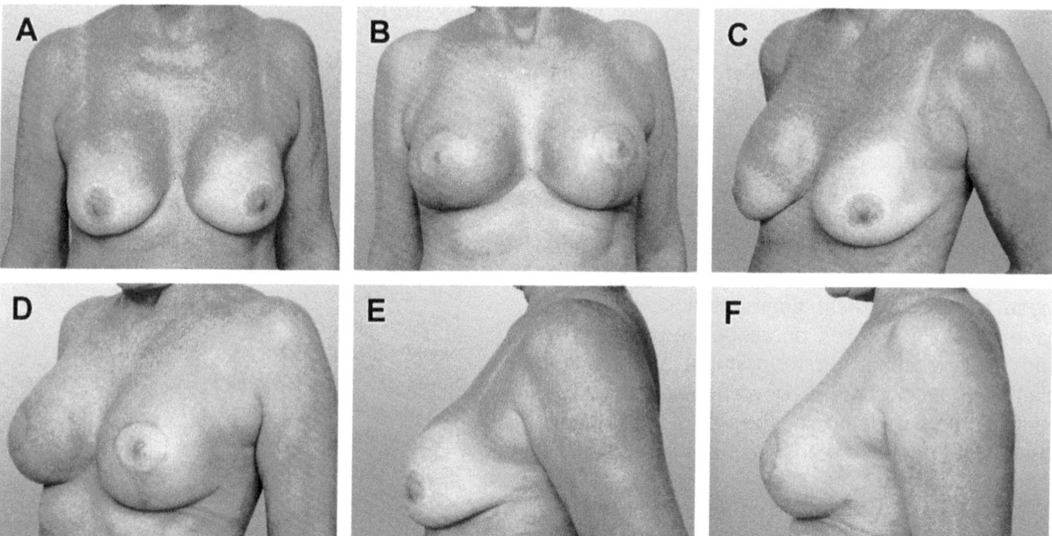

Fig. 8. (*A–F*) (Case 7) Preoperative frontal view, left oblique view, and left view of a 59-year-old patient with previous subglandular breast augmentation, breast ptosis, and extracapsular implant rupture (*A, C, E*). Postoperative (1 year) frontal view, left oblique view, and left view following bilateral implant with Allergan Style 510 MX (335 g) associated with autologous fat grafting, showing a very good outcome (*B, D, F*).

injection, the injected area is carefully reshaped to adapt the outline of the desired surface.

Postoperative Care

All patients received intravenous antibiotics, and oral antibiotics were continued for 48 hours. Immobilization with an occlusive dressing should be used for 3 days in order to improve scarring. An elastic band or strap should be used over the superior poles of the breasts for 2 to 4 weeks in order to avoid superior displacement of the implants, keep the newly created inframammary fold in the desired position, and expand the tissues in the inferior pole of the breast. In terms of postoperative care, one of the most important goals is obtaining adequate adherence between the tissues and implants. Therefore, early massaging or mobilization of the breasts (which may lead to accumulation of liquid around the implants) should be avoided for at least 3 weeks. It is crucial that patients avoid physical activities for a period of time following implantation to minimize the risk of implant rotation, displacement, seroma, and other complications. As the breast edema diminishes, tension of the band requires some adjustment, and patients are seen at appropriate intervals to supervise implant position and band tension.

Results

Results following this procedure have been very acceptable to the authors' patients. Complications and surgical revisions have been rare. The results from the study have verified that most complications occur in the initial postoperative period. Fortunately, all these complications were minor and predictable and did not affect the final esthetic result. The level of satisfaction was assessed after a minimal period of 6 months after the procedure. This period is important because the breast shape continues to change, and remaining edema is a potential cause of volume distortion and asymmetry. Satisfactory esthetic results were obtained, with maintenance of a natural breast shape. At this time, most patients were either very satisfied or satisfied with their results. Implant displacement and major complications were not observed. The final result was generally good, and a soft transition between the subcutaneous tissue and implant edge was observed in all cases. As of this writing, no capsular contraction has been observed in the authors' study; however, a larger number of patients and a longer follow-up period are necessary to draw significant conclusions. Examples of clinical results are illustrated in **Figs. 3–8**.

SUMMARY

Advances in autologous fat-grafting techniques and form-stable implants have led to an important improvement in esthetic outcomes for augmented breasts. The most frequent use is in the medial and lateral chest wall, where thin tissue provides inadequate coverage and leads to implant visibility. This technique can play a useful role in breast augmentation, and the results of the authors' experience demonstrate that is a simple and predictable procedure. Most complications were minor and did not interfere with the esthetic outcome. The ideal esthetic result must provide a natural contour and achieve adequate size and projection. In the authors' experience, to achieve these results in breast augmentation, surgeons have increasingly relied on associate procedures and materials such as form-stable silicone implants and fat grafting. Preoperative patient evaluation is crucial to determine the size of the implant, the implant pocket dimensions, and the future inframammary fold.

Regardless of the esthetic benefits, the association of autologous fat grafting and form-stable breast implants in primary and secondary surgeries presents some limitations. The need for previous training and surgical skills are the main negative aspects. Financial limitations are reported, and longer operative time is also mentioned as a relative disadvantage. Although this latter aspect is partially true, it seems logical that additional operative time is not so significant once experience is acquired. Autologous fat grafting can be considered an essential tool for breast shaping and additional soft tissue coverage because of its simplicity, low morbidity, and long-term results.

Editorial Comments by Bradley P. Bengtson, MD

Dr Goes is one of the greatest modern day thinkers, researchers, histopathologists and plastic surgeons of this generation. Practicing in Brazil he has had access to technologies and devices that we are just in our infancy using here in the US and has an incredible experience with soft-tissue support of the breast, highly cohesive shaped implants and fat transfer. He places form stable devices in a subfascial plane which is intriguing because of maximal adherence on both sides of the device. I personally believe that the majority of issues we see with textured shaped devices: rotation, double capsule, delayed seroma likely initiate on the posterior aspect of the device which lies on the more rigid chest wall. Placing the implant more superficial does however create more potential edge palpability and rippling in very thin patients. Dr Goes addresses this by combining fat transfer in both primary and revision breast surgery with excellent results and minimal adverse events.

REFERENCES

1. American Society of Plastic Surgeons. 2013 cosmetic plastic surgery statistics. Available at: http://www.plasticsurgery.org/news/plastic-surgery-statistics/2013.html. Accessed May 8, 2014.
2. International Society of Plastic Aesthetic Surgery. International survey on aesthetic cosmetic procedures performed in 2009. Available at: http://www.isaps.org/files/html-contents/Analysis_iSAPS_Survey2009.pdf. Accessed October, 2011.
3. Solomon JA, Barton FE. Augmentation mammaplasty. Selected Read Plast Surg 1997;8:1–11.
4. Spear SL, Bulan EJ, Venturi ML. Breast augmentation. Plast Reconstr Surg 2004;114:73–81.
5. Lista F, Ahmad J. Evidence-based medicine: augmentation mammaplasty. Plast Reconstr Surg 2013;132(6):1684–96.
6. Adams WP Jr, Mallucci P. Breast augmentation. Plast Reconstr Surg 2012;130:597e–611e.
7. Handel N, Cordray T, Gutierrez J, et al. A long-term study of outcomes, complications, and patient satisfaction with breast implants. Plast Reconstr Surg 2006;117:757–67.
8. Tebbetts JB. Dual plane breast augmentation: optimizing implant–soft-tissue relationships in a wide range of breast types. Plast Reconstr Surg 2001;107:1255–61.
9. Vazquez B, Given KS, Houston GC. Breast augmentation: a review of subglandular and submuscular implantation. Aesthetic Plast Surg 2007;11:101–5.
10. Ramirez OM, Heller L, Tebbetts JB. Dual-plane breast augmentation: avoiding pectoralis major displacement. Plast Reconstr Surg 2002;110:1198–2003.
11. Spear SL, Schwartz J, Dayan JH, et al. Outcome assessment of breast distortion following submuscular breast augmentation. Aesthetic Plast Surg 2009;33:44–8.
12. Graf RM, Bernardes A, Auersvald A, et al. Subfascial endoscopic transaxillary augmentation mammaplasty. Aesthetic Plast Surg 2000;24:216–22.
13. Graf RM, Bernardes A, Rippel R, et al. Subfascial breast implant: a new procedure. Plast Reconstr Surg 2003;111:904–11.
14. Goes JC, Landecker A. Optimizing outcomes in breast augmentation: seven years of experience with the subfascial plane. Aesthetic Plast Surg 2003;27:178–86.
15. Jinde L, Jianliang S, Xiaoping C, et al. Anatomy and clinical significance of pectoral fascia. Plast Reconstr Surg 2006;118:1160–557.
16. Munhoz AM, Fells K, Arruda EG, et al. Subfascial transaxillary breast augmentation without endoscopic assistance: technical aspects and outcome. Aesthetic Plast Surg 2006;30:503–12.
17. Serra-Renom J, Garrido MF, Yoon T. Augmentation mammaplasty with anatomic soft, cohesive silicone

implant using the transaxillary approach at a subfascial level with endoscopic assistance. Plast Reconstr Surg 2006;116:640–50.
18. Benito-Ruiz J. Subfascial breast implant. Plast Reconstr Surg 2004;113:1088–91.
19. Stoff-Khalili MA, Scholze R, Morgan WR, et al. Subfascial periareolar augmentation mammaplasty. Plast Reconstr Surg 2004;114:1280–9.
20. Ventura OD, Marcello GA. Anatomic and physiologic advantages of totally subfascial breast implants. Aesthetic Plast Surg 2005;29(5):379–83.
21. Hunstad JP, Webb LS. Subfascial breast augmentation: a comprehensive experience. Aesthetic Plast Surg 2010;34(3):365–73.
22. Tijerina VN, Saenz RA, Garcia-Guerrero J. Experience of 1000 cases on subfascial breast augmentation. Aesthetic Plast Surg 2010;34(1):16–22.
23. Bircoll M. Cosmetic breast augmentation utilizing autologous fat and liposuction techniques. Plast Reconstr Surg 1987;79:267–71.
24. Bircoll M, Novack BH. Autologous fat transplantation employing liposuction techniques. Ann Plast Surg 1987;18:327–9.
25. Drever JM. Lipocontouring in breast reconstructive surgery. Aesthetic Plast Surg 1996;20:285–9.
26. Spear SL, Wilson HB, Locjwood MD. Fat injection to correct contour deformities in the reconstructed breast. Plast Reconstr Surg 2005;116:1300–5.
27. Coleman SR, Saboeiro A. Fat grafting to the breast revisited: safety and efficacy. Plast Reconstr Surg 2007;119:775–85.
28. Missana MC, Laurent I, Barreau L, et al. Autologous fat transfer in reconstructive breast surgery: indications, technique and results. Eur J Surg Oncol 2007;33:685–90.
29. Zheng DH, Li QF, Lei H, et al. Autologous fat grafting to the breast for cosmetic enhancement: experience in 66 patients with long-term follow up. J Plast Reconstr Aesthet Surg 2008;61:792–8.
30. Delay E, Garson S, Tousson G, et al. Fat injection to the breast: technique, results, and indications based on 880 procedures over 10 years. Aesthet Surg J 2009;29:360–76.
31. Del Vecchio D. Breast reconstruction using non-operative pre expansion and mega-volume fat grafting: a case report. Ann Plast Surg 2009;62:523–7.
32. Kanchwala SK, Glatt BS, Conant EF, et al. Autologous fat grafting to the reconstructed breast: the management of acquired contour deformities. Plast Reconstr Surg 2009;124:409–14.
33. Illouz YG, Sterodimas A. Autologous fat transplantation to the breast: a personal technique with 25 years of experience. Aesthetic Plast Surg 2009;33:706–15.
34. Auclair E. Apport du lipomodelage extraglandulaire dans les augmentations mammaires à visée esthétique (note technique). Ann Chir Plast Esthét 2009;54:491–5 [in French].
35. Auclair E, Blondeel P, Del Vecchio DA. Composite breast augmentation: soft-tissue planning using implants and fat. Plast Reconstr Surg 2013;132(3):558–68.
36. Li FC, Chen B, Cheng L. Breast augmentation with autologous fat injection: a report of 105 cases. Ann Plast Surg 2014;73(Suppl 1):S37–42.
37. Gutowski KA, ASPS Fat Graft Task Force. Current applications and safety of autologous fat grafts: a report of the ASPS fat graft task force. Plast Reconstr Surg 2009;124:272.
38. American Society of Plastic Surgeons. Fat Transfer/Fat Graft and Fat Injection: ASPS Guiding Principles, January, 2009. Available at: http://www.plasticsurgery.org/Documents/medical-professionals/health-policy/guiding-principles/ASPS-Fat-Transfer-Graft-Guiding-Principles.pdf. Accessed July 17, 2013.
39. Tebbetts JB. Does fascia provide additional meaningful coverage over a breast implant? Plast Reconstr Surg 2004;113:777–82.
40. Heitmann C, Schreckenberger C, Olbrisch RR. A silicone implant filled with cohesive gel: advantages and disadvantages. Eur J Plast Surg 1998;21:329–32.
41. Bogetti P, Boltri M, Balocco P, et al. Augmentation mammaplasty with a new cohesive gel prosthesis. Aesthetic Plast Surg 2000;24:440–4.
42. Heden P, Jernbeck J, Hober M. Breast augmentation with anatomical cohesive gel implants. Clin Plast Surg 2001;28:531–2.
43. Brown MH, Shenker R, Silver SA. Cohesive silicone gel breast implants in aesthetic and reconstructive breast surgery. Plast Reconstr Surg 2005;116:768–79.
44. Hedén P, Boné B, Murphy DK, et al. Style 410 cohesive silicone breast implants: safety and effectiveness at 5 to 9 years after implantation. Plast Reconstr Surg 2006;118:1281–7.
45. Hedén P, Bronz G, Elberg JJ, et al. Long-term safety and effectiveness of style 410 highly cohesive silicone breast implants. Aesthetic Plast Surg 2009;33:430–6.
46. Bengtson BP, Van Natta BW, Murphy DK, et al, Style 410 U.S. Core Clinical Study Group. Style 410 highly cohesive silicone breast implant core study results at 3 years. Plast Reconstr Surg 2007;120(7 Suppl 1):40S–8S.
47. Cunningham B. The mentor core study on silicone MemoryGel breast implants. Plast Reconstr Surg 2007;120(7 Suppl 1):19S–29S [discussion: 30S–32S].
48. Góes JC. Breast implant stability in the subfascial plane and the new shaped silicone gel breast implants. Aesthetic Plast Surg 2010;34(1):23–8.
49. Maxwell GP, Van Natta BW, Murphy DK, et al. Natrelle style 410 form-stable silicone breast implants: core study results at 6 years. Aesthet Surg J 2012;32:709–17.

50. Lista F, Tutino R, Khan A, et al. Subglandular breast augmentation with textured, anatomic, cohesive silicone implants: a review of 440 consecutive patients. Plast Reconstr Surg 2013;132(2):295–303.
51. Baeke JL. Breast deformity caused by anatomical or teardrop implant rotation. Plast Reconstr Surg 2002; 109:2555–64 [discussion: 2568].
52. Nipshagen MD, Beekman WH, Esmé DL, et al. Anatomically shaped breast prosthesis in vivo: a change of dimension? Aesthetic Plast Surg 2007; 31(5):540–3.
53. Schots JM, Fechner MR, Hoogbergen MM, et al. Malrotation of the McGhan Style 510 prosthesis. Plast Reconstr Surg 2010;126:261–5.
54. Largo RD, Tchang LA, Mele V, et al. Efficacy, safety and complications of autologous fat grafting to healthy breast tissue: a systematic review. J Plast Reconstr Aesthet Surg 2014;67:437–48.
55. Hidalgo DA. Breast augmentation: choosing the optimal incision, implant, and pocket plane. Plast Reconstr Surg 2000;105:2202–10.
56. Gir P, Brown SA, Oni G, et al. Fat grafting: evidence-based review on autologous fat harvesting, processing, reinjection, and storage. Plast Reconstr Surg 2012;130:249–60.
57. Saint-Cyr M, Rojas K, Colohan S, et al. The role of fat grafting in reconstructive and cosmetic breast surgery: a review of the literature. J Reconstr Microsurg 2012;28(2):98–107.
58. Rosing JH, Wong G, Wong MS, et al. Autologous fat grafting for primary breast augmentation: a systematic review. Aesthetic Plast Surg 2011;35:882–90.
59. American Society of Plastic Surgeons. Fat Transfer/Fat Graft and Fat Injection: ASPS Guiding Principles, January, 2009. Available at: http://www.plasticsurgery.org/Documents/medical-professionals/health-policy/guiding-principles/ASPS-Fat-Transfer-Graft-Guiding-Principles.pdf. Accessed June 23, 2012.
60. ASPRS Ad-Hoc Committee on New Procedures. Report on autologous fat transplantation, September 30, 1987. Plast Surg Nurs 1987;7:140–1.
61. Asken S. Autologous fat transplantation: micro and macro techniques. Am J Cosmet Surg 1987;4: 111–21.
62. Condé-Green A, Amorim NF, Pitanguy I. Influence of decantation, washing and centrifugation on adipocyte and mesenchymal stem cell content of aspirated adipose tissue: a comparative study. J Plast Reconstr Aesthet Surg 2010;63:1375–81.
63. Fulton JE, Parastouk N. Fat grafting. Dermatol Clin 2001;19:523–30.
64. Kononas TC, Bucky LP, Hurley C, et al. The fate of suctioned and surgically removed fat after reimplantation for soft-tissue augmentation: a volumetric and histologic study in the rabbit. Plast Reconstr Surg 1993;91:763–8.
65. Coleman S. Structural fat grafting. Plast Reconstr Surg 2005;115:1777–8.
66. Pinski KS, Roengik HH. Autologous fat transplantation: long-term follow-up. J Dermatol Surg Oncol 1992;18:179–84.
67. Khater R, Atanassova P, Anastassov Y, et al. Clinical and experimental study of autologous fat grafting after processing by centrifugation and serum lavage. Aesthetic Plast Surg 2009;33:37–43.
68. Rohrich RJ, Sorokin ES, Brown SA. In search of improved fat transfer viability: a quantitative analysis of the role of centrifugation and harvest site. Plast Reconstr Surg 2004;113:391–5.
69. Ramon Y, Shoshani O, Peled IJ, et al. Enhancing the take of injected adipose tissue by a simple method for concentrating fat cells. Plast Reconstr Surg 2005;115:197–201.
70. Codner MA, Mejia JD, Locke MB, et al. 15-year experience with primary breast augmentation. Plast Reconstr Surg 2011;127(3):1300–10.
71. Munhoz AM, Aldrighi C, Ono C, et al. The influence of subfascial transaxillary breast augmentation in axillary lymphatic drainage patterns and sentinel lymph node detection. Ann Plast Surg 2007;58(2): 141–9.

Transaxillary Subfascial Augmentation Mammaplasty with Anatomic Form-Stable Silicone Implants

Alexandre Mendonça Munhoz, MD, PhD[a,b,*],
Rolf Gemperli, MD, PhD[c,d],
João Carlos Sampaio Goes, MD, PhD[c,e]

KEYWORDS

• Breast augmentation • Silicone implant • Form stable implant • Transaxillary approach • Subfascial • Outcome • Complications • High cohesive implant

KEY POINTS

- The transaxillary approach to breast augmentation is a successful technique that not only provides an inconspicuous incision but also offers the advantages of adequate placement of the inframammary crease and subfascial dissection under direct visualization.
- In the upper breast pole, the pectoral fascia helps to decrease visualization of the edges of the implant and provides soft-tissue coverage over the anatomic implant. The technique avoids the negative aspects of the submuscular position and provides a more comfortable recovery than the total submuscular pocket.
- An important characteristic of anatomic cohesive gel implants is their form-stable nature and their ability to maintain shape in all positions without significant deformation. This form-stable characteristic results from a higher degree of cross-linking within the gel.
- Ideal primary candidates are those who have significant hypomastia/amastia, are thin without sufficient soft tissue to adequately cover the implant, and have an absent or high inframammary fold. Patients who require greater volume in the lower breast and want to avoid visible incision scars on their chests also benefit from the present technique.

Funding Sources/Financial Disclosures: This work was not supported by any external funding. Drs J.C. Sampaio Goés and A.M. Munhoz are consultants to Allergan Corporations. Dr R. Gemperli is consultant to Ethicon and Johnson & Johnson Corporations.
Contributors' Statement: A.M. Munhoz is principal investigator of this study. J.C. Sampaio Goés and R. Gemperli are coinvestigators. The principal investigator made significant contributions to the conception and design of this study. J.C. Sampaio Goés and R. Gemperli made substantial contributions to the acquisition, analysis, and interpretation of data. A.M. Munhoz drafted the article. All authors revised the article for intellectual content, gave final approval of the version to be published, and have sufficiently participated in the work to take public responsibility for appropriate portions of the content.
[a] Department of Plastic Surgery, Hospital Sírio-Libanês, Rua Dona Adma Jafet, 115 - Bela Vista, São Paulo - SP 01308-050, Brazil; [b] Breast Plastic Surgery, Department of Plastic Surgery, University of São Paulo School of Medicine and Instituto do Câncer do Estado de São Paulo, Avenida Doutor Arnaldo, 251 - Cerqueira César, São Paulo - SP 01255-000, Brazil; [c] Department of Plastic Surgery, Hospital Albert Einstein, Avenida Albert Einsten, 627/701 - Morumbi, São Paulo - SP 05652-900, Brazil; [d] Department of Plastic Surgery, University of São Paulo School of Medicine, São Paulo, Brazil; [e] Breast Surgery and Plastic Surgery Department, Instituto Brasileiro do Controle do Câncer, Av. Alcântara Machado, 2576 - Móoca, São Paulo - SP 03102-002, Brazil
* Corresponding author. Rua Mato Grosso, 306 cj. 1706 – Higienópolis, São Paulo, São Paulo 01239-040, Brazil.
E-mail address: munhozalex@uol.com.br

Clin Plastic Surg 42 (2015) 565–584
http://dx.doi.org/10.1016/j.cps.2015.06.016

INTRODUCTION

Breast augmentation has become one of the most frequently performed aesthetic surgical procedures, with more than 290,000 of these surgeries performed in 2013.[1] Over time, improvements in surgical techniques and different implant designs have led to improvements in safety and esthetic outcomes. The introduction of the latest-generation form-stable silicone gel implants and new surgical approaches have improved outcomes and established a new era of breast augmentation.[2–4]

The transaxillary approach for breast augmentation (TBA) is a well-known procedure, and its main benefits are related to the absence of incisions on the breast and the ability to place the implant within the submuscular and subglandular plane (Solz H, personal communication, 2005).[5–16] Described initially for a submuscular pocket with blunt dissection,[5] the procedure is not without drawbacks, including implant displacement, muscular distortion, and postoperative pain.[17–21] Although TBA has been available for many years, critics have emphasized its limits in attaining precise positioning of the anatomic implant in the lower pole of the breast. However, in the authors' experience, the major advantages have been the absence of scars in the breast region, avoidance of breast ductal transection, and low probability of sensory nerve injury. In addition, endoscopic assistance has enhanced TBA by allowing better placement of the silicone implant inferiorly and improved management of the inframammary crease.[9,11,12,14]

An alternative implant pocket is gaining popularity because of the better postoperative recovery it provides compared with submuscular approaches and because it avoids distortion when the pectoral muscle is contracted.[10,22–29] Introduced in the 1990s, the subfascial technique is helpful for creating a support structure for the upper pole of the implant, which avoids inferior displacement and palpation of the implant edges.[12,22,23] In addition, with the advent of the subfascial technique, the potential benefits of TBA to patients, such as axillary incision and shorter recovery time, have become clearer. Consequently, because of the association of both procedures, subfascial TBA seems to have gained new popularity.[12]

Silicone breast implants have advanced in recent decades with the introduction of new textures and anatomically shaped implants.[30–38] With advances in implant technology involving different types of textures and gel cohesion, more satisfactory outcomes with lower complication rates can be achieved. Usually, these implants are anatomically shaped with less fullness at the upper pole compared with round implants. Because of their high cohesiveness, these latest-generation implants maintain their shape with less gel bleeding and decreased rippling and wrinkling.

This article provides an overview of the use of subfascial TBA in primary breast augmentation with form-stable implants. Although breast augmentation is a well-studied procedure, previous reports concerning the TBA subfascial technique are limited, especially those associated with the latest generation of form-stable breast implants.[11–13] In addition, there are few detailed clinical reports that specifically address the operative planning, outcomes, and complications following TBA using form-stable implants.[11] Therefore, a detailed description of the authors' technique, including preoperative evaluation and intraoperative care of patients undergoing primary breast augmentation, is provided herein.

AXILLARY APPROACH

Introduced in the 1970s, TBA has become a popular technique for breast augmentation because the scar is placed in a less visible position, hidden in an aesthetically acceptable area, and this technique permits an adequate positioning of the new inframammary crease (Solz H, personal communication, 2005)[5–16] (**Figs. 1** and **2**). In patients with a small areola or a poorly defined inframammary fold, TBA may be particularly advantageous.[10–12]

Since the introduction of TBA techniques in clinical practice in 1973,[5] they have undergone significant modifications. The submuscular position was first introduced to provide optimal implant coverage; however, the drawbacks were breast asymmetry, implant displacement, and pain.[5–7] In this technique, one-third of the upper implant was placed under the pectoralis major and two-thirds of the implant was placed over the rectus sheath, serratus, and oblique muscle. However, in the early stages of TBA, technical limitations were related to aspects of the blind technique, including difficult hemostasis and traumatic dissection, and technical limitations in creating an adequate pocket.[14]

Subfascial TBA was first introduced by Wright and Bevin.[6] They emphasized the importance of the junction of the pectoral fascia with the rectus abdominis and the external oblique fascia. However, at that time, one of the main concerns was the possibility of unfavorable outcomes in terms of implant edge visibility. This aspect was more evident in thin patients with less soft-tissue coverage, whereby a sharp transition could be seen in the upper pole.[7,10] With the goal of improving aesthetic outcomes, alternative

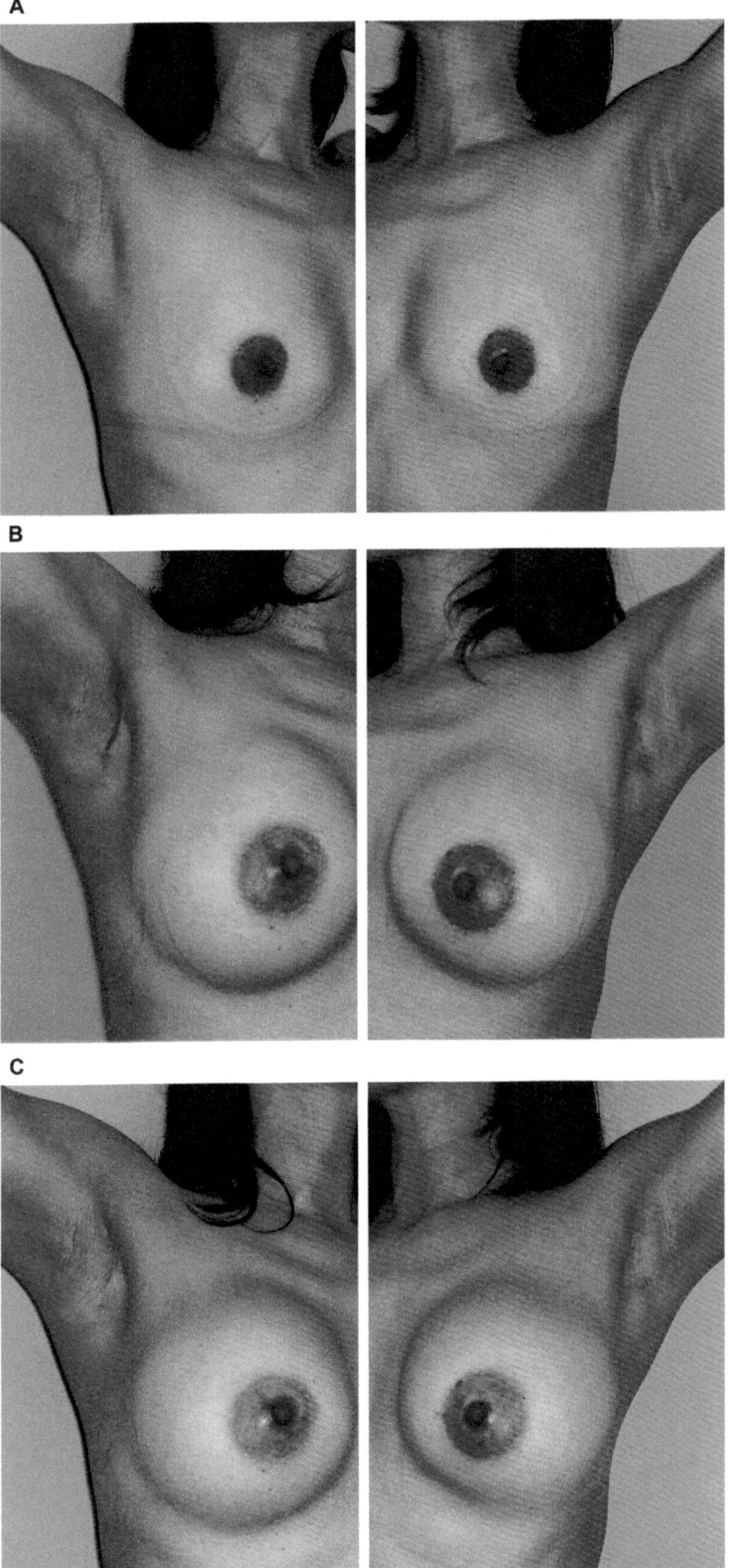

Fig. 1. Axillary incision outcome. (*A*) Preoperative view, left and right axilla. (*B*) Four months postoperative appearance, left and right axilla. (*C*) One year postoperative appearance, left and right axilla.

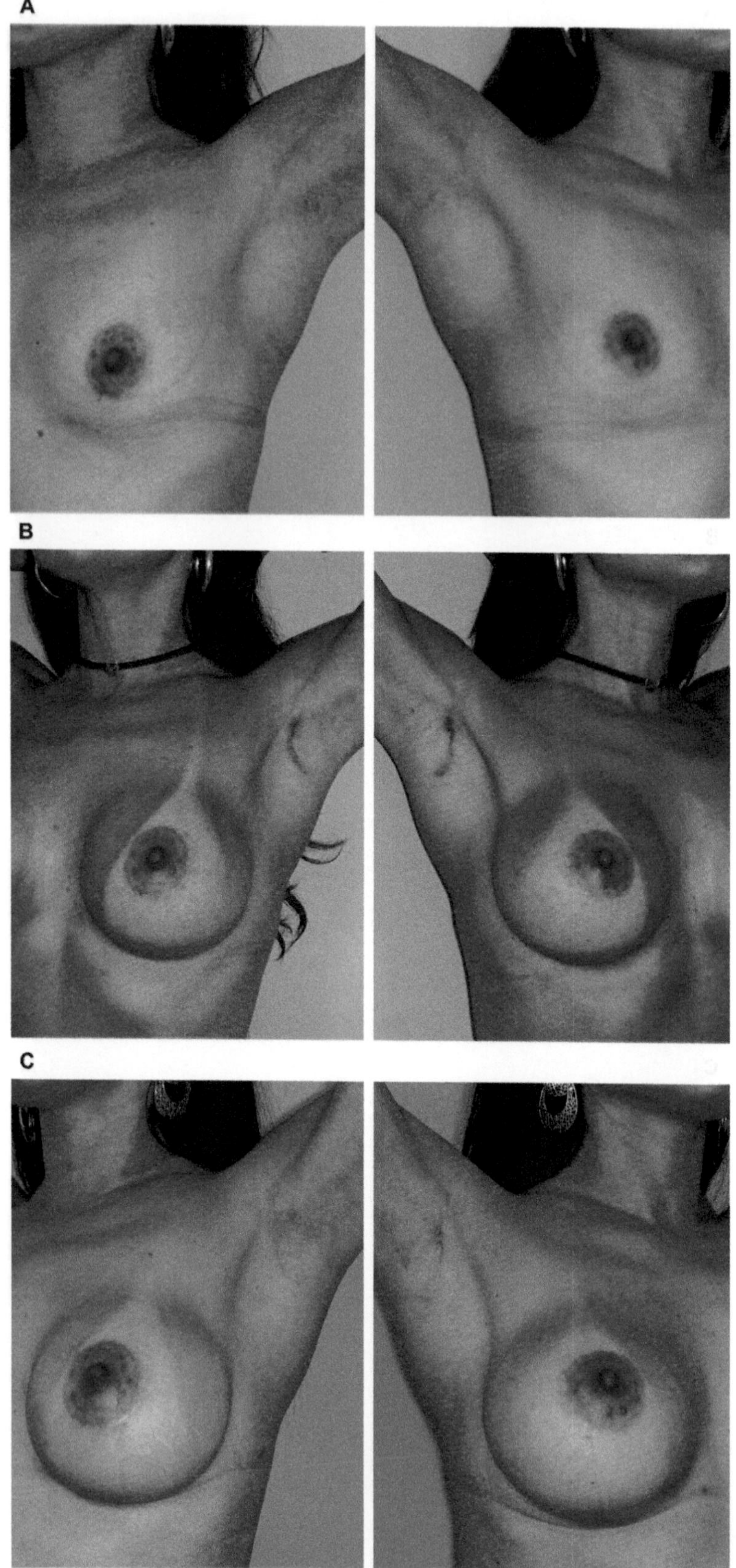

Fig. 2. Axillary incision outcome. (*A*) Preoperative view, left and right axilla. (*B*) Six months postoperative appearance, left and right axilla. (*C*) One year postoperative appearance, left and right axilla.

techniques for the implant pocket have been described.

To minimize the risk of implant contour deformity, Tebbets[7] introduced dual-plane TBA, whereby the subpectoral plane was associated with the subglandular plane. According to the investigator, the implant pocket permits varying degrees of submuscular and subglandular placement individualized for each patient, depending on breast tissue characteristics. During the 1980s and 1990s, in the United States, TBA was frequently associated with saline-filled implants because of the US Food and Drug Administration moratorium. Following the introduction of high-cohesive, anatomically shaped implants in Europe and Latin America, clinical application of TBA was not supported by most surgeons. In fact, technical limitations during implant placement of this shaped high-cohesive gel and the risk of implant rotation made the inframammary incision mandatory in the early 1990s.

Almost 20 years after the first description of TBA, Ho[39] described the endoscope-assisted transaxillary approach to breast augmentation to control hemostasis and confirm pocket location. In medial and lateral dissection, some researchers have suggested blunt dissection rather than using endoscopy.[14,16,39] However, the authors believe that the blind technique did not guarantee adequate hemostasis and accurate pocket dissection and implant placement. In a study of 232 TBA procedures, Sim[14] used sharp electrocautery dissection even in the medial and lateral dissections and not blunt dissection.

Reintroduced by Graf and colleagues,[12] the subfascial TBA technique is particularly attractive to surgeons who have been seeking alternative planes, with the advantages and reduced drawbacks of the subglandular and submuscular planes (**Box 1**). Despite the controversy concerning the suboptimal soft-tissue coverage provided by the subfascial approach and the limits of pectoral fascia thickness,[10,40] some clinical studies have demonstrated satisfactory outcomes in selected patients.[10–14] The benefits of the subfascial pocket are additional soft-tissue coverage and the avoidance of the limitations of the submuscular position. In the authors' experience, the pectoral fascia is a well-defined structure in the upper thorax, which is useful in minimizing the appearance of the edges of the implant.[10] As other investigators have observed, the fascia is a strong, distinct layer that can be easily identified on axillary approach.[22–28] This layer has a significant strength that becomes apparent during intraoperative manipulation, and when approximated, provides continuous fascial coverage over a round and anatomically shaped implant (**Fig. 3**).

As a consequence of advances in breast augmentation procedures, the subfascial plane has come to be associated with the axillary approach.[10–13] Basically, most prior clinical studies have used endoscopic assistance, which provides better visualization of the muscular fascia and the pectoralis muscle.[11,12,14,16] Regardless of adequate hemostasis and the precise dissection of soft-tissue attachments, endoscopic assistance is not reproducible like other techniques.[10] The need for previous training and surgical skills are the main disadvantages. Adequate endoscopic surgical training is involved, sometimes requiring time away from one's practice. In addition, costs are also observed as a limitation, and it may be necessary to invest in equipment that may not always be available in regular hospitals.[15] Furthermore, longer operative time is also mentioned as a relative disadvantage. Although this last aspect is partially true, it seems logical that the additional operative time is not so significant once experience is acquired[10] (**Box 2**).

Despite the advantages of endoscopic TBA, some surgeons are satisfied with their results using nonendoscopic techniques (Solz H, personal communication, 2005).[10,25,41] Solz described blunt pocket dissection with the finger and utilization of a customized breast dissector (personal communication, 2005). Benito-Ruiz[25] observed that the endoscope is not routinely necessary and can be used just to check the correct plane of dissection. This investigator mentioned the use of a cold light retractor after dissection, without any bleeding. Hidalgo[41] pointed out that the TBA approach does not usually require endoscopy but emphasized that the procedure is more accurate when this technique is applied. Niechajev, in a study following 140 cases of TBA, stopped routinely performing endoscopic inspection but kept endoscopic equipment available in case of

Box 1
Advantages of transaxillary approach for breast augmentation

- Final scar (less visible position)
- Patients who oppose visible scarring on the breast or nipple
- Adequate definition of the inframammary fold
- Adequate position of the inframammary fold
- Surgical access to subfascial, subglandular, and submuscular pockets

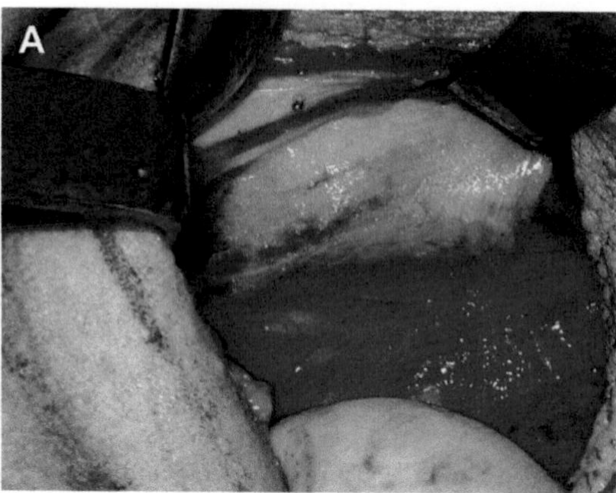

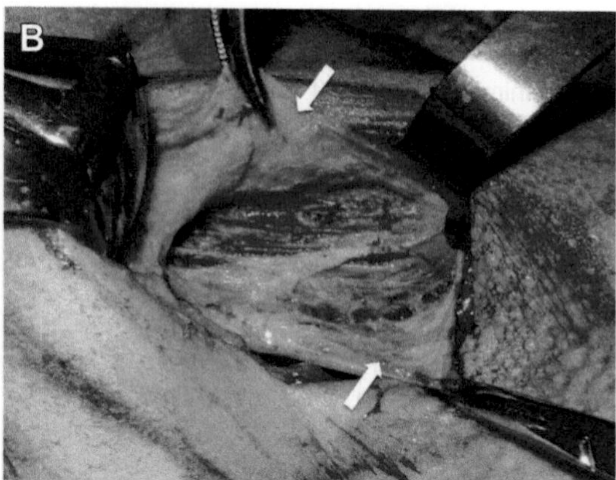

Fig. 3. Intraoperative view of the pectoral fascia. An incision is made in the axillary fold, and the superficial fascia of the pectoralis major muscle is identified (*A*) and opened through an incision parallel to the lateral border of the muscle (*B*).

unexpected difficulties in creating the pocket or unexpected bleeding.[15]

In the authors' experience,[10] TBA was performed in a manner similar to that proposed by Graf and colleagues,[12] except without endoscopy. The pectoral fascia was incised, and the dissection continued through the subfascial plane. Similar to the method proposed by Solz (personal communication, 2005), this plane was directly dissected with a finger, and the distal end of the fascia was detached with a breast dissector under direct view. This maneuver was restricted to the previous skin marks to create an adequate and precise pocket for the form-stable implant and to avoid breast asymmetry. TBA frequently required lowering the inframammary fold, the dimension of which was directly related to implant volume (**Fig. 4**). In most cases, the original fold was lowered to center the implant behind the nipple-areola complex. This step was necessary to prevent the implant from creating excessive upper-pole fullness and a downward-pointing nipple-areola complex. Care must be taken to not lower the fold excessively to accommodate an anatomically shaped implant, to avoid pseudoptosis or inframammary fold asymmetry.

Box 2
Disadvantages of transaxillary approach for breast augmentation

- Necessity of previous training and surgical skills
- Longer learning curve
- Customized instruments (eg, retractors, dissectors, light)
- Equipment, costs (for endoscopic approach)
- Secondary augmentation/capsulectomy (technical limitation)

Compared with other techniques, subfascial TBA has some limitations. Because the incision is located in a remote region, secondary procedures and implant replacement may be difficult, and an inframammary incision may be necessary. Another important aspect concerns oncologic safety. Pathologic analysis of axillary lymph nodes provides crucial information for adjuvant therapies in breast cancer, and sentinel lymph node biopsy has been proposed as an alternative in selected cases.[42–44] Therefore, the authors advocate minimal undermining in the lateral aspect of the breast to avoid interruption of the lymphatics between the breast tissue and the lower axilla. The authors' observations have demonstrated that the lymphatic channels can be preserved and that sentinel lymph node mapping is feasible with this technique.[45–47]

THE SUBFASCIAL TECHNIQUE

Despite the lack of consensus concerning the surgical pocket, the decision is frequently determined by patient preference, the surgeon's experience, and the anatomy of the breast.[3,4,10,41] Despite the reliability of the subglandular pocket, placing the silicone implant next to the glandular tissue may lead to an unsatisfactory result in terms of implant visibility, which is especially noticeable in thin patients with smaller breasts and soft-tissue coverage, whereby a sharp transition can be seen in the limits of the implant.[22–28]

To improve aesthetic results, alternative surgical options for the implant pocket have been described.[3,4] Among these, the submuscular technique was first introduced to contribute optimal

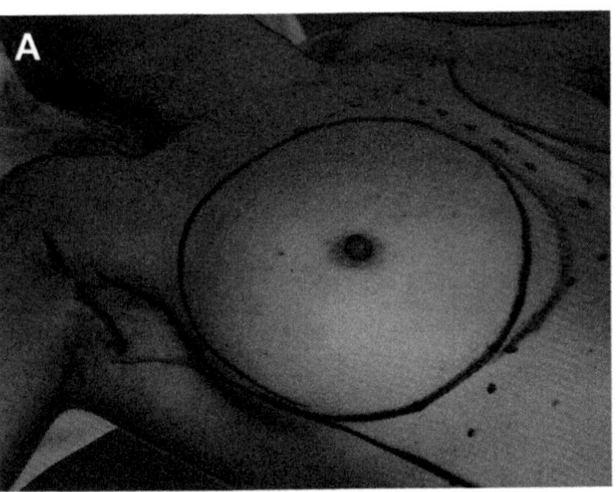

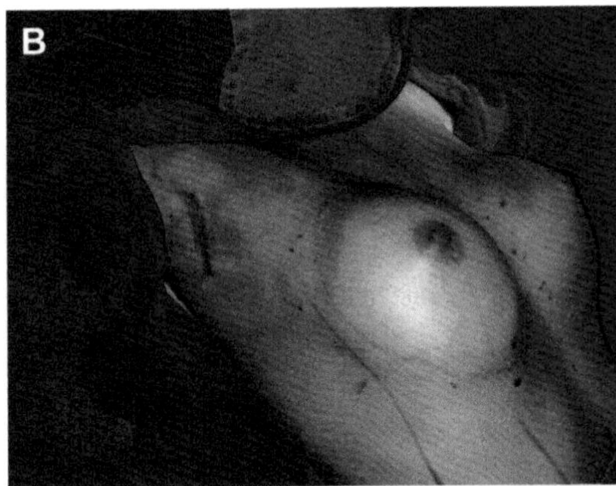

Fig. 4. (*A, B*) Intraoperative view. TBA frequently requires lowering the inframammary fold, and its size is directly related to the implant volume. This is necessary to prevent the implant from creating excessive upper-pole fullness and a downward-pointing nipple-areola complex.

implant coverage[17–20]; however, the main drawbacks are implant distortion, morbidity, and postoperative pain.[18,21] To minimize the risk of implant contour deformity, Tebbets[18] introduced dual-plane augmentation, whereby the submuscular pocket was associated with the subglandular plane. In the dual-plane procedure, the implant pocket permits varying degrees of submuscular and subglandular placement depending on the breast anatomy and soft-tissue characteristics. The advantages of the dual-plane technique are related to lesser implant visibility and reduced superior implant migration compared with complete submuscular placement.[18,20] However, as observed by other investigators, sometimes a flattening effect of the implant below the pectoralis muscle and implant animation still develop, with unsatisfactory long-term results.[21]

Introduced in the 1990s, the subfascial technique is especially attractive for plastic surgeons who have been searching for alternative planes.[12,22,23] The pectoral fascia is a distinct layer that can be identified and has adequate strength that becomes apparent during intraoperative manipulation. According to some investigators, when the subglandular pocket is created, the fibers connecting the deep layer of the superficial fascia and the superficial layer of the deep pectoralis muscle fascia are divided.[23,27,28] Otherwise, when the subfascial pocket is created, these important attachments are preserved, lessening the possibility of subsequent breast ptosis and maintaining better implant positioning.[10,23]

Despite these advantages, some researchers have observed that the average thickness of the pectoral fascia is approximately less than 1 mm.[24,28] It has been the authors' experience that the fascia is a strong, distinct layer that can be easily visualized on intraoperative dissection (see **Fig. 3**).[10,12,23] Another important point is the creation of a support structure for the upper pole of the implant. In a clinical study of subfascial breast augmentation, Tijerina and colleagues[29] observed that upper displacement of the implant is avoided because the fascia forces the implant downward. The subfascial pocket makes the upper pole of the implant more natural, avoiding contact with the skin or subcutaneous tissue.[10,23,29] In addition, the dissected anterior-pectoral fascia with the curved limit of the upper pole fits the upper curved edge of the implant, creating a muscle-fascia system that surrounds and adheres to the implant. In the upper pole, the pectoral fascia is helpful in minimizing visualization of the edges of the implant and provides an adequate support system for the implant's superior pole[23] (**Box 3**).

The advantages of the subfascial pocket are supplementary soft-tissue coverage and avoiding the limitations of the submuscular position. Some studies have demonstrated satisfactory aesthetic

Box 3
Advantages of subfascial approach for breast augmentation

- Improved upper pole contour
- Support structure for the upper/lower pole of the implant
- No implant edge visibility and palpability
- No muscular dynamics over the implant
- Keeps the implant in place

results after subfascial breast augmentation in selected patients.[10–13,22–29] In addition, this technique provides faster postoperative recovery than the total submuscular pocket, without breast animation when the pectoral muscle is contracted.

FORM-STABLE IMPLANTS

Silicone gel breast implants have advanced in recent decades with the introduction of new texturized surfaces and anatomic (or teardrop-shaped) implants.[30–38,48] Despite recent progress in terms of silicone technology, breast implant manufacturers continue to research and make advances in implant design resulting in lower complication rates, better aesthetic outcomes, and more consistent results.

Cohesive gel implants, unlike traditional silicone gel implants, are form stable, meaning that if the implant ruptures, the gel remains restricted inside the shell. The authors have been using a highly cohesive, form-stable implant available in Brazil since the 1990s for aesthetic and reconstructive breast surgery (Style 410, Allergan, Inc, Irvine, CA, USA). This silicone gel-filled breast implant is designed with a low-diffusion silicone elastomer shell (Intrasheil™ barrier technology) and also features a Biocell™ surface texture, which promotes tissue adherence to reduce implant rotation and capsular contracture.[33–38] The Style 410 is available in a wide range of shapes (a matrix involving 12 combinations of implant height and projection ratios that extend across a range of base widths) so that the surgeon can select an implant appropriate to each patient's anatomy.

The authors observed significant benefits of placing the Style 410 implant in the subfascial pocket, from preservation of the teardrop configuration to projection. Another important point is related to the low rate of wrinkling/rippling for form-stable implants. One single-center Swedish study of a sample of 163 subjects (70% had augmentation [n = 112], 15% had reconstruction [n = 25], and 15% had revision [n = 26]) observed high patient satisfaction with the Style 410 shaped, form-stable gel implant.[35] A low rate of wrinkling for the Style 410 devices, only 5%, was observed. It has been the authors' experience that these implants maintain the shape and fill of the upper pole while resisting folding, thus decreasing the incidence of wrinkling[34,35] (**Box 4**).

Additional aesthetic benefits can be achieved with the use of anatomically shaped form-stable implants. The clinical features of some breast deformities, including insufficient lower pole or breast base, lack of skin in the lower pole, short nipple-to-inframammary fold distance, and inframammary fold, can be more appropriately treated with these shaped implants (see **Box 7**). The anatomic cohesive gel implants can maintain their shape in all positions and resist deformation. Compared with traditional low-cohesive round implants, these shaped implants are designed to more closely resemble the shape and dimensions of a normal breast. This aspect can be especially helpful in a breast that presents abnormal shape and a tight skin envelope in the lower pole.[49] In summary, the choice of implant is based on objective measurements of breast height and width and an assessment of the degree of tissue deficiency in the lower pole of the breast.

Box 4
Advantages of form-stable implant

- Upper pole shape and contour
- High cohesive gel (less gel bleed)
- Gel stability (less rippling)
- Tissue adherence and implant stability (Biocell)
- Wide range of shapes (a matrix involving 12 combinations of implant height and projection)

Despite the positive aspects of these form-stable implants in terms of shape and gel stability, highly cohesive anatomically shaped implants have their drawbacks. Malrotation of shaped implants has been observed from the beginning of their clinical use.[50,51] Schots and colleagues,[51] in a study following a series of 73 augmentation mammaplasty procedures using Style 510 implants, described 12 patients (8.2%) self-reporting unilateral malrotation after a mean period of 10 months (range, 3–19 months); 7 patients required surgery. The investigators interrupted the use of the Style 510 implant for primary breast augmentations. Baeke[50] described his experience with anatomic saline implants in both the subglandular and submuscular positions. He predicted the risk of malrotation to be at least 14% in this sample (**Box 5**).

To avoid implant rotation and to ensure implant stability, it is important to create a tight pocket; this can be accomplished by using the exact dimensions of the implant's width and height, which aids in avoiding implant movement and/or displacement.[48] The pocket should be adjusted to the implant size, and if an implant has insufficient volume compared with the volume of the pocket, rotation occurs. If necessary, the pocket may be adjusted with some internal sutures to achieve an appropriate match between the implant and pocket volume (**Box 6**).

Box 5
Form-stable implants rotation/displacement causes

- No capsule adherence
- Large subfascial pocket (especially on the lateral pole)
- Seroma, hematoma
- Double capsule
- Postoperative massage/physical exercises
- Pseudosynovial metaplasia

SURGICAL PLANNING/TECHNIQUE

Patient Selection

Primary augmentation

Adequate patient selection during the preoperative appraisal is crucial for achieving satisfactory outcomes. Ideal candidates are those with significant hypomastia/amastia, lack of or minimal ptosis, and a minimally defined inframammary fold. The technique is also more indicated for patients with a small nipple-areolar complex (ie, patients who are not candidates for periareolar augmentation) and for those who are especially opposed to visible scarring on the breast. Because the inframammary crease can be accurately lowered, small degrees of ptosis can be treated during TBA by extended dissection of the pectoral fascia. A pinch test result of less than 2 cm is considered a relative contraindication to subfascial placement and an indication for submuscular placement. The form-stable structure of anatomic implants is particularly advantageous for patients with deficient lower breast poles and short areola-to-fold distance. Patient preference regarding shape in the upper pole (in other words, more natural appearance) can also be considered for TBA using the present technique (**Box 7**).

Box 6
Surgical procedures to avoid form-stable implant displacement/rotation after TBA

- Subfascial plane
- Implant superior edge limitation with muscular-fascia system
- Tight and precise subfascial pocket
- Postoperative immobilization
- No physical activities and massage
- Elastic band/strap over the superior pole (4 weeks)

Preoperative Evaluation/Implant Selection

Before surgery, with the patient sitting and her arms at her sides, the skin marks are drawn: current inframammary sulcus, anterior axillary line, the limits of the pocket, and the future inframammary fold. This marking allows accurate centering of the implant. Slight pressure is applied with the hand on top of the gland to mark the inferior limit of the pocket. For small implants (less than 250 mL), the new inframammary fold is located 0.5 to 1 cm below, and for large implants (more than 305 mL), 1.5 to 2 cm may be necessary to achieve a satisfactory position (**Figs. 5** and **6**). To mark the medial limit of the pocket, slight pressure is applied on the gland while taking it medially until the border is seen; then it is marked. The superior limit of the pocket depends on the diameter of the implant. The axillary incision is marked with the patient's arms raised. Usually the deepest natural fold is chosen, with the incision placed along the fold. For small implants, 2 to 2.5 cm is adequate; for large implants, a length of 3.5 to 4.5 cm is necessary. It is important to maintain the incision within the limits of the axilla, never crossing outside the lateral edge of the pectoralis major muscle (**Fig. 7**).

Implant size is chosen together with the patient, considering factors such as height and weight, thoracic cage, degree of ptosis, and thickness of subcutaneous tissue in the upper and the lower pole. Breast and thoracic cage asymmetries are identified, incorporated into the preoperative design, and corrected as much as possible. The limits of the dissection are delineated, depending on breast anatomy of the breast and size of the implant.

Box 7
Subfascial TBA and form-stable implants

- Severe hypomastia/amastia
- Thin patients (body mass index <20)
- Less upper pole coverage
- Pinch test result of greater than 2 cm
- Deficient lower breast pole/short areola-to-fold distance
- Insufficient breast base
- Paucity of skin in the lower pole
- Inframammary fold

Patient selection: primary augmentation.

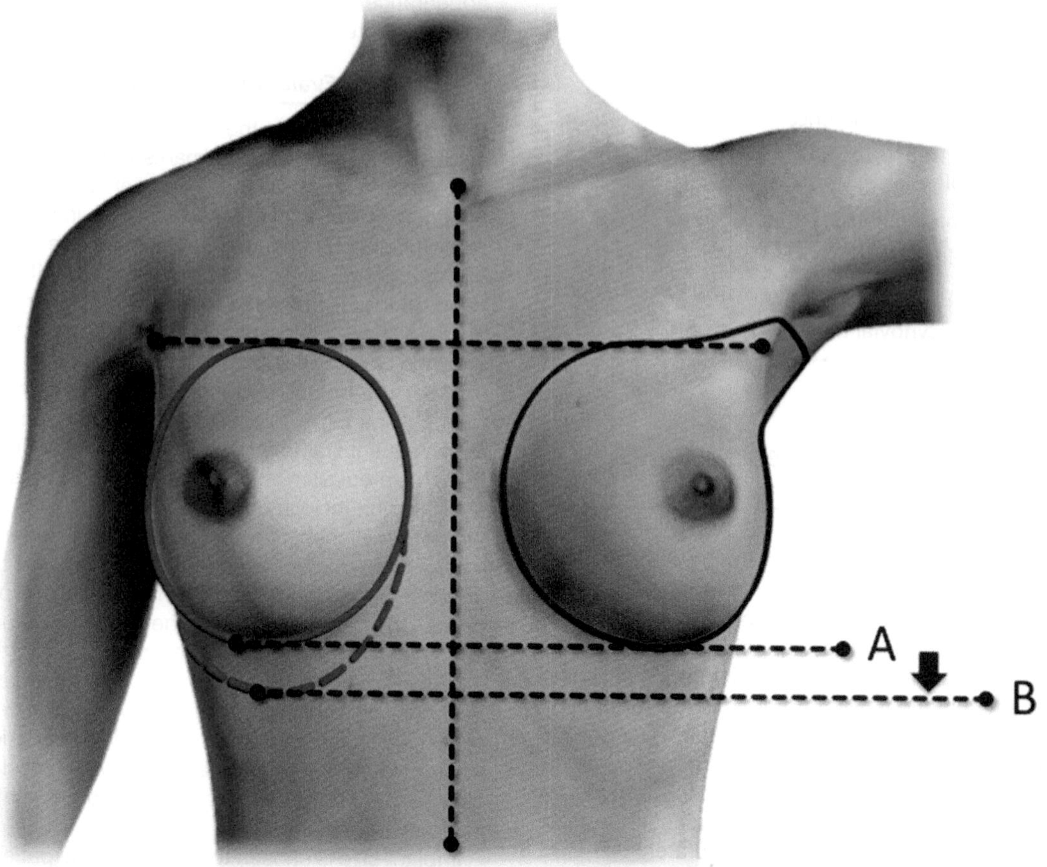

Fig. 5. Preoperative planning. With the patient sitting and her arms placed at her sides, the skin marks are drawn: current inframammary sulcus (*A*), anterior axillary line, the limits of the pocket, and future inframammary fold (*B*). For small implants (less than 250 mL), the new inframammary fold is located 0.5 to 1 cm below, and for large implants (more than 305 mL), 1.5 to 2 cm may be necessary to achieve a satisfactory position.

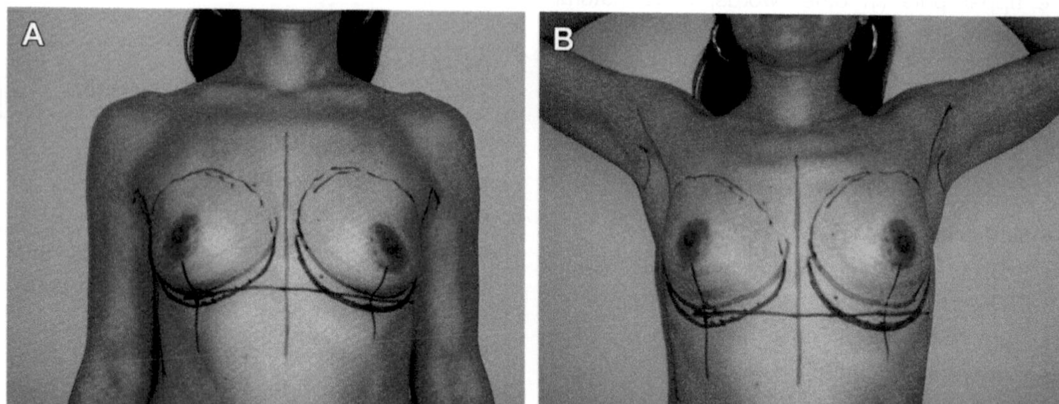

Fig. 6. (*A*, *B*) Preoperative view of a 29-year-old patient with symmetric hypomastia. Preoperative skin marks are drawn: current inframammary sulcus, anterior axillary line, the limits of the pocket, and future inframammary fold.

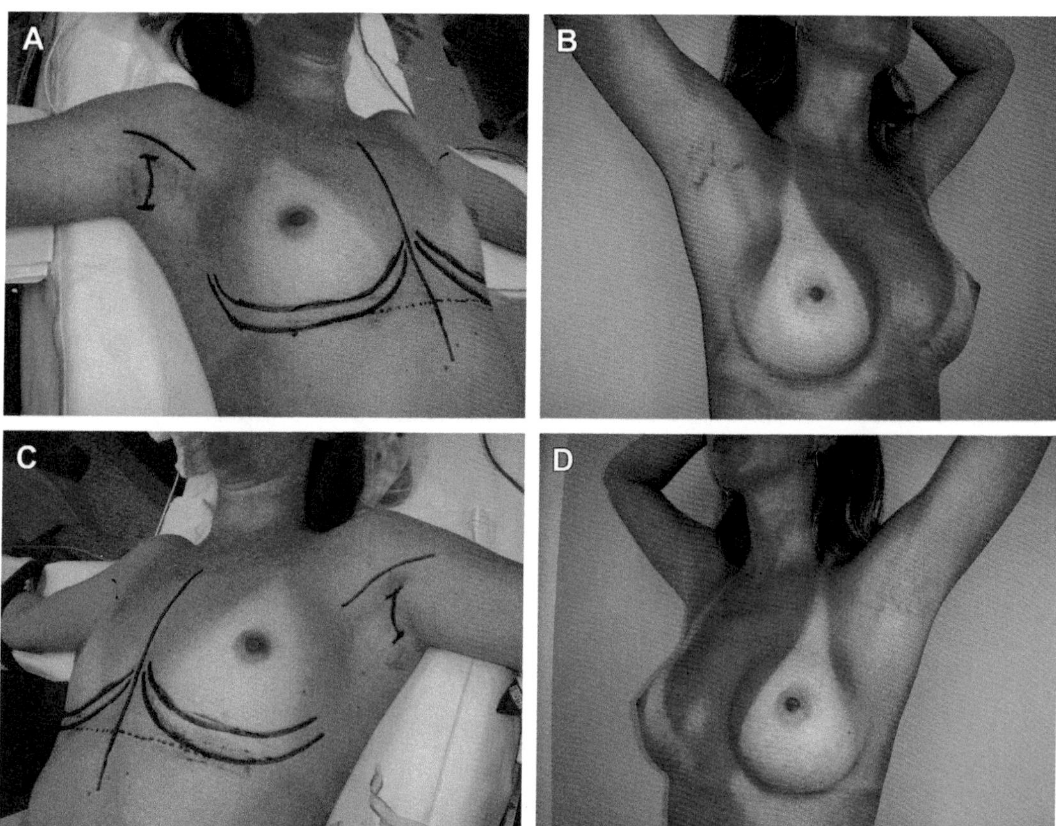

Fig. 7. (*A, B*) Preoperative view of axillary incision. The incision is marked with the patient under general anesthesia and the arms abducted at 90°. Usually the deepest natural fold is chosen, and the incision is placed along the fold. (*C, D*) Postoperative (1 year) view of the same clinical case. It is important to maintain the incision within the limits of the axilla, never crossing outside the lateral edge of the pectoralis major muscle.

Surgical Technique

Subfascial transaxillary approach for breast augmentation dissection

The operative procedure begins with the patient under general anesthesia. With the patient's arms abducted at 90°, an incision is made and the superficial fascia of the pectoralis muscle is identified and opened. The initial dissection is performed parallel to the skin for approximately 2 to 4 cm until the lateral border of the pectoralis muscle. The fascia is identified and then incised radially (perpendicular to the skin incision) and vertically until the pectoralis muscle is reached. Dissection of the implant pocket is then performed in the well-defined subfascial plane using electrocautery with cauterization of the main perforators. With the aid of customized retractors, subfascial dissection continues on the pectoralis muscle beneath the fascia, moving toward the upper, medial, and lateral breast pole. Usually, sharp cautery dissection is used under direct visualization to release the pectoral fascia from the 11-o'clock to the 4-o'clock position. To do so, the dissection is started in the upper-medial breast pole and progressively moved toward the intermediate pole in the lateral direction up to the lateral-inferior breast quadrants, in a staged release of the subfascial pocket. At this stage, it is important to avoid long dissections and the formation of long tunnels (**Fig. 8**). The glandular tissue is lifted away from the chest, consequently elevating the gland and muscular fascia, facilitating the passage between them and the retractors. The attachments between the fascia and the skin at level of the fold must be disrupted to avoid deformities such as high-riding implants and double-bubble contours in the lower breast. The boundaries of the pocket and the new inframammary fold are checked with the use of dissectors and enlarged if necessary (**Fig. 9**). Undermining should not extend laterally beyond the lateral breast border because of innervation of the nipple areola complex and to avoid implant displacement after surgery. Medially, the dissection then proceeds laterally

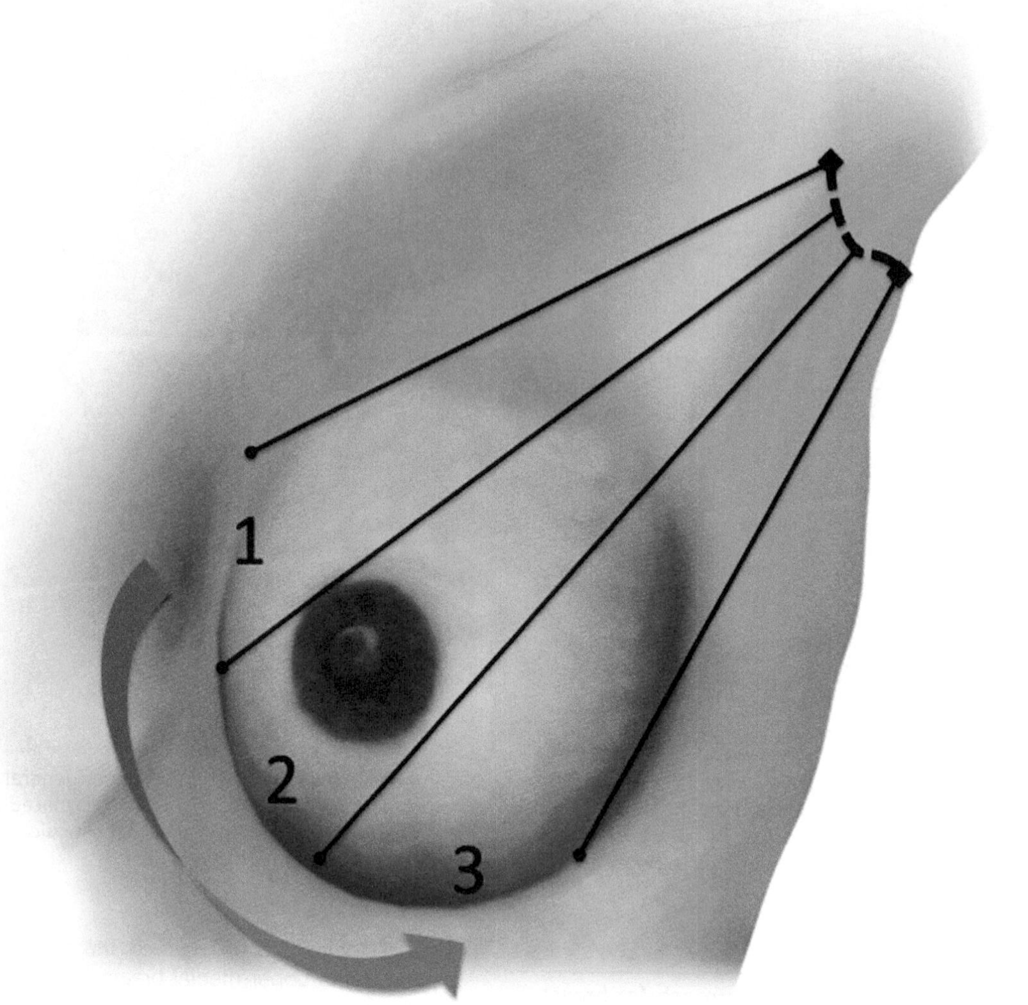

Fig. 8. Intraoperative staged release of subfascial pocket. Usually, sharp cautery dissection is used under direct visualization to release the pectoral fascia from the 11-o'clock to the 4-o'clock position, upper-medial to inferior-lateral pole of the breast.

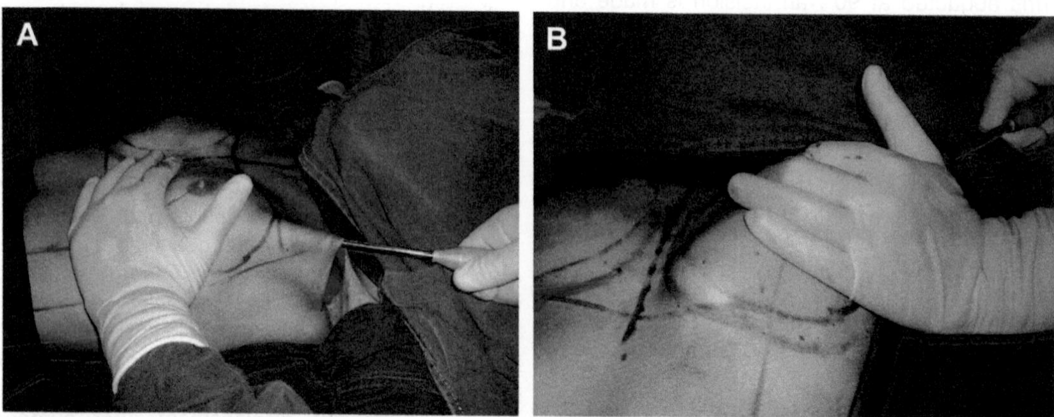

Fig. 9. (*A*, *B*) Intraoperative view. The boundaries of the pocket and the new inframammary fold are checked with the use of the dissectors, and enlarged if necessary.

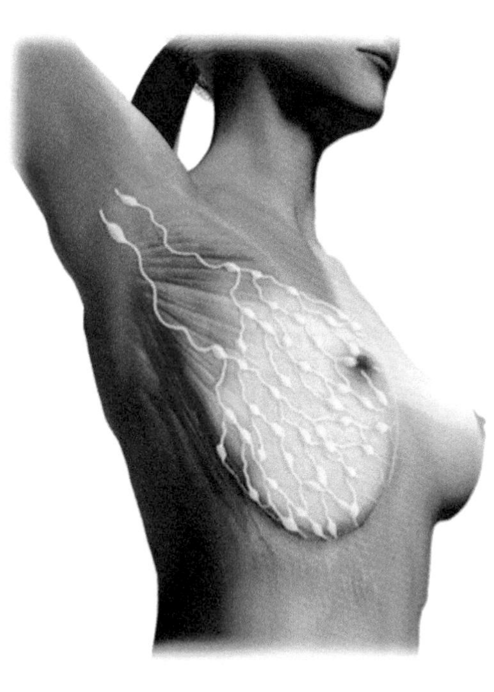

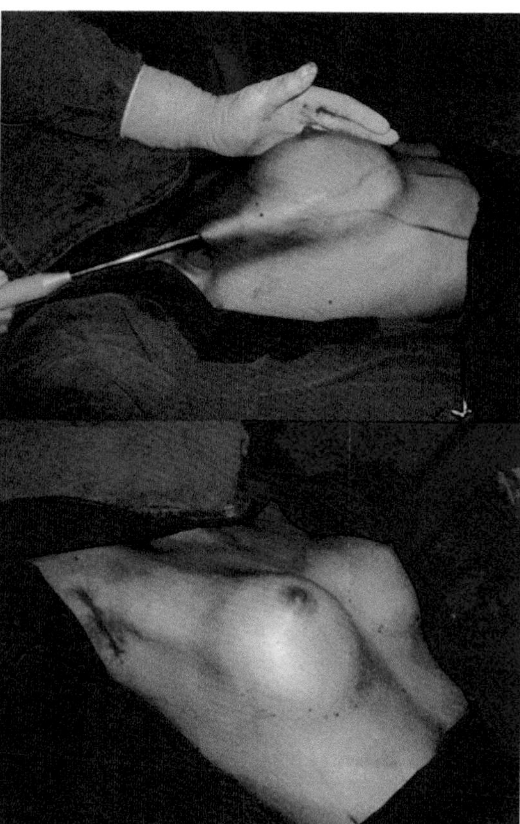

Fig. 10. Intraoperative dissection of the lateral pole of the breast and lymphatic channels. Laterally, dissection should be limited to the anterior axillary line to avoid lateral displacement of the implant and injury to the lateral cutaneous nerves and the lymphatic channels.

approximately 1 to 2 cm to the sternal border, depending on the preoperative markings. Lateral dissection should be limited to the anterior axillary line to avoid lateral displacement of the implant, and to avoid injury to the lateral cutaneous nerves and lymphatic channels, the lateral aspect of the pocket dissection should also be minimized (**Fig. 10**).[10,15] Before implant insertion and following meticulous hemostasis, the pocket is irrigated with antibiotic solution (80 mg gentamicin + 500 mg cephazolin + 500 mL saline). The silicon form-stable gel implants are placed in the

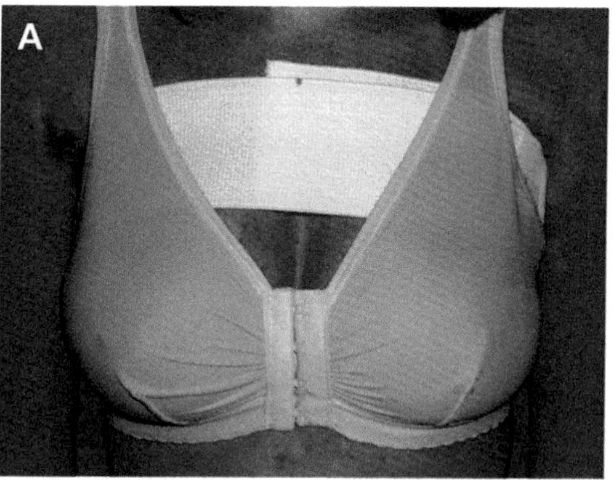

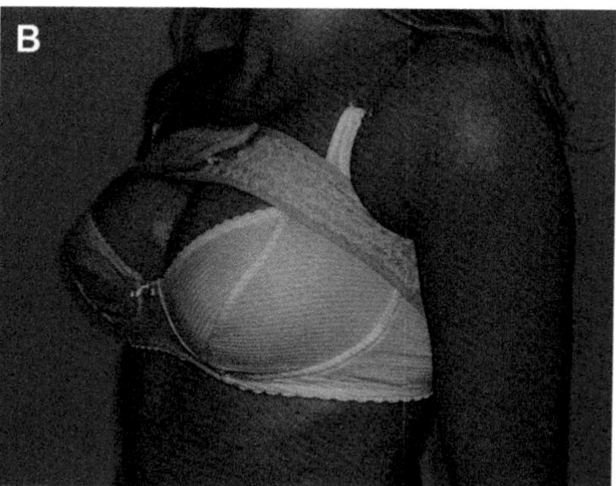

Fig. 11. (*A*, *B*) Postoperative view. An elastic band or strap should be used over the superior poles of the breasts for 4 weeks to avoid superior displacement of the implants, maintaining the newly created inframammary fold in the appropriate position.

subfascial location, and the patient is positioned upright to assess implant position and breast shape. Layered wound closure is done using nonabsorbable sutures in the pectoral fascia, subcutaneous and subdermal planes, and absorbable subcuticular running sutures. No suction drains are used. At the end of the surgery, an elastic band is used over the superior breast poles to avoid superior displacement of the implants.

Postoperative Care

All patients receive intravenous antibiotics, and oral antibiotics are continued for 48 hours. An

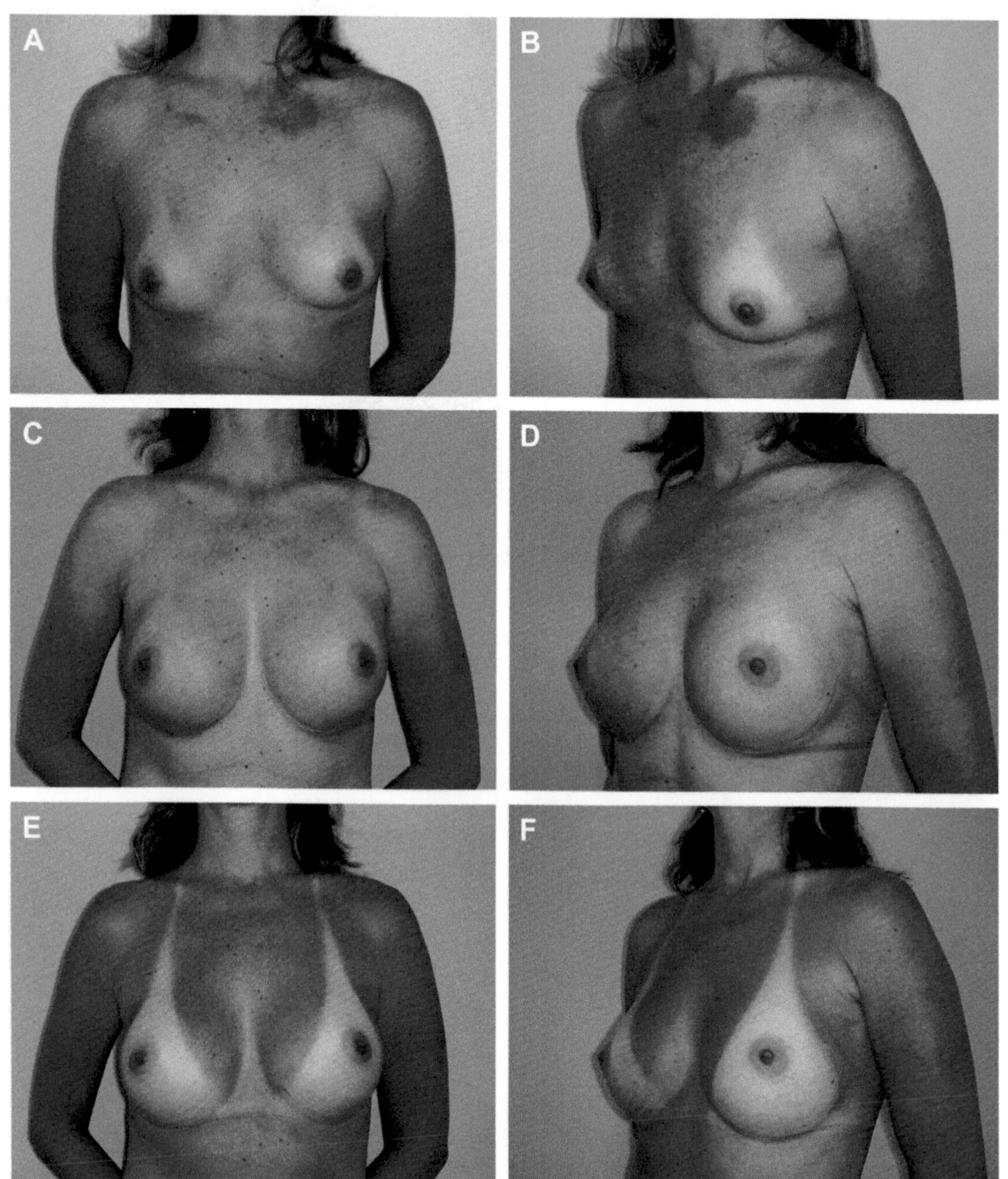

Fig. 12. (*A*, *B*) Preoperative frontal and left oblique view of a 31-year-old patient with hypoplastic breasts with an asymmetrical inframammary fold position. (*C*, *D*) Three months postoperative appearance with very good outcome. Bilateral 255-mL Natrelle Style 410 MF implants were used. (*E*, *F*) Four years postoperative appearance with good symmetry and projection.

elastic band or strap should be used over the superior poles of the breasts for 4 weeks to avoid superior displacement of the implants and keep the newly created inframammary fold in the appropriate position (**Fig. 11**). Care must be taken to obtain adequate adherence between the soft tissues and form-stable implant. Consequently, early massaging or mobilization of the breasts (which may lead to accumulation of liquid around the implants) should be avoided for at least 3 weeks. It is important to avoid physical activities for some time (usually 6 weeks) to reduce the risk of implant rotation, displacement, and seroma.

Results

Results following TBA with form-stable implants have been satisfactory with maintenance of a natural breast shape. Complications and surgical revisions have been rare. All these complications were minor, predictable, and did not affect the final aesthetic outcome. The results verified that most complications occur in the initial postoperative period and are directly related to the axillary incision. Axillary upper-inner arm subcutaneous banding was observed in 10% of the patients, representing almost 35% of total complications. According to Young and Bindrup,[52] transient axillary subcutaneous banding after TBA may be attributed to local inflammation of the cutaneous nerves. Other researchers have attributed banding to possibly sclerosed lymphatic channels or to local thrombophlebitis.[53–55] In the authors' sample, the patients were instructed to perform a local massage with satisfactory results after some weeks. Contrary to the suggestion by Young and Bindrup,[52] the authors do not advocate early arm stretching maneuvers to avoid implant displacement and rotation.

Transient sensory loss of the inner aspect of the arm was observed in 5% of patients, all of whom achieved total recovery within 3 to 4 months after the procedure. In fact, intercostobrachial nerve damage has been reported as a potential complication of the TBA technique.[56,57] Previous clinical studies noted a 1% to 24% incidence of sensory loss in patients; however, the true incidence of intercostobrachial injury is not defined.[57] Similar to the method proposed by Tebbetts,[18] the authors did not dissect near the nerve, and the axillary fat was always preserved. The subcutaneous tissue was undermined parallel to the skin and superficially to the axillary fat as far as the lateral aspect of the pectoralis muscle to avoid nerve injury. Despite the transient paresthesias observed, and the technique used (similar to Tebbetts), the authors believe that with meticulous axillary dissection, the incidence of nerve injury may decrease.

Implant displacement and major complications were not observed. At the time of this writing, most patients were either very satisfied or satisfied with their results. The final results were generally good, and a soft transition between the

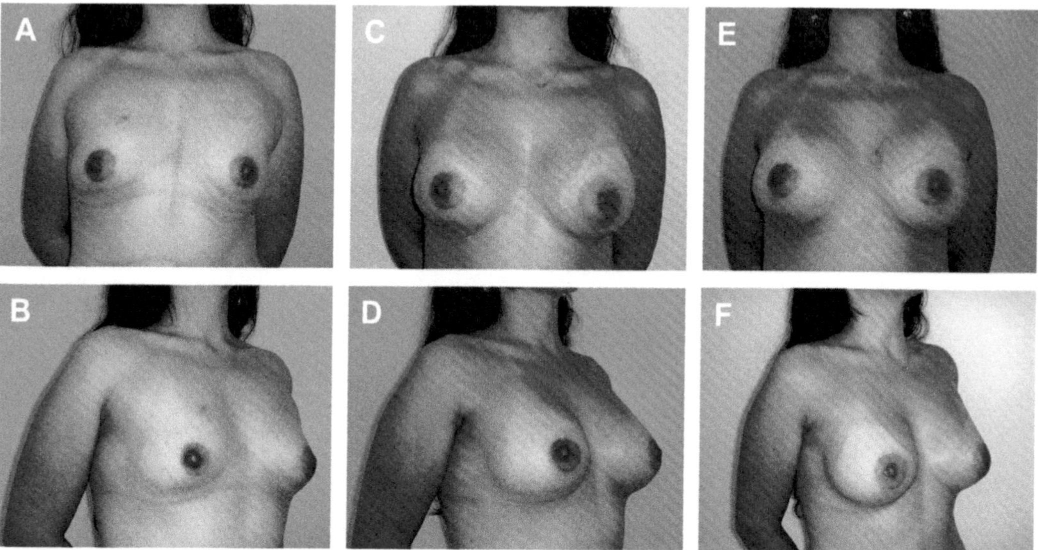

Fig. 13. (*A, B*) Preoperative frontal and right oblique view of a 27-year-old patient with hypoplastic breasts with deficient lower breast poles and short areola-to-fold distance. (*C, D*) Two months postoperative appearance with very good outcome. Bilateral 290-mL Natrelle Style 410 MX implants were. (*E, F*) Five years postoperative appearance with good symmetry and projection.

subcutaneous tissue and implant edge was observed in all cases. At this time, no capsular contraction has been observed; however, a larger number of patients and longer follow-up period are necessary to draw significant conclusions. Examples of clinical results are illustrated in **Figs. 12–16**.

SUMMARY

Recent progress in surgical techniques and form-stable implants has led to important improvements in aesthetic outcomes after breast augmentation. The authors feel that subfascial TBA can play a useful role in breast augmentation, and their

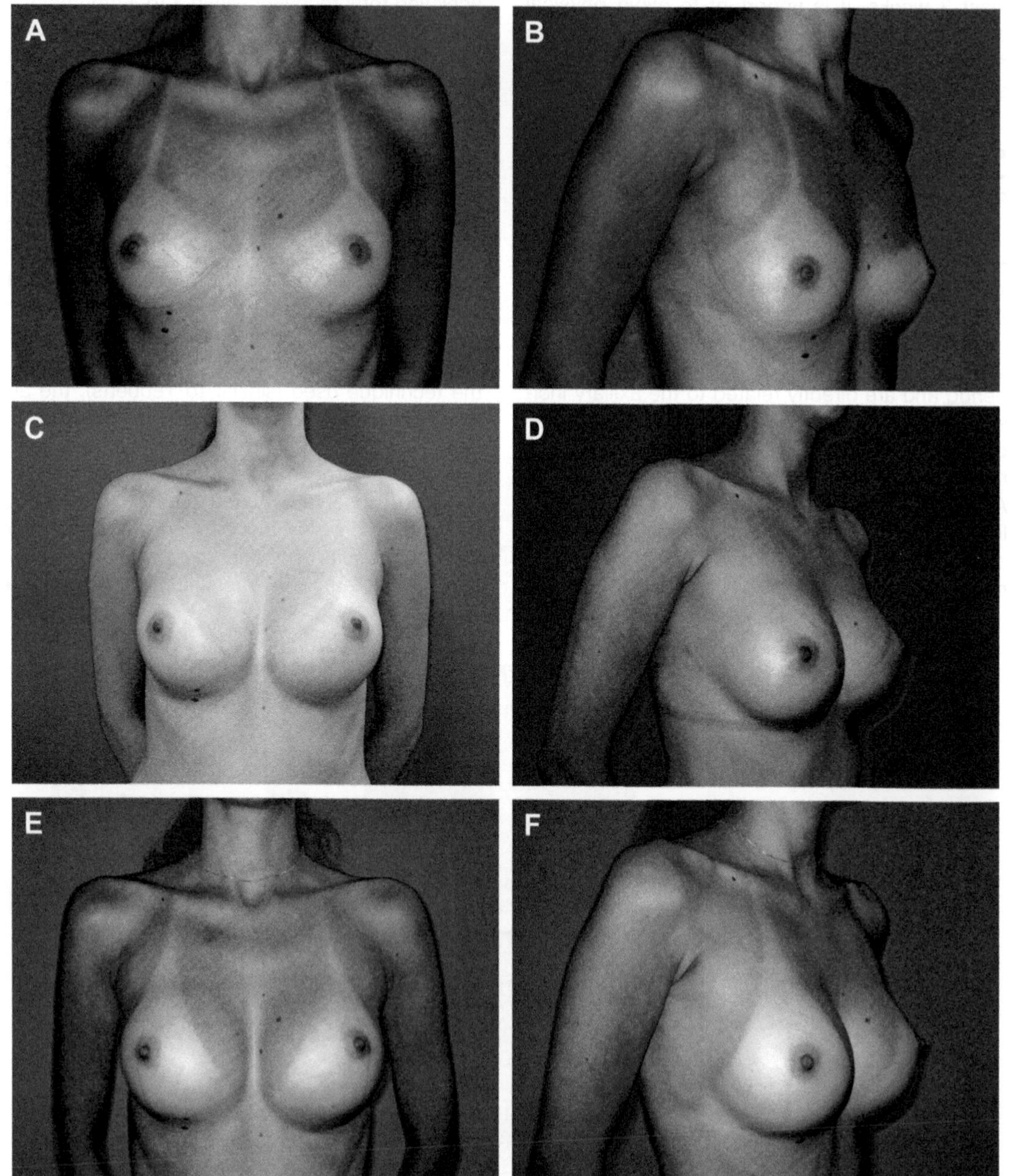

Fig. 14. (*A, B*) Preoperative frontal and right oblique view of a 19-year-old patient with symmetric hypoplastic breasts and a minimally defined inframammary fold. (*C, D*) Five months postoperative appearance with very good outcome. Bilateral 225-mL Natrelle Style 410 MF implants were used. (*E, F*) Six years postoperative appearance with good symmetry and projection.

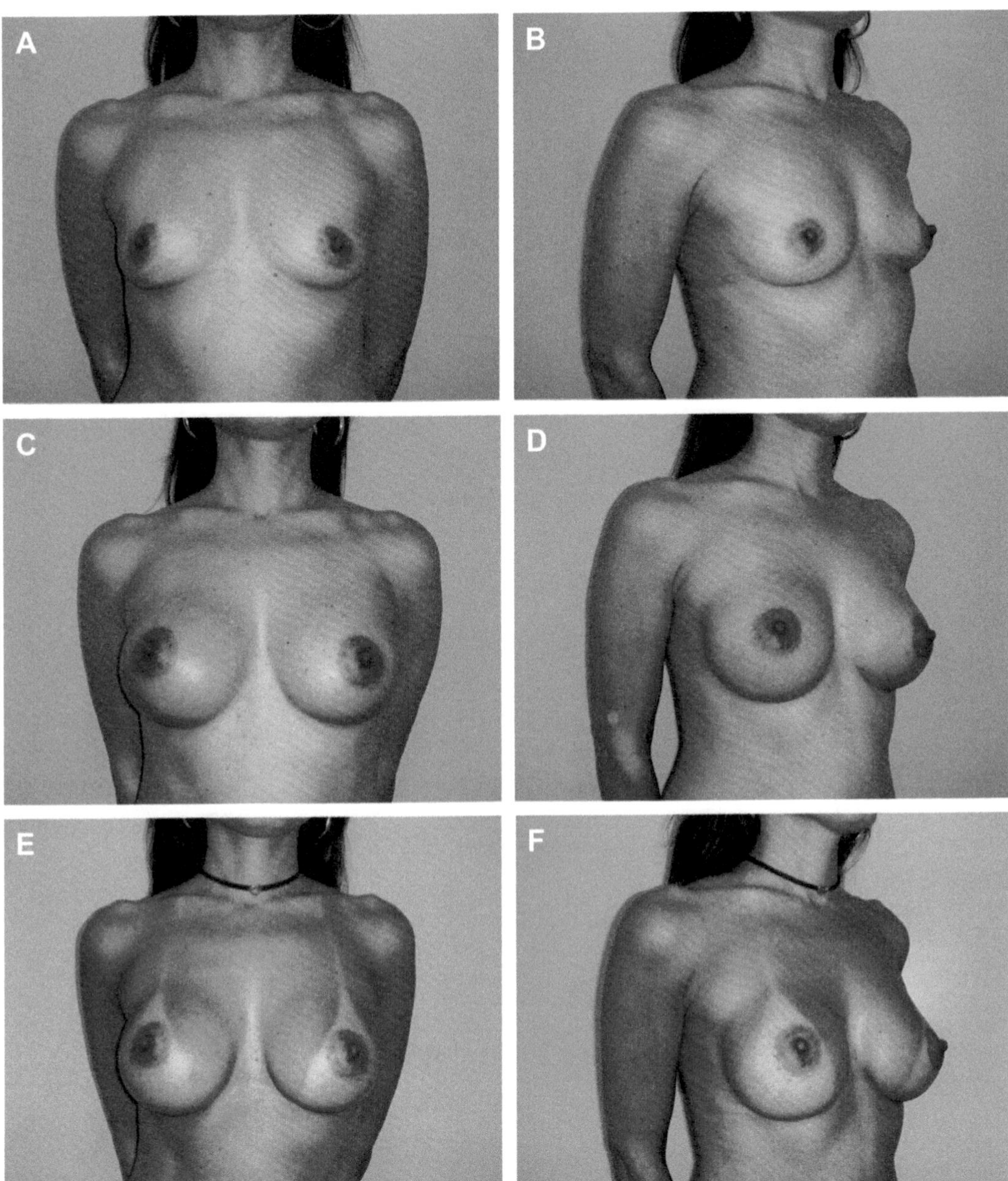

Fig. 15. (*A, B*) Preoperative frontal and right oblique view of a 30-year-old patient with symmetric hypoplastic breasts. (*C, D*) Two months postoperative appearance with a very good outcome. Bilateral 295-mL Natrelle Style 410 MF implants were used. (*E, F*) Six years postoperative appearance with good symmetry and projection.

results demonstrate that it is a simple and reproducible technique; nevertheless, important technical steps must be planned before the procedure. Preoperative patient evaluation is crucial to determine the size of the implant, the dimensions of the implant pocket, and the future inframammary fold. The success of this technique depends on patient selection, adequate technique, and careful postoperative management. The ideal aesthetic result must provide natural contours and achieve adequate size and projection. Because the final scar in located in the axilla, thus avoiding visible signs of surgery in the breast region, TBA provides outstanding aesthetic results. With the help of customized retractors, the surgeon can meticulously dissect the subfascial implant pocket, resulting in adequate control over bleeding and form-stable implant placement

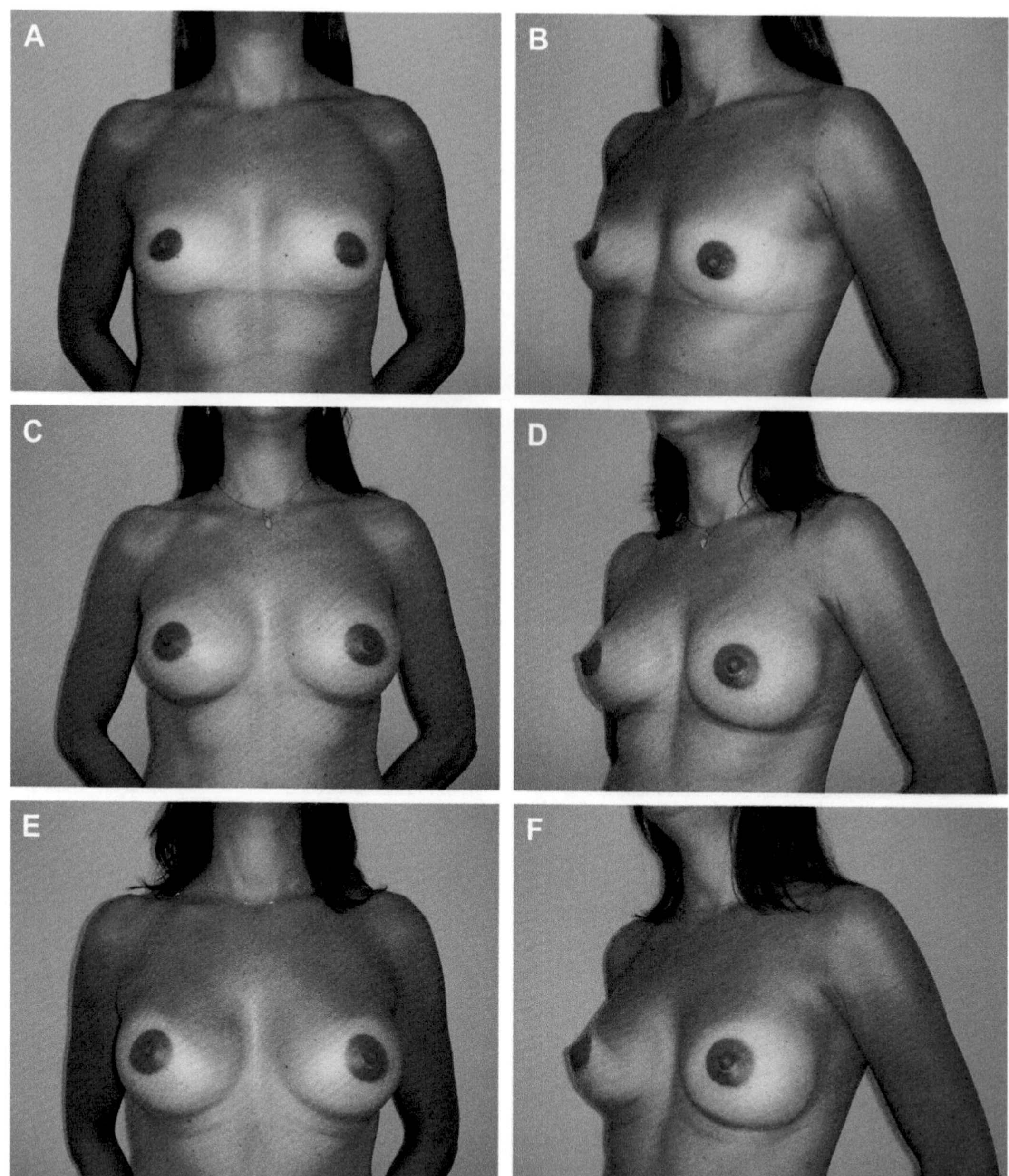

Fig. 16. (*A*, *B*) Preoperative frontal and left oblique view of a 35-year-old patient with symmetric hypoplastic breasts and a minimally defined inframammary fold. (*C*, *D*) Four months postoperative appearance with very good outcome. Bilateral 325-mL Natrelle Style 410 MF implants were used. (*E*, *F*) Two years postoperative appearance with good symmetry and projection.

and positioning. Regardless of the aesthetic benefits in terms of incision location, the association of TBA and form-stable breast implants in primary breast augmentation presents some limitations. The need for previous training and surgical skills are the main drawbacks. Although TBA requires a longer learning curve, with adequate training, the present technique can take approximately the same time to perform as augmentation through other incisions. Therefore, it has been our experience that the technique and the outcomes of TBA with form-stable implants are now comparable to those using the inframammary and periareolar approaches.

Editorial Comments by Bradley P. Bengtson, MD

In Dr Goes second chapter, he describes the subfascial placement of the implant through a Transaxillary Approach. In the US Style 410 Highly Cohesive Silicone Gel Core Study approximately 87% of devices were placed through the inframammay fold with only 0.4% of patients having their devices placed through the axilla. With new techniques and technology such as funnels and sleeves this approach may be facilitated although in my limited experience the incision may need to be placed slightly lower in the axilla and longer depending on the implant size.

REFERENCES

1. American Society of Plastic Surgeons. 2013 cosmetic plastic surgery statistics. Available at: http://www.plasticsurgery.org/news/plastic-surgery-statistics/2013.html. Accessed May 8, 2014.
2. Spear SL, Bulan EJ, Venturi ML. Breast augmentation. Plast Reconstr Surg 2004;114:73–81.
3. Lista F, Ahmad J. Evidence-based medicine: augmentation mammaplasty. Plast Reconstr Surg 2013;132(6):1684–96.
4. Adams WP Jr, Mallucci P. Breast augmentation. Plast Reconstr Surg 2012;130:597e–611e.
5. Hoehler H. Breast augmentation: the axillary approach. Br J Plast Surg 1973;26:373–7.
6. Wright JH, Bevin AG. Augmentation mammaplasty by the transaxillary approach. Plast Reconstr Surg 1976;58:429.
7. Tebbetts JB. Transaxillary subpectoral augmentation mammaplasty: long-term follow-up and refinements. Plast Reconstr Surg 1984;74:636.
8. Smith JW, Shaw LW, Friedland JA. Endoscopic transaxillary subpectoral augmentation mammaplasty: a comparative analysis of endoscopic versus non-endoscopic transaxillary subpectoral augmentation mammaplasty using smooth saline implants. Plast Surg Forum 1998;21:127.
9. Pacella SJ, Codner MA. The transaxillary approach to breast augmentation. Clin Plast Surg 2009;36(1):49–61.
10. Munhoz AM, Fells K, Arruda EG, et al. Subfascial transaxillary breast augmentation without endoscopic assistance: technical aspects and outcome. Aesthetic Plast Surg 2006;30:503–12.
11. Serra-Renom J, Garrido MF, Yoon T. Augmentation mammaplasty with anatomic soft, cohesive silicone implant using the transaxillary approach at a subfascial level with endoscopic assistance. Plast Reconstr Surg 2006;116:640–50.
12. Graf RM, Bernardes A, Auersvald A, et al. Subfascial endoscopic transaxillary augmentation mammaplasty. Aesthetic Plast Surg 2000;24:216–22.
13. Aygit AC, Basaran K, Mercan ES. Transaxillary totally subfascial breast augmentation with anatomical breast implants: review of 27 cases. Plast Reconstr Surg 2013;131(5):1149–56.
14. Sim HB. Transaxillary endoscopic breast augmentation. Arch Plast Surg 2014;41(5):458–65.
15. Niechajev I. Improvements in transaxillary breast augmentation. Aesthetic Plast Surg 2010;34(3):322–9.
16. Momeni A, Padron NT, Bannasch H, et al. Endoscopic transaxillary subpectoral augmentation mammaplasty: a safe and predictable procedure. J Plast Reconstr Aesthet Surg 2006;59(10):1076–81.
17. Handel N, Cordray T, Gutierrez J, et al. A long-term study of outcomes, complications, and patient satisfaction with breast implants. Plast Reconstr Surg 2006;117:757–67.
18. Tebbetts JB. Dual plane breast augmentation: optimizing implant–soft-tissue relationships in a wide range of breast types. Plast Reconstr Surg 2001;107:1255–61.
19. Vazquez B, Given KS, Houston GC. Breast augmentation: a review of subglandular and submuscular implantation. Aesthetic Plast Surg 2007;11:101–5.
20. Ramirez OM, Heller L, Tebbetts JB. Dual-plane breast augmentation: avoiding pectoralis major displacement. Plast Reconstr Surg 2002;110:1198–2003.
21. Spear SL, Schwartz J, Dayan JH, et al. Outcome assessment of breast distortion following submuscular breast augmentation. Aesthetic Plast Surg 2009;33:44–8.
22. Graf RM, Bernardes A, Rippel R, et al. Subfascial breast implant: a new procedure. Plast Reconstr Surg 2003;111:904–11.
23. Goes JC, Landecker A. Optimizing outcomes in breast augmentation: seven years of experience with the subfascial plane. Aesthetic Plast Surg 2003;27:178–86.
24. Jinde L, Jianliang S, Xiaoping C, et al. Anatomy and clinical significance of pectoral fascia. Plast Reconstr Surg 2006;118:1160–557.
25. Benito-Ruiz J. Subfascial breast implant. Plast Reconstr Surg 2004;113:1088–91.
26. Stoff-Khalili MA, Scholze R, Morgan WR, et al. Subfascial periareolar augmentation mammaplasty. Plast Reconstr Surg 2004;114:1280–9.
27. Ventura OD, Marcello GA. Anatomic and physiologic advantages of totally subfascial breast implants. Aesthetic Plast Surg 2005;29(5):379–83.
28. Hunstad JP, Webb LS. Subfascial breast augmentation: a comprehensive experience. Aesthetic Plast Surg 2010;34(3):365–73.
29. Tijerina VN, Saenz RA, Garcia-Guerrero J. Experience of 1000 cases on subfascial breast augmentation. Aesthetic Plast Surg 2010;34(1):16–22.

30. Heitmann C, Schreckenberger C, Olbrisch RR. A silicone implant filled with cohesive gel: advantages and disadvantages. Eur J Plast Surg 1998;21:329–32.
31. Bogetti P, Boltri M, Balocco P, et al. Augmentation mammaplasty with a new cohesive gel prosthesis. Aesthetic Plast Surg 2000;24:440–4.
32. Heden P, Jernbeck J, Hober M. Breast augmentation with anatomical cohesive gel implants. Clin Plast Surg 2001;28:531–2.
33. Brown MH, Shenker R, Silver SA. Cohesive silicone gel breast implants in aesthetic and reconstructive breast surgery. Plast Reconstr Surg 2005;116:768–79.
34. Hedén P, Boné B, Murphy DK, et al. Style 410 cohesive silicone breast implants: safety and effectiveness at 5 to 9 years after implantation. Plast Reconstr Surg 2006;118:1281–7.
35. Hedén P, Bronz G, Elberg JJ, et al. Long-term safety and effectiveness of Style 410 highly cohesive silicone breast implants. Aesthetic Plast Surg 2009;33:430–6.
36. Bengtson BP, Van Natta BW, Murphy DK, et al, Style 410 U.S. Core Clinical Study Group. Style 410 highly cohesive silicone breast implant core study results at 3 years. Plast Reconstr Surg 2007;120(7 Suppl 1):40S–8S.
37. Maxwell GP, Van Natta BW, Murphy DK, et al. Natrelle Style 410 form-stable silicone breast implants: core study results at 6 years. Aesthet Surg J 2012; 32:709–17.
38. Lista F, Tutino R, Khan A, et al. Subglandular breast augmentation with textured, anatomic, cohesive silicone implants: a review of 440 consecutive patients. Plast Reconstr Surg 2013;132(2):295–303.
39. Ho LC. Endoscopic assisted transaxillary augmentation mammaplasty. Br J Plast Surg 1993;46:332–6.
40. Tebbetts JB. Does fascia provide additional meaningful coverage over a breast implant? Plast Reconstr Surg 2004;113:777–82.
41. Hidalgo DA. Breast augmentation: choosing the optimal incision, implant, and pocket plane. Plast Reconstr Surg 2000;105:2202–10.
42. Krag D, Weaver D, Ashikaga T, et al. The sentinel node in breast cancer - a multicenter validation study. N Engl J Med 1998;339:941.
43. Huang GJ, Hardesty RA, Mills D. Sentinel lymph node biopsy in the augmented breast: role of the transaxillary subpectoral approach. Aesthet Surg J 2003;23:184.
44. Gray RJ, Forstner-Barthell AW, Pockaj BA, et al. Breast-conserving therapy and sentinel lymph node biopsy are feasible in cancer patients with previous implant breast augmentation. Am J Surg 2004;188:122.
45. Munhoz AM, Aldrighi C, Buschpiegel C, et al. The feasibility of sentinel lymph node detection in patients with previous transaxillary implant breast augmentation: preliminary results. Aesthetic Plast Surg 2005;29:163.
46. Munhoz AM, Aldrighi CM, Aldrighi JM. Could the way of approaching the implantation of silicone breast prostheses alter the investigation of the sentinel lymph node in eventual cancer of the breast? Rev Assoc Med Bras 2005;51(5):244–5.
47. Munhoz AM, Aldrighi C, Ono C, et al. The influence of subfascial transaxillary breast augmentation in axillary lymphatic drainage patterns and sentinel lymph node detection. Ann Plast Surg 2007;58(2): 141–9.
48. Góes JC. Breast implant stability in the subfascial plane and the new shaped silicone gel breast implants. Aesthetic Plast Surg 2010;34(1):23–8.
49. Panchapakesan V, Brown MH. Management of tuberous breast deformity with anatomic cohesive silicone gel breast implants. Aesthetic Plast Surg 2009;33(1):49–53.
50. Baeke JL. Breast deformity caused by anatomical or teardrop implant rotation. Plast Reconstr Surg 2002; 109:2555–64 [discussion: 2568].
51. Schots JM, Fechner MR, Hoogbergen MM, et al. Malrotation of the McGhan Style 510 prosthesis. Plast Reconstr Surg 2010;126:261–5.
52. Young RV, Bindrup JR. Transaxillary submuscular augmentation and subcutaneous fibrous bands. Plast Reconstr Surg 1997;99:257.
53. Maximovich SP. Fibrous bands following subpectoral endoscopic breast augmentation. Plast Reconstr Surg 1996;97:1304.
54. Laufer E. Fibrous bands following subpectoral endoscopic breast augmentation. Plast Reconstr Surg 1997;99:257.
55. Dowden RV. Subcutaneous fibrous banding after transaxillary subpectoral endoscopic breast augmentation. Plast Reconstr Surg 1997;99:257.
56. Ghaderl B, Hoenig JM, Dado D, et al. Incidence of intercostobrachial nerve injury after transaxillary breast augmentation. Aesthet Surg J 2002;22:26.
57. Temple WJ, Ketcham AS. Preservation of the intercostobrachial nerve during axillary dissection for breast cancer. Am Surg 1985;150:585.

Surgical Approaches to Breast Augmentation

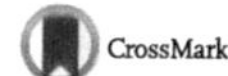

The Transaxillary Approach

Louis L. Strock, MD*

KEYWORDS

• Transaxillary breast augmentation • Transaxillary endoscopic breast augmentation
• Endoscopic breast augmentation • Breast implants • Breast augmentation

KEY POINTS

- The transaxillary approach to breast augmentation has the advantage of allowing breast implants to be placed with no incisions on the breasts.
- The approach has been criticized because of a general perception of a lack of technical control compared with the more widely favored inframammary approach.
- This article presents the transaxillary approach from the perspective of the technical control gained with the aid of an endoscope, which allows precise creation of the tissue pocket with optimal visualization.
- The components and aspects of technique that allow optimal technical control are covered in detail, in addition to postoperative processes that aid in stabilizing the device position and allow consistent and predictable outcomes.

Video of a transaxillary endoscopic breast augmentation procedure, with moderate-plus profile, smooth-wall silicone gel implants (325 mL) and partial subpectoral tissue pocket, accompanies this article at http://www.plasticsurgery.theclinics.com/

The transaxillary approach to breast augmentation has the appeal of allowing breast implants to be placed with no incisions on the breast. However, the technique has met with long-standing resistance among plastic surgeons because of a perceived lack of technical control compared with the more universally accepted inframammary approach. This resistance is likely the result of the earliest reports of the technique that relied on blunt dissection performed in a largely blind fashion.[1,2] There have been recent reports, however, that suggest this to be a reliable technique in large, single-surgeon experiences with long-term follow-up.[3,4] In addition, higher patient satisfaction scores have been associated with use of the transaxillary incisions compared with visible-incision approaches, suggesting that this approach may warrant a more careful evaluation.[4,5]

The addition of endoscopic assistance, as reported by Price and colleagues[6] in 1994, allowed for direct tissue visualization and provided an improved level of technical control previously unseen with the transaxillary approach.[7] This series detailed the use of endoscopic assistance in the placement of saline implants in a partial subpectoral pocket, at a time when silicone gel breast implants were under restriction by the Food and Drug Administration in the United States. Strock[8–11] has

Disclosure: Consultant Mentor Worldwide (Johnson & Johnson); Investigator for Mentor CPG and Allergan 410 Studies.

Department of Plastic Surgery, UT Southwestern Medical Center, 5323 Harry Hines Boulevard, Dallas, TX 75390, USA
* Private Practice, 800 Eighth Avenue, Suite 606, Fort Worth, TX 76104, USA
E-mail address: llstrock@gmail.com

Clin Plastic Surg 42 (2015) 585–593
http://dx.doi.org/10.1016/j.cps.2015.06.014

reported on the technique of transaxillary placement of smooth silicone gel devices in a partial subpectoral pocket with endoscopic assistance. Additional reports from multiple investigators around the world have shown consistent and predictable outcomes with multiple device types through a transaxillary endoscopic approach.[12–15] The author outlines his current approach to transaxillary breast augmentation, with emphasis on technical refinements that provide consistent technical control with this approach.

PREOPERATIVE PLANNING

The incisions are marked preoperatively with the patient in a sitting position. The incision design and length differ depending on the type of device to be used. For saline devices, a 2.5-cm incision is made in an existing skin crease in the apex of the axilla. For silicone gel devices, a 5-cm incision is made, also centered in the axillary apex. The markings are started with a small mark made in the center of the axillary apex, in an existing skin crease. This mark is extended anteriorly toward the posterior aspect of the pectoralis major muscle, stopping just short of the posterior muscle border. From the initial mark in the center of the axillary apex, the incision is extended in a posterior direction, beveled superiorly, which allows the incision to not be visible when the patient stands with her hands on her waist[8,11,16] (**Fig. 1**A). Alternatively, a straight incision can occasionally be used when a small volume device is to be placed in a patient with a long skin fold in the axilla.

Additional markings focus on the inframammary fold, to define its preexisting level and shape, compared with the intended level and shape created during tissue pocket dissection and device placement. These markings are made with the patient in the sitting position preoperatively, and confirmed with the patient in the supine position at the start of the procedure. This method allows for a precise ability to confirm technical accuracy and symmetry intraoperatively following device placement[8] (see **Fig. 1**B).

PATIENT POSITIONING AND SETUP

Following the induction of general anesthesia, the patient is positioned supine with the arms out at 90° on secure arm boards. Quick-acting muscle relaxation is used for the procedure. The operating room bed is positioned with enough space in front of the anesthesia machine to allow the surgeon to conduct most of the procedure standing above the patient' shoulder on each side. The patient is then prepped and draped in a sterile fashion, and Tegaderm™ dressings are applied to cover the nipple areolar complexes before the start of the procedure.[17] All additional equipment, including the suction, cautery, and endoscopic tower, is positioned at the foot of the bed to allow free transition between the sides of the patient (**Fig. 2**A).

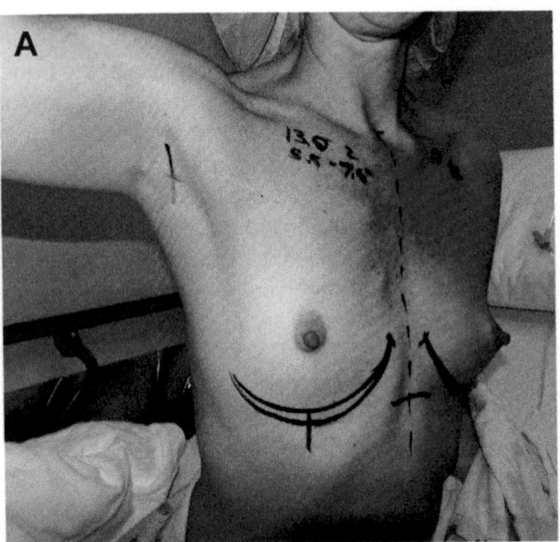

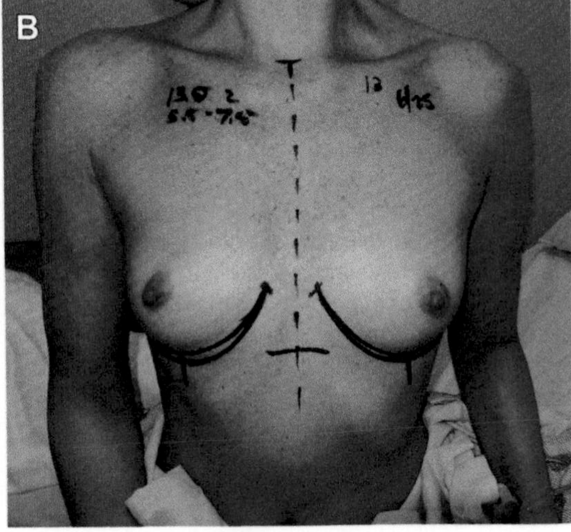

Fig. 1. (*A*) The incision markings are shown, starting with an initial mark at the axillary apex, with anterior extension placed to a point just behind the posterior pectoralis major border. The overall orientation of this segment is governed by an existing skin crease. The posterior extension is oriented in a slightly superior direction to make this less visible when the patient has her hands on her waist. (*B*) Anterior preoperative markings of a 33-year-old patient. The initial markings show the anatomic midline, preoperative inframammary fold, and intended level and shape of the proposed inframammary fold. Note that there is a fold asymmetry to be addressed with a slightly different release technique on each side. The ideal breast width, tissue thickness, and measurements of nipple to fold at rest and at stretch are also shown.

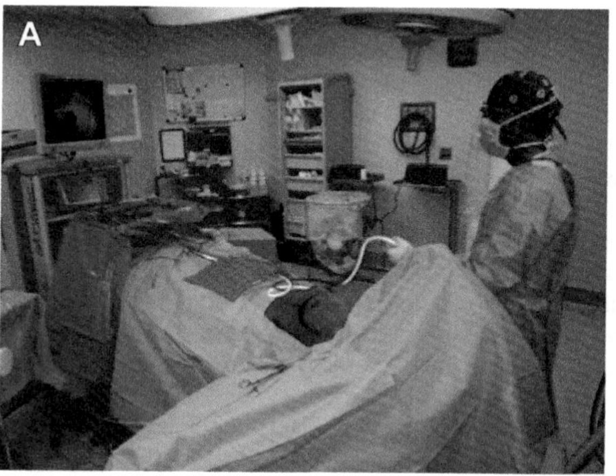

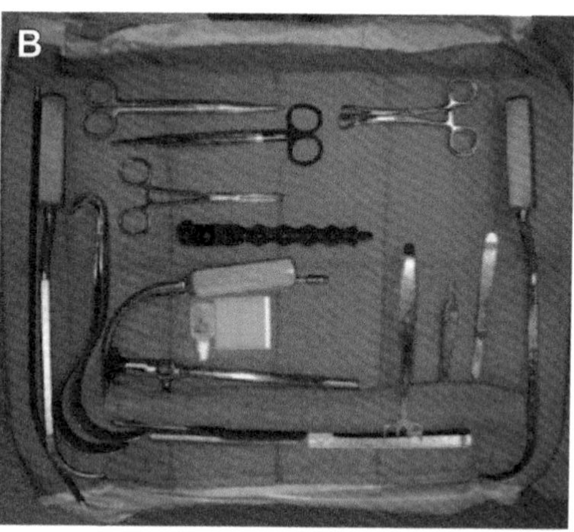

Fig. 2. (*A*) The patient is positioned with the arms out at 90°. This position allows most the procedure to be performed with the surgeon standing above the shoulder on each side. The operating room setup is based on all equipment being placed at the foot of the bed, to minimize any changes needed from side to side. (*B*) Endoscopic instrumentation.

Instrumentation for the procedure includes a needle-tip electrocautery, a 4-prong skin hook, blunt-tip facelift scissors, a 25-mm (1-inch) fiberoptic retractor, two 25-mm Deaver retractors, and a pair of mirror-image Agris-Dingman dissectors (see **Fig. 2**B). The basic endoscopic setup is that described by Price and colleagues,[6] and consists of a 10-mm 30° angled endoscope with matching endoscopic retractor with combination suction cautery handle. The cautery is foot switched (Snowden-Pencer™/ Cardinal Health- Dublin, OH). Although there are numerous cautery rod shapes available, the author prefers the J shape with the curve of the J oriented laterally on each side. The rods are designed so that the suction opening is above the spatulated cautery tip. The endoscopic tower and xenon light source are those that are routinely available in most surgery centers and hospitals.[6,8]

PROCEDURE

Incision and Initial Dissection

The incision is made in the axillary apex per preoperative marking, using a scalpel to the deep dermis. The incision is then completed into the subcutaneous plane using a needle-tipped electrocautery in cut mode (**Fig. 3**A). Dissection is then performed in the immediate subcutaneous plane, with a thin skin flap created in the direction of the lateral border of the pectoralis major muscle. A 4-prong skin hook is used to retract, with the correct thickness of the skin flap confirmed repeatedly during the dissection. This technique prevents damage to the axillary contents, the intercostobrachial nerve, and the skin flap (see **Fig. 3**B). The 4-prong skin hook is then replaced as the dissection proceeds anteriorly, and is replaced with a fiberoptic retractor 25 mm (1 inch) wide. This retractor is used to identify the lateral

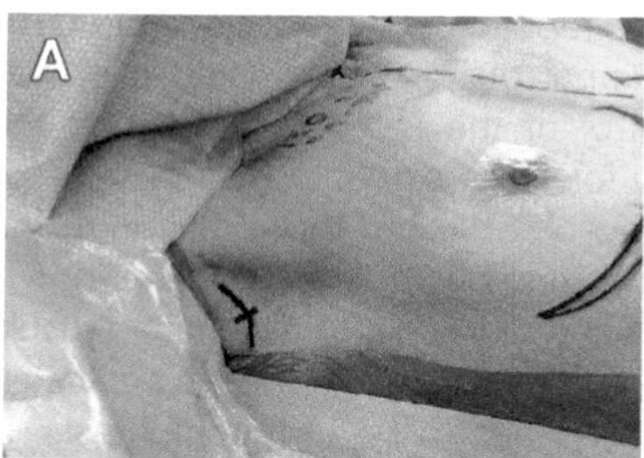

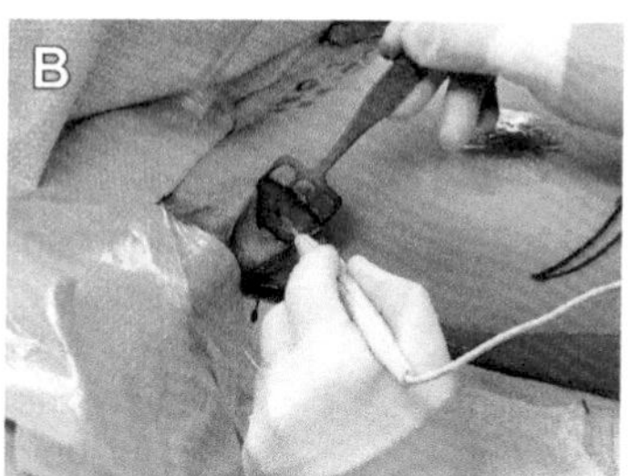

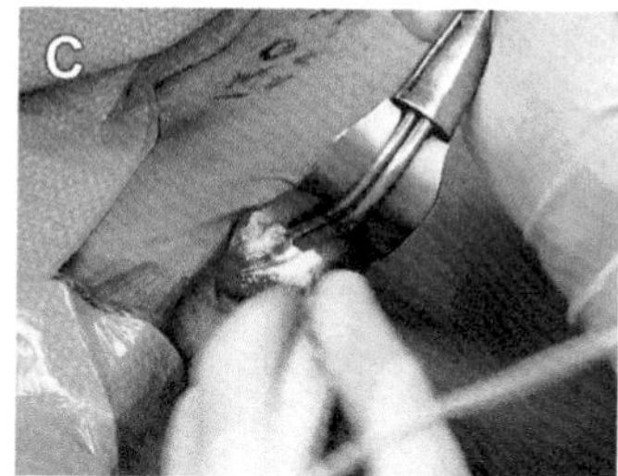

Fig. 3. (*A*) Incision markings. (*B*) A thin skin flap is raised in the immediate subcutaneous plane, with the dissection extending anteriorly toward the lateral border of the pectoralis major muscle. The thickness of the flap is repeatedly checked to prevent damage to the skin or axillary contents. (*C*) A fiberoptic retractor is inserted to continue the dissection to identify the lateral border of the pectoralis major muscle, allowing for entry into the subpectoral space under direct vision.

edge of the pectoralis major muscle. Once the lateral muscle edge has been identified, the subpectoral space is entered under direct vision (see **Fig. 3**C). A clean tissue plane is identified and developed between the pectoralis major muscle above and the pectoralis minor muscle below. The author prefers a finger-sweep–type approach to enlarge the initial area of the subpectoral space, with hemostasis then carefully confirmed with the aid of the fiberoptic retractor. Alternatively, this can all be done sharply, but the author has noted little advantage in this area. The key point is that the initial tissue dissection is performed to minimize blood staining to the tissues of the subpectoral space.[8–11]

Creation of the Optical Cavity

A central concept to the creation of the tissue pocket begins with creation of an optical cavity before release of the pectoralis major muscle. Although this was reported initially as a blind and blunt maneuver using a tissue dissector, the author prefers a sharp technique to minimize blood staining and provide an optimal view when the muscle division is performed with the aid of the endoscope.[6,8] This approach is critical to facilitate the optimal tissue visualization that is at the heart of the precise endoscopic control needed for creation of the tissue pocket.

The endoscopic retractor is then inserted just beneath the undersurface of the pectoralis major muscle, directed toward the medial release point of the inframammary fold. The 10-mm, 30° angled endoscope is then placed in the retractor sheath on the undersurface of the retractor handle (**Fig. 4**). With the technique as described to this point, the first endoscopic view is an areolar plane on the undersurface of the pectoralis major muscle (**Fig. 5**A). The correct orientation of the endoscopic camera is confirmed externally before insertion of the suction cautery handle. Sharp dissection is then performed using the cautery in the areolar plane that is just below the undersurface of the pectoralis major muscle, until a rib is identified at the base of the optical cavity. Identification of a rib helps to ensure creation of the correct plane in a safe fashion that avoids inadvertent entry into the chest cavity. Creation of the optical cavity is then completed by sharp dissection of this areolar plane until the undersurface of the body of the pectoralis major muscle has been visualized. Any accessory slips of the pectoralis major muscle are divided using the cautery, carefully controlling bleeding in a prospective fashion. Thus, the entire optical cavity and the undersurface of the main body of the pectoralis major muscle are clearly visible with minimal or no blood staining of tissues.[8,11]

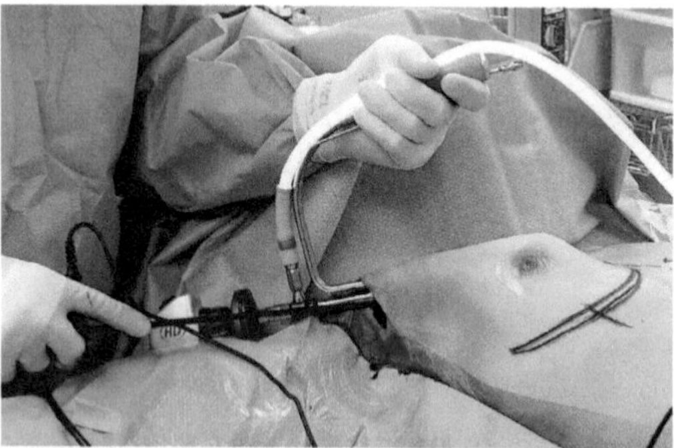

Fig. 4. The endoscopic retractor has a sheath to hold the 10-mm 30° angled endoscope, permitting endoscopic visualization as a partial subpectoral tissue pocket is created.

Pectoralis Major Muscle Release

The release of the main body of the pectoralis major muscle is started internally at a level corresponding with the external marking at the most medial extent of the inframammary fold. Correlation of the location of external markings relative to internal anatomy is carefully confirmed (see **Fig. 5**B). Much attention is directed toward avoidance of overdissection of the pectoralis major muscle medially and in the area of the inframammary fold. Any division of the main body of the pectoralis major muscle above the external reference marking at the medial inframammary fold is avoided. As the muscle release proceeds from medial to lateral, the level of the release and curve of the intended fold are carefully confirmed. As a rule of thumb, the muscle is released 1 to 1.5 cm above the existing fold to maintain preexisting inframammary fold position. If the release is at the preexisting fold level, the inframammary fold level will be lowered. The tissue release is performed through the prepectoral fascia, but can be individualized according to the specific needs of the patient.[8,18] The internal level and shape of the tissue release are repeatedly rechecked and correlated with external markings to maintain proper technical control of the level and shape of the inframammary fold. The extent of dual-plane separation can also be adjusted to the needs of the specific patient situation[8,16,19] (see **Fig. 5**C).

After completion of the pectoralis major muscle release, the adequacy of the release is evaluated for tissue layer uniformity and hemostasis is confirmed. Agris-Dingman dissectors are used to confirm the adequacy of the peripheral extent of the tissue pocket, carefully avoiding trauma to rib cage periosteum in the process. This process is particularly helpful in evaluating the level, shape,

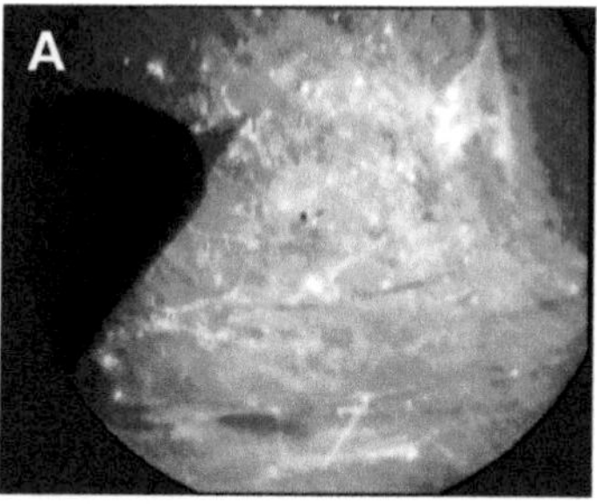

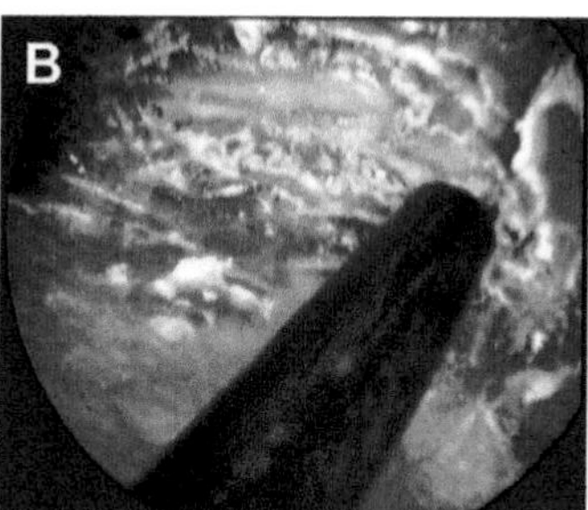

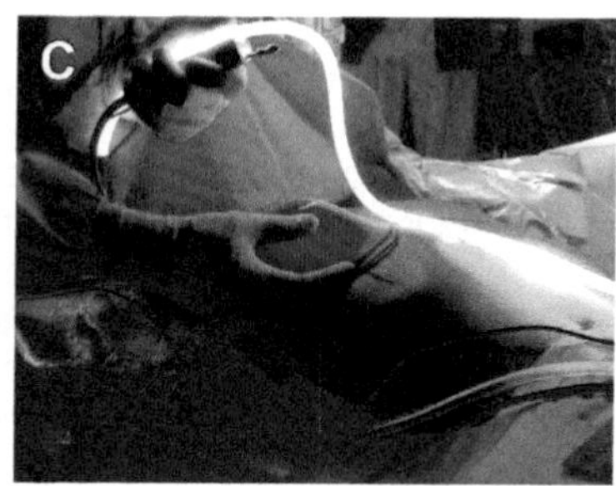

Fig. 5. Endoscopic view of the right breast tissue pocket. For orientation, medial is left and lateral is right. The pectoralis major muscle is above and the rib cage is below. (*A*) Following placement of the endoscope, the areolar plane between the pectoralis major is dissected sharply using electrocautery. Identifying a rib is an important aid to maintaining correct orientation. (*B*) The main body of the pectoralis muscle is released from medial to lateral (left to right). Repeated confirmation of the correct level of the tissue release is the key to control of level and shape of the proposed inframammary fold. (*C*) Transillumination can be helpful in assessing that the release has created the intended degree of dual-plane soft tissue release and that the inframammary fold is at the correct level.

and uniformity of the tissue release along the inframammary fold, with areas marked for refinement as needed.[8–11] Measurements are taken of the tissue pocket and compared with external measurements, and a device is selected (**Fig. 6**A). The endoscope is then reinserted to recheck hemostasis and complete any refinements in the tissue release that may be needed under direct vision. The tissue pocket is evaluated to ensure that the pocket has been created in a fashion that is optimal for the breast implant device selected. The tissue pocket is then irrigated with saline, antibiotic, and local anesthetic solutions.

Device Placement

The adequacy of the entrance to the soft tissue tunnel between the incision and the tissue release is evaluated and optimized in preparation for device placement. The fiberoptic retractor is used to recheck hemostasis in this area. The patient is then placed in a 45° sitting position. Two 25-mm Deaver retractors are placed, 1 parallel to the clavicle in the upper part of the incision, and the second parallel to the lateral chest wall, such that the retractors are perpendicular to one another (see **Fig. 6**B). The assistant holds these retractors in place from the opposite side of the patient to allow the surgeon to prepare the implant for placement.[8–11]

The device is brought into the operating field, and antibiotic solution is placed into the contained holding the implant. The surgeon's outer gloves are replaced. The device can then be placed directly into the tissue pocket by carefully holding 1 hand below the device to prevent it from rubbing against the skin during placement. The upper hand is used to guide the implant into the tissue pocket using a rolling technique along the side of the device until the device is correctly inserted into the

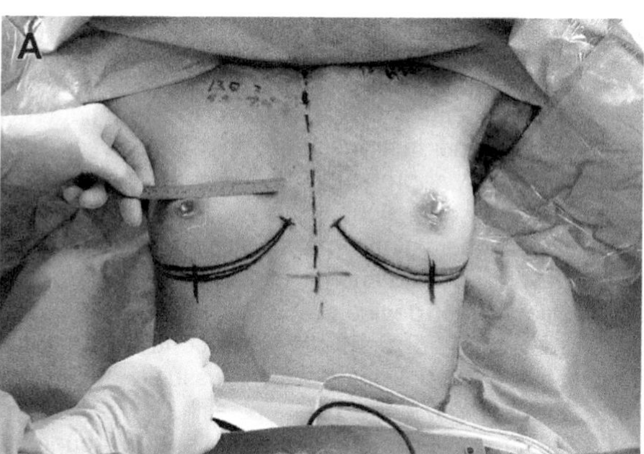

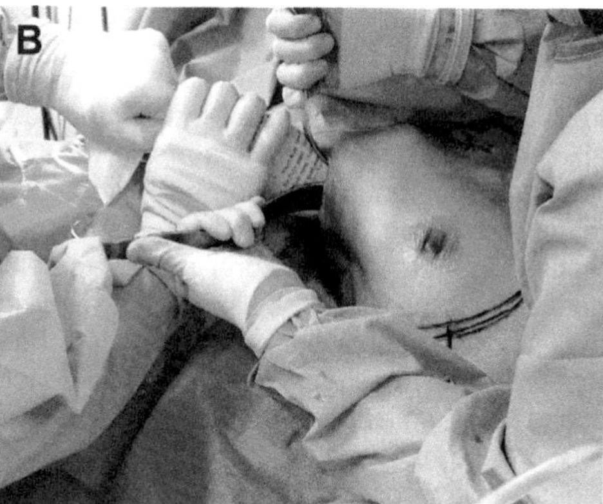

Fig. 6. (*A*) Following creation of the tissue pocket, a measurement of the ideal breast width is confirmed to allow specific device selection. (*B*) The implant is placed with the aid of an insertion sleeve, which can help to minimize contact between the device and the patient's skin and subcutaneous tissue during breast implant placement.

tissue pocket. However, the author prefers to use an insertion sleeve to attempt to greatly reduce or eliminate contact between the device and the patient's skin. Alternate techniques of skin draping and coverage have been described to accomplish similar protection of the implant from skin contamination risk during placement (see **Fig. 6**B).

The patient is placed in 80° and 45° sitting positions to assess the shape of the augmented breast. Minor refinements can be performed using the Agris-Dingman dissectors as needed, with great care taken to avoid significant contact with the breast implant and rib periosteal surfaces. Experience with the technique helps to minimize the needs for significant refinements of this type. The patient is then returned to the supine position and an identical procedure is performed on the contralateral side. On completion of the second side, the patient is placed in a 45° sitting position and measurements are rechecked to confirm symmetric distances from the sternal notch to midbreast meridian at the inframammary fold, and from the nipple to inframammary fold. The patient is then returned to the supine position, hemostasis in the axillary areas is reconfirmed, the incision areas irrigated with local anesthetic solution, and multilayer skin closures are performed. Drains are not routinely used except for shaped gel devices. Twenty-five-millimeter microfoam tape (3-M Healthcare, St Paul MN) is placed in 2 layers, followed by a pressure dressing.[20] The dressing is left in place until the first or second day postoperatively, and is replaced with a bra and elastic wrap for the first week (**Fig. 7**). Specific bra support is maintained for 8 weeks to help stabilize breast implant position.[8–10] Preoperative and postoperative photographs are shown in **Fig. 8** and in Video 1.

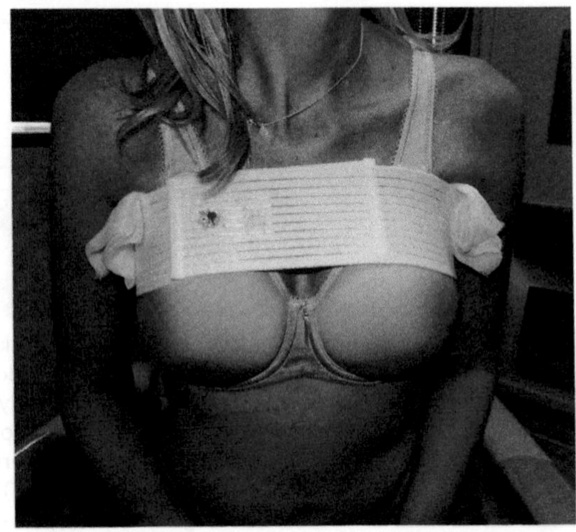

Fig. 7. This patient is shown 2 days after transaxillary endoscopic breast augmentation using silicone gel implants. She is wearing a combination of a supportive bra and pectoral band, used by the author to help stabilize breast implant position in the early postoperative period.

Clinical Results

The transaxillary approach to breast augmentation has been shown to be a reliable technique for breast implant placement over many years, as established by multiple investigators in the United States and internationally. Barnett[18] presented an anatomic solution to many early problems by suggesting an extended pectoral sweep to release the pectoral fascia and thus prevent high-riding implants and double-bubble deformities. Proponents of the nonendoscopic approach include Huang and colleagues[3] and Gryskiewicz and LeDuc,[4] and have published large single-surgeon series with low complication and reoperation rates. Huang[3] compared available data on transaxillary breast augmentation outcomes in his series with endoscopic series and showed significant reductions in reoperations and malpositions in the endoscopic group, with no differences in contracture and hematoma between study groups. Gryskiewicz and LeDuc[4] also showed better patient satisfaction scores reported by patients after transaxillary augmentation compared with an inframammary group.[4]

The addition of endoscopic assistance was introduced by Price and colleagues,[6] and was further popularized by Eaves and colleagues[7] and Bostwick and colleagues.[21] Additional patient series using an endoscopic-assisted approach have been reported by Serra-Renom and colleagues,[13] Giordano and colleagues,[14] Aygit and colleagues,[15] and Tebbetts.[16] Although these investigators reported differing approaches to tissue plane, incision design, and device type, all have reported excellent outcomes with low complication rates. Momeni and colleagues[5] reported a series of 78 patients who underwent breast augmentation using either a transaxillary endoscopic or inframammary approach. Although both patient groups had low complication rates, patient satisfaction was higher in the transaxillary group.[22] Strock[8] described refinements of technique to allow for silicone gel device placement using endoscopic assistance for consistent and controlled creation of the partial subpectoral tissue pocket (see **Fig. 8**; **Figs. 9** and **10**).

A review of the available literature suggests that, although the transaxillary approach is met with continued resistance, this technique can be performed with consistent outcomes and technical

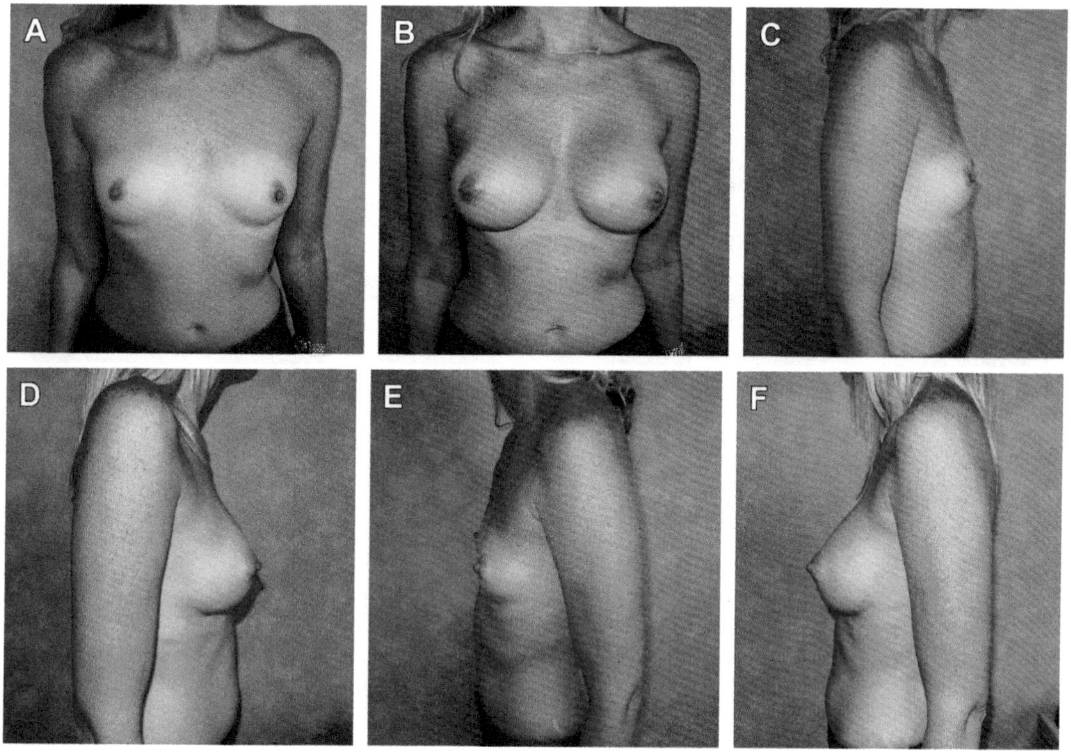

Fig. 8. (*A, C, E*) This 33-year-old woman presented for breast augmentation. She was noted to have a moderate tissue envelope with mild asymmetry. (*B, D, F*) Nine months after placement of 12.3-cm base width, 325-mL, moderate-plus profile, smooth-wall silicone gel implants in a partial subpectoral pocket using a transaxillary endoscopic approach.

control. However, a notable exception to this was shown in a recent article that attempted to study the effect of incision choice on outcomes in primary breast augmentation, which concluded that the axillary approach had a 13-fold higher risk of contracture than the inframammary approach.[22] However, a closer analysis of these retrospective data shows a much smaller number of transaxillary patients relative to the overall series, with 5 of the 6 transaxillary contractures reported as Baker II, which is frequently difficult to distinguish from a superior malposition issue that would be a much more powerful predictor for a need for revision procedures.[4] Although agreeing with the conclusions of the study in his commentary, Adams[23] suggested that more consistent methodology is needed in attempting to report on capsular contracture.

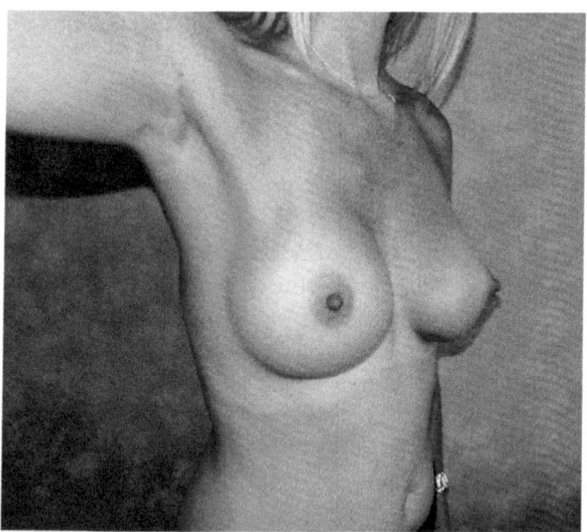

Fig. 9. This patient is shown at 9 months postoperatively, with the arm elevated. These incisions typically become difficult to see by about 9 months postoperatively.

The available literature suggests that there are many surgeons worldwide who remain dedicated to this approach, and reports consistent outcomes both with and without endoscopic assistance. Lista and Ahmad[24] suggested, in their review entitled "Evidence-based Medicine: Augmentation Mammaplasty," that use of either the inframammary or transaxillary incision was the preferred approach. Although Lista and Ahmad[24] did not distinguish between the endoscopic and nonendoscopic transaxillary approaches, this author favors the addition of endoscopic assistance to provide visibility and technical control during

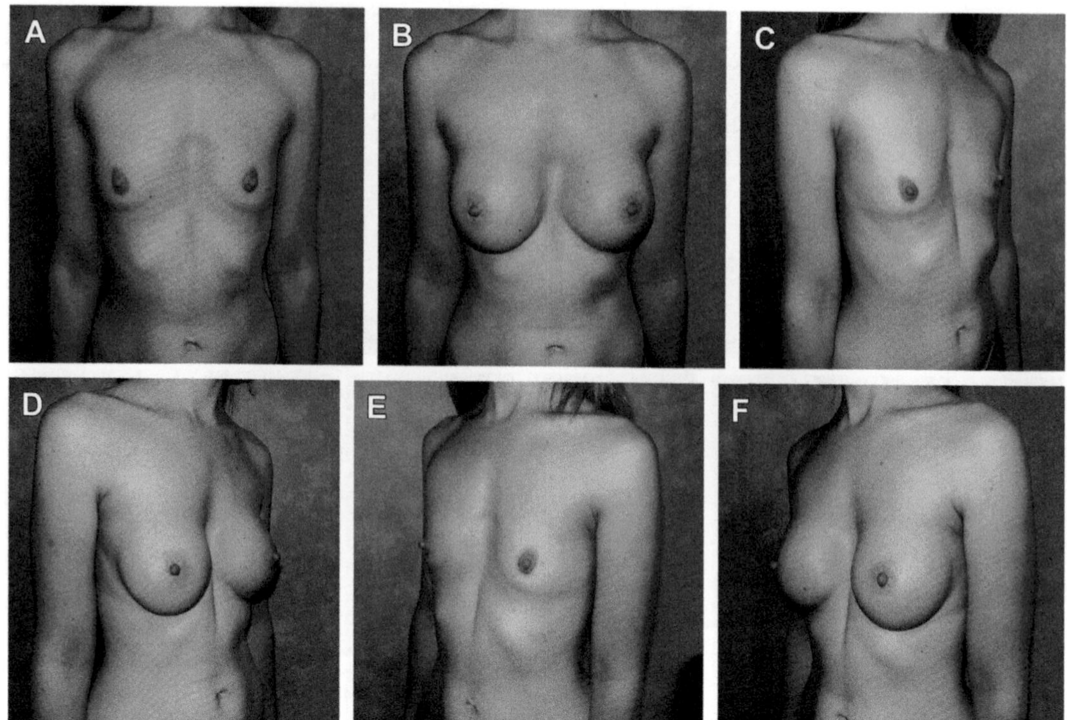

Fig. 10. (*A, C, E*) This 29-year-old woman presented for breast augmentation. She was noted to have thin tissue, poorly defined inframammary folds, and significant rib cage asymmetry. (*B, D, F*) Her result is shown following placement of 11.7-cm base width, 275-mL, moderate-plus profile, smooth-wall silicone gel on the right, and 11.7-cm, 350-mL, high-profile, smooth-wall silicone gel implant on the left. Both devices were placed in a partial subpectoral pocket using a transaxillary endoscopic approach.

creation of the tissue pocket, which allows outcomes similar to the inframammary approach, which is most widely practiced worldwide.[8–11,24]

Editorial Comments by Bradley P. Bengtson, MD

Dr Strock is one of the masters and greatest advocates of the Transaxillary Approach to breast augmentation. He walks through his approach in a very thorough and step-wise fashion with excellent and consistent results. His routine is to use endoscopic assistance which I agree goes a long way in reducing complications particularly fold and lateral malposition that were as high as 18% when I performed this procedure without endoscopic control. To deliver consistent outcomes with minimal complications, the surgical principles remain the same regardless of the surgical incision performed: adequate visualization, prospective hemostasis, precise pocket dissection, and no touch implant technique to minimize biofilm. Dr Strock has truly mastered this approach.

SUPPLEMENTARY DATA

Supplementary data related to this article can be found online at http://dx.doi.org/10.1016/j.cps.2015.06.014.

REFERENCES

1. Wright JH, Bevin AG. Augmentation mammaplasty by the transaxillary approach. Plast Reconstr Surg 1976;58(4):429–33.
2. Tebbetts JB. Transaxillary subpectoral augmentation mammaplasty: long-term follow-up and refinements. Plast Reconstr Surg 1984;74(5):636–47.
3. Huang GJ, Wichmann JL, Mills DC. Transaxillary subpectoral augmentation mammoplasty: a single surgeon's 20-year experience. Aesthet Surg J 2011;31(7):781–801.
4. Gryskiewicz J, LeDuc R. Transaxillary nonendoscopic subpectoral augmentation mammoplasty: a 10-year experience with gel vs saline in 2000 patients–with long-term patient satisfaction measured by the Breast-Q. Aesthet Surg J 2014;34(5):696–713.

5. Momeni A, Padron NT, Fohm M, et al. Safety, complications, and satisfaction of patients undergoing subpectoral breast augmentation via the inframammary and endoscopic transaxillary approach. Aesthetic Plast Surg 2005;29:558–64.
6. Price CI, Eaves FF, Nahai F, et al. Endoscopic transaxillary subpectoral breast augmentation. Plast Reconstr Surg 1994;94(5):612–9.
7. Eaves FF, Bostwick J, Nahai F. Augmentation mammaplasty. In: Bostwick J, editor. Endoscopic plastic surgery. 1st edition. St. Louis: Quality Medical Publishers; 1995. p. 357–400.
8. Strock LL. Transaxillary endoscopic silicone gel breast augmentation. Aesthet Surg J 2010;30(5): 745–55.
9. Strock LL. Transaxillary breast augmentation. In: Spear SL, editor. Surgery of the breast: principles and art. 3rd edition. Philadelphia: Elsevier; 2010. p. 1290–9.
10. Strock LL. Surgical technique: transaxillary approach. In: Atlas of breast augmentation. McGraw-Hill; 2011.
11. Strock LL. Surgery spotlight: transaxillary endoscopic breast augmentation. Chicago: Plastic Surgery Education Network (PSEN); 2012.
12. Graf RM, Bernardes A, Auersvald A, et al. Subfascial endoscopic transaxillary augmentation mammaplasty. Aesthetic Plast Surg 2000;24:216–20.
13. Serra-Renom JM, Garrido MD, Yoon TS. Augmentation mammoplasty with anatomic, cohesive silicone implant using transaxillary approach at a subfascial level with endoscopic assistance. Plast Reconstr Surg 2005;116:640.
14. Giordano PA, Roif M, Laurent B, et al. Endoscopic transaxillary breast augmentation: clinical evaluation of a series of 306 patients over a 9-year period. Aesthet Surg J 2007;27(1):47–54.
15. Aygit AC, Basaran K, Marcan ES. Transaxillary totally subfascial breast augmentation with anatomical breast implants: review of 27 cases. Plast Reconstr Surg 2013;131:1149.
16. Tebbetts JB. Axillary endoscopic breast augmentation: processes derived from a 28-year experience to optimize outcomes. Plast Reconstr Surg 2006; 118(7S):53S–80S.
17. Collis N, Mirza S, Stanley PR, et al. Reduction of potential contamination of breast implants by use of "nipple shields". Br J Plast Surg 1999;52:445.
18. Barnett A. Transaxillary subpectoral augmentation in the ptotic breast: augmentation by disruption of the extended pectoral fascia and parenchymal sweep. Plast Reconstr Surg 1990;86(1):76.
19. Tebbetts JB. Dual plane breast augmentation: optimizing implant-soft-tissue relationships in a wide range of breast types. Plast Reconstr Surg 2006; 118(7S):81S, 1255.
20. Maxwell GP, Falcone PA. Eighty four consecutive breast reconstructions using a textured silicone tissue expander. Plast Reconstr Surg 1992;89(6): 1022–35.
21. Bostwick J, Eaves FF, Nahai F. Endoscopic breast augmentation. Aesthet Surg J 1996;16:11.
22. Jacobson JM, Gatti MD, Schaffner AD, et al. Effect of incision choice on outcomes in primary breast augmentation. Aesthet Surg J 2012;32(4):456–62.
23. Adams WP. Commentary on: effect of incision choice on outcomes in primary breast augmentation. Aesthet Surg J 2012;32(4):463–4.
24. Lista F, Ahmad J. Evidence-based medicine: augmentation mammoplasty. Plast Reconstr Surg 2013;132:1684.

Clinical Applications of Barbed Suture in Aesthetic Breast Surgery

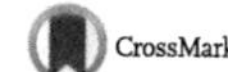

Ryan T.M. Mitchell, MD, FRCSC[a],
Bradley P. Bengtson, MD[a,b,*]

KEYWORDS

- Barbed suture • Sutures • Incision closure techniques • Wound closure techniques
- Surgical Specialties Quill suture • Covidien V-Loc suture • Ethicon Stratafix suture
- Breast incision closure

KEY POINTS

- In primary and revisional breast surgery, incisions are limited, and it often feels like trying to operate through a "mail slot"!
- In these limited access applications barbed technology is extremely useful by facilitating suturing internally in limited spaces without the need for tying knots.
- This limited access application and increased speed and efficiency of incisional closures are the main applications and benefits of using these barbed devices.
- The future development of barbed sutures technology along with the number of applications continues to grow.

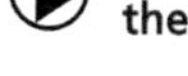

Videos of 2-layer closure techniques accompany this article at http://www.plasticsurgery.theclinics.com/

BACKGROUND

The breadth of literature regarding barbed suture applications in plastic surgical procedures signifies the importance of this article Barbed suture applications in breast surgery is growing dramatically as surgical practitioners are becoming more familiar with the advantages of this new suture technology. Barbed suture devices were first implemented by plastic surgeons for the use in various minimally invasive techniques for facial rejuvenation.[1] Although the initial devices had their share of pitfalls, the most noticeable advantage in their implementation was a reduction in procedural time.[2] With the increase of bariatric procedures, there has been a similar increase in the number of body-contouring procedures in order to address the significant skin redundancies related to massive weight loss of the breast and body. In an effort to improve operative efficiency, the implementation of barbed suture technologies has increased to streamline the closure of large skin resection margins of the body and also the breast, particularly breast reductions and mastopexy procedures. A common theme to the advantages of this modality of tissue closure is the speed and ease of placement. Often either deep suture material is not required or fewer deep approximation points are necessary, which subsequently reduces the operative closure time.[3] In addition, complications associated with more conventional suture material related to knot slippage or breakage,

[a] Bengtson Center for Aesthetics and Plastic Surgery, 555 MidTowne Street, NE, Suite 110, Grand Rapids, MI 49503, USA; [b] Department of Surgery, School of Medicine, Michigan State University, East Lansing, MI, USA
* Corresponding author. Bengtson Center for Aesthetics and Plastic Surgery, Grand Rapids, MI.
E-mail address: drm@bengtsoncenter.com

Clin Plastic Surg 42 (2015) 595–604
http://dx.doi.org/10.1016/j.cps.2015.06.003

suture extrusion or spitting, and infection may be reduced. Furthermore, tension may also be more uniformly distributed along the wound, and the barbed nature of the suture prevents tissue sliding with more than 20 points of fixation per square inch. Some have even suggested that the final scar result is subjectively improved from a clinical perspective as a result of a reduction of tissue-related ischemia, less suture extrusion, and locking of the tissues more tightly through the barbing, although this is difficult to prove clinically when Monocryl-type sutures are used.[4–9]

Three main barbed suture device companies are currently being used for soft tissue closure in breast, body contouring, and other soft tissue closure procedures in the United States. A bidirectional self-retaining suture (Quill SRS, now Surgical Specialties, Vancouver, British Columbia, Canada) uses a helically distributed back-cut spaced distance of 5.08 mm apart on a variety of monofilament sutures of both the absorbable (polyglycolic acid/polycaprolactone [Monoderm]) and polydioxanone (PDO) along with nonabsorbable (nylon and polypropylene) (**Figs. 1** and **2**). The barb cut in the strand reduces the diameter of the suture such that a 3-0 suture has the corresponding strength

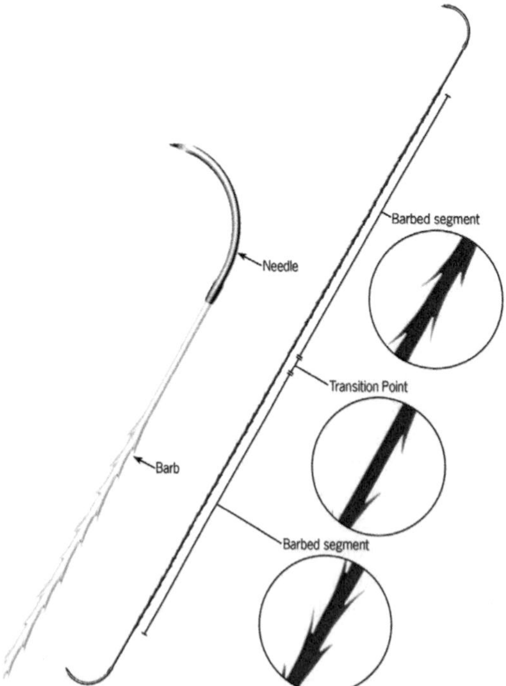

Fig. 1. The standard barbed suture is depicted with barbed segments oriented to lock the soft tissues into position and prevent back-tracking or sliding of the suture. The swaged on needles and transition zone centrally are also shown.

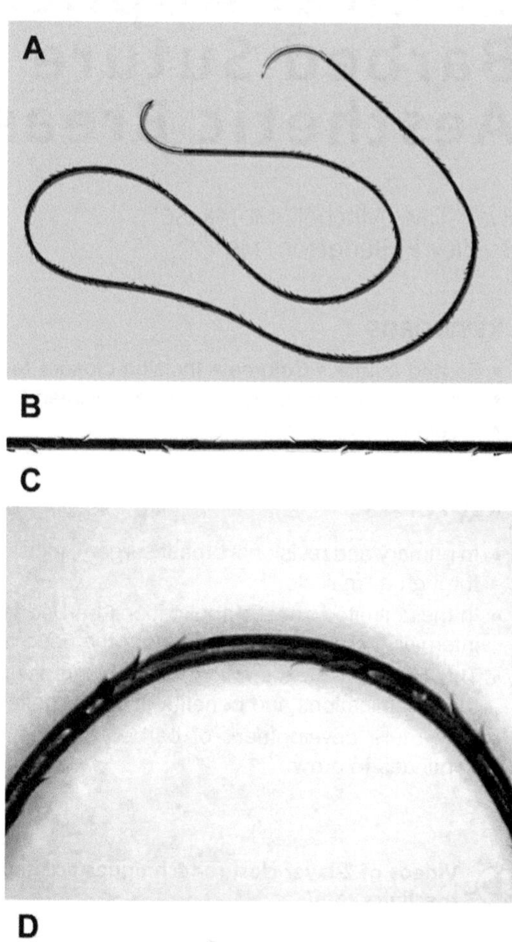

Fig. 2. (*A–D*) Progressively increasing magnification of the barbed suture technology. (*Courtesy of* Angiotech Pharmaceuticals, Inc, Vancouver, British Columbia, © 2015; with permission.)

of a 4-0 standard monofilament suture. Quill suture is available in both bidirectional and unidirectional formats.

Surgical Specialties licensed their Quill technology to Johnson & Johnson/Ethicon in 2012, who is also marketing and distributing their barbed suture under the trade name Stratafix (Somerville, NJ, USA). Quill and Stratifix 3-0 suture have a tensile strength of a 4-0 suture, while V-Loc keeps the 1:1 ratio of standard suture, so that a 3-0 Monocryl is the same diameter as a 3-0 V-Loc.

The third suture device is the Covidien V-Loc (**Fig. 3**) wound closure system (Covidien, Mansfield, MA, USA), which consists of a dual-angled back-cut spaced helically with 20 barbs per centimeter in a unidirectional orientation. Similar to the

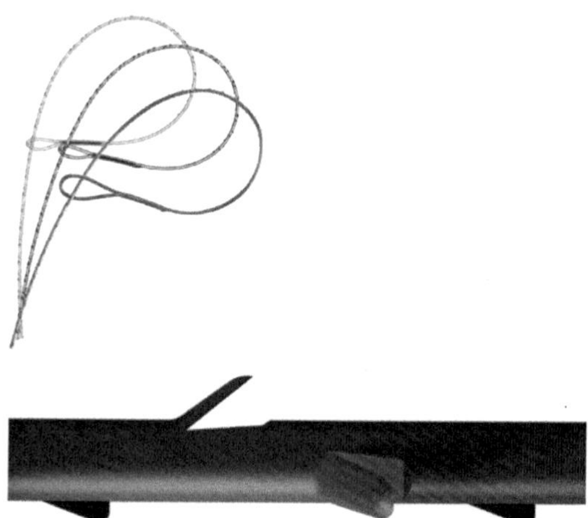

Fig. 3. The Covidien V-Loc suture. It is a unidirectional design with a slightly different barb cut and orientation (Product brochure: http://www.covidien.com/surgical/products/wound-closure/barbed-sutures#resources). (*Courtesy of* Medtronic, Minneapolis, MN; with permission.)

Quill device, the back cut into the suture reduces the diameter such that a 3-0 V-Loc device has a corresponding strength profile of a 4-0 standard monofilament suture.

CLINICAL APPLICATIONS

Internal cost studies performed by the authors have shown that for most breast procedures the net cost of using barbed versus standard sutures is essentially equivalent. For instance, the cost of using one 2-0 Vicryl and two 3-0 Monoderm for a bilateral breast augmentation is cost equivalent to using two 3-0 and 4-0 Monocryl sutures. In addition, surgery time is expensive, approaching $100 per minute in large hospital settings; thus, any saving in Operating Room time may result in a significant overall cost savings. Additional advantages, such as time savings and closure techniques, have also been well outlined.[10]

TWO-LAYER BREAST AUGMENTATION CLOSURE

The authors' longest and most used closure application with barbed suture is the 2-layer breast closure in primary augmentation and revisional breast surgery. The authors have used this specific closure method for the past 5 years in more than 1200 breast procedures. It is fast and efficient and works well with first assistants, residents, and fellows, or dual surgeons. The authors have not experienced any wound breakdown, skin dehiscence, or suture track infections since its implementation. Their average standard primary breast augmentation time is averages 35 minutes, skin to skin, with the incision closure time less than 5 minutes.

Following the breast augmentation and checking for pocket and implant symmetry, the deep closure is performed setting the inframammary fold, if the inframammary fold incision is being used, with either a 2-0 polydioxanone suture (PDS) or 2-0 Vicryl, placing the suture into the deep fascia directly in the fold and then through the breast fascia of the lower skin flap followed by the upper breast skin flap. Charles Randquist has termed this the "Baby-Sitter Stitch." The authors place 1 or 2 of these sutures followed by running the deep fascia. A more superficial bite is taken directly over these 1 to 2 deep sutures to potentially avoid damaging the underlying device. The fascia is run under direct vision, allowing for a more uniform tightly approximated closure and avoiding the potential knuckling of the device that patients may palpate between interrupted sutures. Two to 3 sutures of this deep closure material (2-0 Vicryl) is then placed to approximate the incision edges just beneath the dermis. Following this, a 2-layer closure of 3-0 Monoderm or similar barbed suture completes the closure (**Fig. 4** and Videos 1 and 2).

Deep closure is typically performed simultaneously on both sides, and if operating with a first assistant, transition to the contralateral side following deep closure next to the device, and superficial barbed suture closure on the right side, as the assistant is closing the patient's left side. The barbed suture skin closure is initiated beginning medially. The bidirection suture is preferred for this application with both sutures being able to be run toward the surgeon and obtaining a strong 2-layer repair. The closure begins internally at the medial crotch of the deep dermis. The free end of the suture is placed beneath an instrument or sponge and held out of the way. The first pass approximates the deep dermis and is then brought out directly through the skin approximately 1 to 2 cm lateral to the lateral incision edge. The next pass begins again suturing toward the surgeon in the superficial dermis, a 3-0 Monoderm or 4-0 Stratifix, or 4-0 V-Loc, for this closure in either a 7 × 7-cm or a 14 × 14-cm length depending on the incision length for either a primary or a revision patient. This second pass is made approximating the dermis directly underneath the epidermal layer in the more superficial plane and also brought out laterally through the skin and both sutures cut flush with the skin and massaged gently, allowing the cut end to migrate subdermally. Again, this closure is very fast and strong, is an efficient use of suture material, and allows the

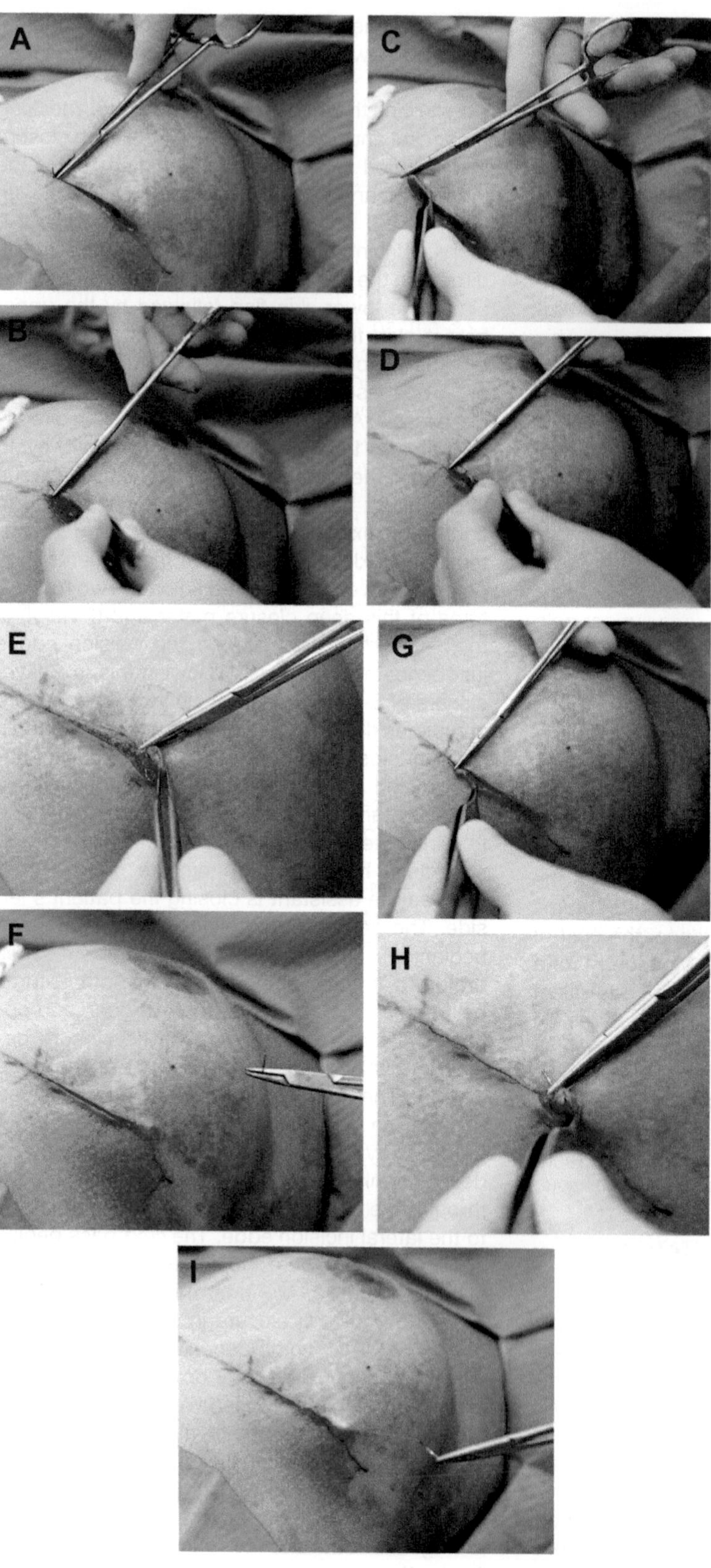

Fig. 4. (*A–I*) The repair sequence is initiated medially backhanding the suture out deeply into the corner of the dermis. A short bite is then taken, and the deep dermal layer is initiated. The deep dermis is then approximated, and the suture is brought out laterally through the skin. The second pass is then initiated at the superficial dermal-epidermal junction, completing the closure with the suture brought out percutaneously through the skin and cut at the skin level. The area is massaged to allow the cut edge of the suture to retract just deep to the dermis.

entire closure to be performed suturing toward the surgeon. More than 600 augmentation closures have been performed with this technique with no suture spitting, dehiscence, or wound healing complications (Bengtson, unpublished data).

BREAST REDUCTION AND MASTOPEXY CLOSURE

Barbed suture material may be used in all types of breast reduction patterns, nipple areolar incisions, and pedicle orientations. Both unidirectional and

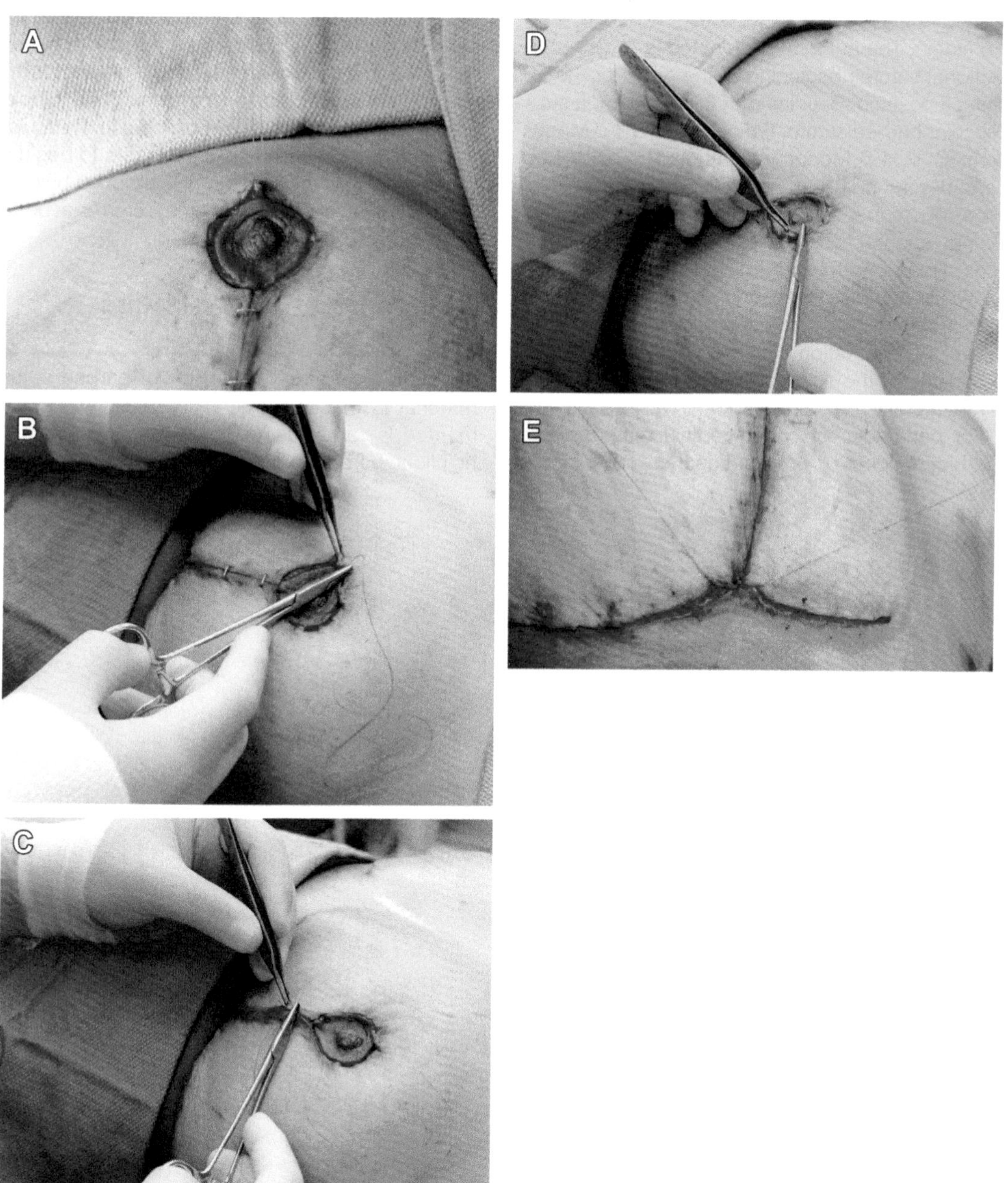

Fig. 5. (*A–E*) For full mastopexy closures, the authors begin at the 12 o'clock position with the bidirectional barbed suture and run each arm, one medially and one around the areola laterally. At the vertical limb, one suture is run in the deep dermis and the second pass at the dermal-epidermal junction to the T region. At this point, one suture is run medially and the other is run laterally and brought out percutaneously through the skin after the closure is complete. It may be helpful to run the contralateral closure from the opposite side of the bed toward yourself.

bidirectional suture orientations may be used to facilitate final closure. A similar theme is consistent with regards to skin closure in these procedures. Once the markings have been incised and the required tissue resected, closure begins with the placement of a unifying suture that will orient the breast into its respective shape. The areola is initially tacked into position at respective positions around the face of a clock (ie, 12, 3, 6, and 9 o'clock). The authors' preference is to use bidirectional sutures beginning at the apex, or the 12 o'clock position. Beginning at this position, a subcuticular barbed suture, typically with a 3-0 Monoderm Quill, 4-0 Monocryl Stratafix, or 3-0 V-Loc barbed suture, is then run around the circumference in a subcuticular fashion, allowing for fine manipulation of tissue tension and locking the tissues in place. With bidirectional suture, the sutures are run in opposite directions and then at different dermal depths, deep and superficial, similar to the 2-layer augmentation closure, and then at the T point, one of the sutures is run medially and one is run laterally (**Fig. 5**).

For periareolar or circumvertical mastopexies, the bidirectional or unidirectional suture may be used. Typically, the authors will run circumferentially 1.5 to 2 times, overlapping the suture for better skin approximation. It may be also of interest, in the case of a noncircular nipple areolar complex postoperatively, the authors have had some success stretching and fracturing the barbs at 1 to 2 weeks postoperatively with some improvement in re-creating the circular diameter versus more oval or a flattened side. Long-term outcomes are pending, but it would be a nice additional benefit to have somewhat of an adjustable suture for this application in helping to create a round nipple-areolar complex if needed. For the use of a unidirectional barbed suture, it is advisable to begin at the extent of the incision margin, although building in smaller areas of overlap may create a better approximated incision (**Figs. 6–8**).[11]

ADDITIONAL BREAST APPLICATIONS

Review of the Literature

Although the history of the use of barbed suture material in Plastic Surgery has been well documented,[12] previous reviews of the literature highlight barbed technology uses in suspension

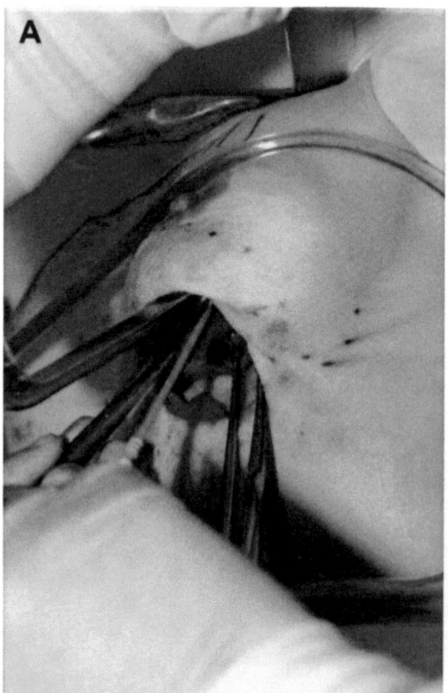

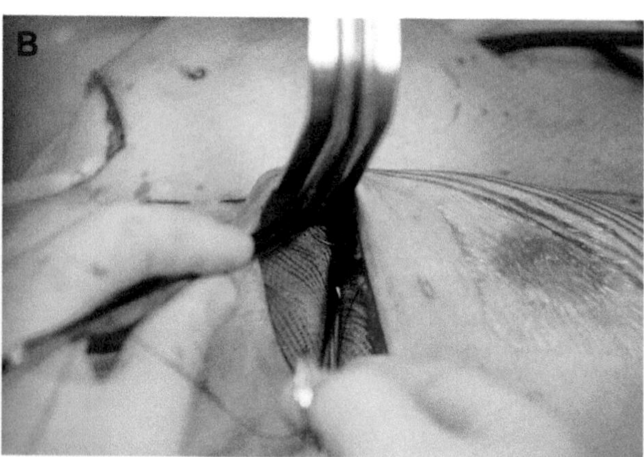

Fig. 6. (*A, B*) In these 2 images, it is evident how barbed suture is having increased applications in both primary augmentation mastopexy and breast reduction surgery in massive weight-loss patients that require significant soft tissue support. In addition, barbed suture is a critical element in breast revision surgery, which has created a new zone of surgery that may be referred to as limited access surgery. It is the surgical area between open surgical procedures and laparoscopic/endoscopic surgery. It requires operating through smaller, limited incisions, and it is here where the barbed suture is extremely beneficial. Trying to operate through these small incisions is like operating through a mail slot.

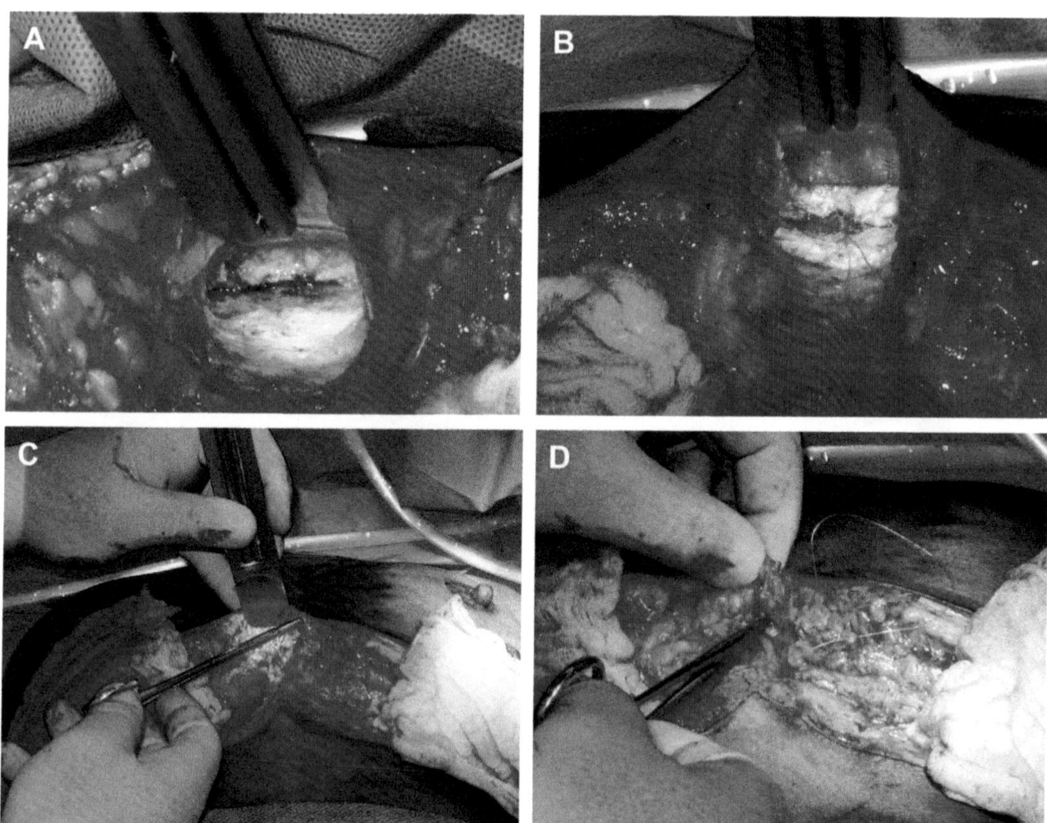

Fig. 7. (*A–D*) This sequence of images shows a case of natural symmastia. Both symmastia that occurs naturally and following breast augmentation or reconstruction have been difficult to treat in the past with one operation. In breast revision, capsular flaps and scaffolds or tissues are helpful in reinforcing pockets and correcting the deformity. In primary cases where symmastia occurs, barbed sutures are critical in that they may be placed percutaneously with multiple rows run down simultaneously, closing down the presternal space. In this patient, liposuction was also performed in the presternal area. It is also importance to come at least 1.5 cm off the midline to help re-establish the proper intermammary distance.

procedures for facial rejuvenation,[5] bariatric surgery,[13] and a significant bulk pertaining to its use in body-contouring procedures.[2,4,11,14–17] With specific regards to its use in the breast, there currently is a paucity of literature depicting barbed suture applications.[18–20] Early literature with respect to breast surgery has focused on the effectiveness of barbed suture material in the closure of donor sites in breast reconstruction.[21–23] Thekkinkattil and colleagues[21] in 2013 evaluated the use of unidirectional barbed suture for quilting of the donor site in a latissimus dorsi myocutaneous flap breast reconstruction compared with nonbarbed material in 50 patients. The implementation of barbed sutures was found to have a similar complication profile with regards to seroma formation and wound concerns as conventional suture materials. Furthermore, there was no significant difference in their secondary outcomes in relation to total duration of surgery, total inpatient stay, and total amount of drain at the donor site.

In comparison with conventional closure devices, barbed sutures have a comparable wound strength and tissue reaction scores in animal models.[24] There have been mixed results with respect to the use of barbed sutures in breast procedures. Jandali and colleagues[23] reported conflicting results. They found that there were time savings associated with the use of barbed sutures as well as an associated cost benefit. However, this came with an increased risk, which trended toward significance with respect to wound dehiscence, infection, and suture extrusion. These initial increased rates of wound dehiscence and suture exposure were related to the PDS/PDO version of suture used superficially. When using the Monocryl/Monoderm version of suture in the dermal and direct subdermal planes, these wound-healing issues have largely been mitigated.

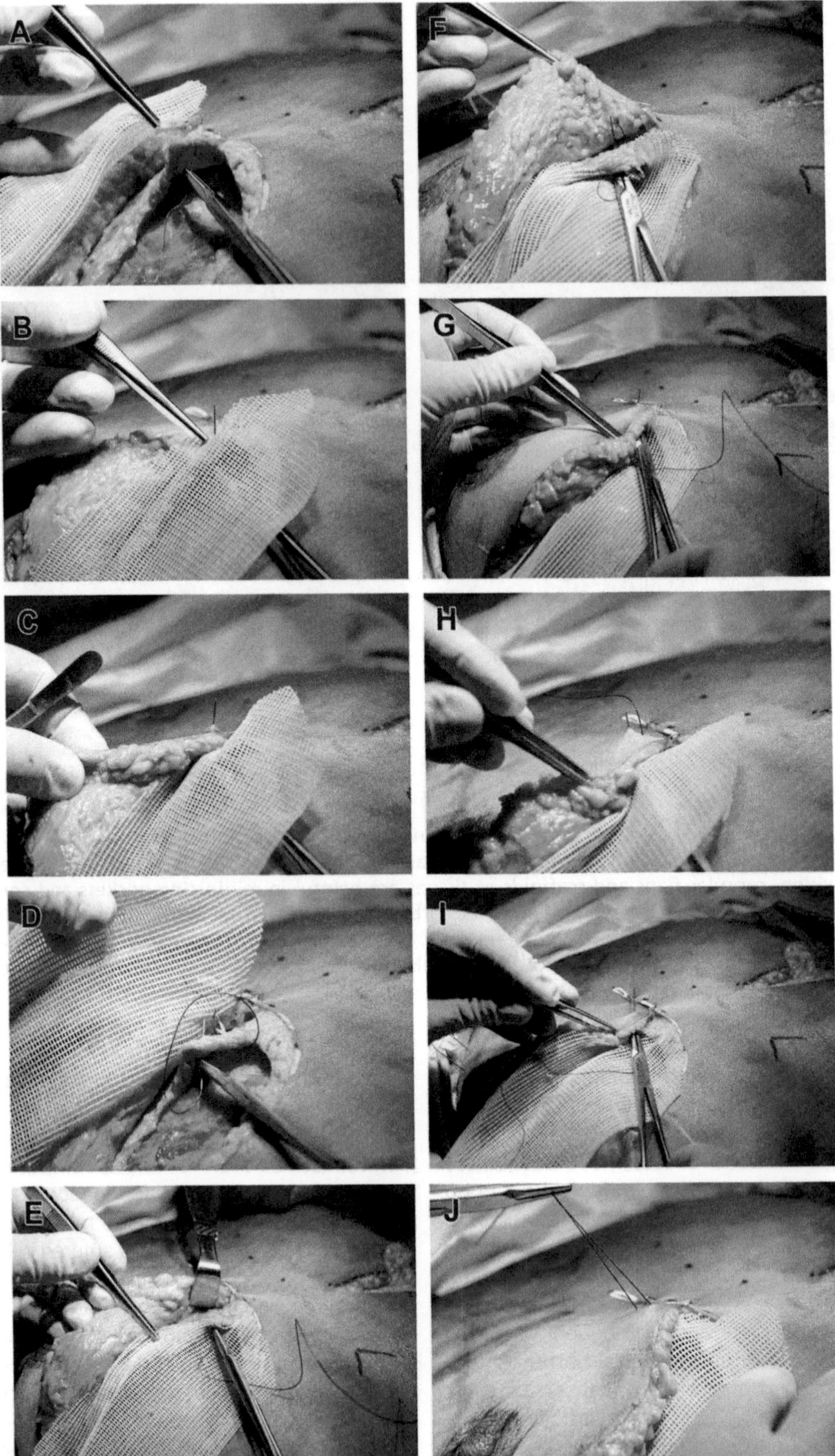

Fig. 8. (*A–J*) This sequence of images depicts one of the main benefits of barbed sutures in the placement of scaffolds or tissues. Parachute or marionette-type sutures are useful but may create suture track infections if left in position or lose their function if removed at the end of the procedure. Barbed suture particularly on a double-armed Keith needle can be placed through the muscle, then through the scaffold or tissue, and then through the breast, and when place medially, centrally, and laterally, will set up the material for the surgeon, who can then more easily inset the scaffold and visualize the templating and finalize the inset.

de Blacam and colleagues[22] compared closure of deep inferior epigastric perforator flap donor sites in breast reconstruction patients. In 142 patients, the initial 71 were closed with conventional suture, and the latter 71 were closed with unidirectional barbed material. They showed no significant difference with respect to wound dehiscence, wound infection, or seroma formation.

Mantarasso and Paul[11] in the very thorough *ASJ Supplement* on barbed suture in September 2013 gave a great overview of barbed technology, and although primarily focused on facial applications, it included 2 brief but significant descriptions on mastopexy and breast reduction closure.[10]

Rubin and colleagues[10] in a multicenter randomized controlled trial compared conventional absorbable sutures to a unidirectional barbed suture for closure of open wounds. They found that the mean dermal closure time was significantly faster in all procedures conducted with barbed sutures, primarily because of the need for fewer deep dermal sutures.

Although the literature in body contouring is expanding within this realm,[2,4,11,14–17] far fewer articles discuss the benefits and surgical techniques using barbed suture with specific reference to the breast. Most of the literature is anecdotal with reference to barbed suture technology. Salzberg[1] discussed his experience with barbed suture in breast reconstruction with and without acellular dermal matrix. Since he started using barbed sutures, he noticed that his operative time decreased, and he was better able to control skin tension on closure by more uniform distribution of vectors along the skin edge. In additional, in immediate and delayed implant-based reconstructions, he places barbed sutures in the insetting of acellular dermal matrix to the pectoral muscle and for definition of the pocket by recreation of the inframammary fold and lateral breast curvature. He has also found barbed suture material useful for autologous reconstruction for closure of the donor and recipient site. The incorporation of barbed material in the periariolar closure of breast cases has also been described.[4] Here, a barbed subcuticular suture evenly distributes tissue tension and prevents tissue slippage, which would result in subsequent widening of the nipple areolar complex. In this article, the authors review of more than 300 cases, leading to the impression that there is a subjective improvement on the appearance of the final scar. The theory is that the barbed sutures eliminate the micromotion associated with traditional suture material in final wound closure. This lack of motion allows for the final appearance of the scar to heal in well and allows for a thin fine line. Furthermore, there is less of a risk of suture spitting and erosion associated with other suture material, particularly in regards to periareolar closure techniques. Paul[11] described the uses of barbed sutures in esthetic surgery. In the breast, he uses a bidirectional device for deep dermal closure of the areola. Starting at the 12 o-clock position, one strand is run clockwise and the other is run counterclockwise. If a vertical and horizontal component is present, the suture can then be run down the vertical incision and along their respective horizontal component within the inframammary fold. For thicker dermal tissue, a second suture in the mid to superficial dermis can be applied.

In conclusion, there is an emerging new area of plastic surgery that has been termed limited access surgery. Often in primary and revisional breast surgery, the incisions are limited, and it often feels like trying to operate through a mail slot! It is in these limited access applications where barbed technology is extremely useful by facilitating suturing internally in limited spaces without the need for tying knots. This limited access application and increased speed and efficiency of closures are the main applications and benefits of using these barbed devices.

The future development of barbed sutures technology along with the number of applications continues to grow. It is hoped that this brief review of clinical applications has been helpful in current practice as well as in spawning new ideas and innovations in the use of barbed suture technology to improve efficiency and patient outcomes.

Editorial Comments by Bradley P. Bengtson, MD

The use of barbed suture has gained significant poularity in the past few years. There continues to be ongoing misinformation about barbed suture use. The Monocryl/Monoderm products, regardless of manufacturer, should be the only type used in the subcuticular or direct subdermal plane. We have had no suture spitting or incision dehiscence in 2-layer augmentation closures in over 1000 consecutive patients. When using PDO or PDS suture, we initially experienced significant wound healing issues. Surgeons need to discriminate between suture types, PDO should not be used in the direct subdermal plane. These barbed sutures may be used in innovative ways in all types of breast surgery with uni-directional or bi-directional suture types and facilitates closures by reducing surgical time, placing fewer knots, and can be used by two surgeons simultaneously. The reduction of surgical time can create significant cost savings intraoperatively.

SUPPLEMENTARY DATA

Supplementary data related to this article can be found online at http://dx.doi.org/10.1016/j.cps.2015.06.003.

REFERENCES

1. Salzberg CA. Barbed sutures in breast reconstruction. Aesthet Surg J 2013;33(3):40S–3S.
2. Moya AP. Barbed sutures in body surgery. Aesthet Surg J 2013;33(3):57S–71S.
3. Paul MD, Budd M. Evaluating the Quill self-retaining system: closure time, cost analysis and current clinical applications. Plast Surg Pract 2009;30–3.
4. Hammond DC. Barbed sutures in plastic surgery: a personal experience. Aesthet Surg J 2013;33(3): 32S–9S.
5. Villa MT, White LE, Alam M, et al. Barbed sutures: a review of the literature. Plast Reconstr Surg 2008; 121(3):102e–8e.
6. Paul MD. Bidirectional barbed sutures for wound closure: evolution and applications. J Am Col Certif Wound Spec 2009;1(2):51–7.
7. Ruff G. Technique and uses for absorbable barbed sutures. Aesthet Surg J 2006;26(5):620–8.
8. Rosen AD. Use of absorbable running barbed suture and progressive tension technique in abdominoplasty: a novel approach. Plast Reconstr Surg 2010;125(3):1024–7.
9. Matarasso A, Pfeifer TM. The use of modified sutures in plastic surgery. Plast Reconstr Surg 2008;122(2):652–8.
10. Rubin JP, Hunstad JP, Polynice A, et al. A multicenter randomized controlled trial comparing absorbable barbed sutures versus conventional absorbable sutures for dermal closure in open surgical procedures. Aesthet Surg J 2014;34(2):272–83.
11. Matarasso A, Paul MD. Barbed Sutures in Aesthetic Plastic Surgery: evolution of thought and process. Aesthetic Surg J 2013;33(3 Suppl 1):17S–31S.
12. Ruff GL. The history of barbed sutures. Aesthet Surg J 2013;33(3):12S–6S.
13. Kassir R, Breton C, Lointier P, et al. Laparoscopic Roux-en-Y gastric bypass with hand-sewn gastrojejunostomy using an absorbable bidirectional monofilament barbed suture: review of the literature and illustrative case video. Surg Obes Relat Dis 2014; 10(3):560–1.
14. Shermak MA. The application of barbed sutures in body contouring surgery. Aesthet Surg J 2013; 33(3):72S–5S.
15. Hurwitz DJ, Reuben B. Quill barbed sutures in body contouring surgery: a 6-year comparison with running absorbable braided sutures. Aesthet Surg J 2013;33(3):44S–56S.
16. Gutowski KA, Warner JP. Incorporating barbed sutures in abdominoplasty. Aesthet Surg J 2013; 33(3):76S–81S.
17. Shermak MA, Mallalieu J, Chang D. Barbed suture impact on wound closure in body contouring surgery. Plast Reconstr Surg 2010;126(5): 1735–41.
18. Hirsch EM, Seth AK, Fine NA. Reconstruction of the inframammary fold using barbed suture. Ann Plast Surg 2014;72(4):388–90.
19. Prucz R, Wheeler C, Edwards J, et al. The use of a barbed self-retaining suture system in the positioning and manipulation of the breast mound during reconstructive and aesthetic breast surgery. Plast Reconstr Surg 2011;128(2):90e–1e.
20. Aveta A, Tenna S, Cagli B, et al. V-Loc suture: a simple wound closure device for areola diameter and shape control in breast reduction and mastopexy. Plast Reconstr Surg 2012;129(6):1004e–5e.
21. Thekkinkattil DK, Hussain T, Mahapatra TK, et al. Feasibility of use of a barbed suture (v-loc 180) for quilting the donor site in latissimus dorsi myocutaneous flap breast reconstruction. Arch Plast Surg 2013;40(2):117–22.
22. de Blacam C, Colakoglu S, Momoh AO, et al. Early experience with barbed sutures for abdominal closure in deep inferior epigastric perforator flap breast reconstruction. Eplasty 2012;12:e24.
23. Jandali S, Nelson JA, Bergey MR, et al. Evaluating the use of a barbed suture for skin closure during autologous breast reconstruction. J Reconstr Microsurg 2011;27(5):277–86.
24. Zaruby J, Gingras K, Taylor J, et al. An in vivo comparison of barbed suture devices and conventional monofilament sutures for cosmetic skin closure: biomechanical wound strength and histology. Aesthet Surg J 2011;31(2):232–40.

Coming of Age

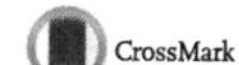

Breast Implant–Associated Anaplastic Large Cell Lymphoma After 18 Years of Investigation

Mark W. Clemens, MD[a,*], Roberto N. Miranda, MD[b]

KEYWORDS

- Breast implant–associated ALCL • Anaplastic large cell lymphoma • Non-Hodgkin lymphoma
- CD30

KEY POINTS

- Breast implant–associated anaplastic large cell lymphoma (BI-ALCL) is a distinct type of T-cell lymphoma involving the capsule or effusion surrounding a breast implant.
- BI-ALCL most commonly presents in two-thirds of cases as a delayed (>1 year) periprosthetic fluid collection and as a capsular mass in one-third of cases. One-in-8 patients presents with lymphadenopathy.
- Optimal screening tools include ultrasound or positron emission tomography (PET)/CT scan with directed fine-needle aspiration. Diagnosis should be made prior to surgical intervention.
- Tissue and fluid specimens from suspected cases should be sent with a clinical history to pathology to rule out anaplastic large cell lymphoma (ALCL).
- Operative treatment should include removal of the implant and resection of the entire capsule as well as complete excision of the disease and involved lymph nodes.
- The role of adjunctive treatments, such as chemotherapy, chest wall radiation, anti-CD30 immunotherapy, and stem cell transplant for advanced disease, is under investigation.

INTRODUCTION

In 2011, the United States Food and Drug Administration (FDA) published a safety communication stating, "Women with breast implants may have a very small but increased risk of developing anaplastic large cell lymphoma (ALCL) in the scar capsule adjacent to an implant."[1] This warning was based on case reports dating back to a sentinel case described by Keech and Creech in 1997.[2] The past 18 years have been marked by a transition from a few case reports of a novel periprosthetic T-cell lymphoma to the current understanding and recognition of BI-ALCL. The association of breast implants with a rare cancer of the immune system has created understandable concern among patients, surgeons, and oncologists; therefore, continued investigation is needed to determine which factors play a role in the

Conflict of Interest: Dr M.W. Clemens has consulted for Allergan Corporation (Irvine, California). All other authors report no conflicts of interest.
Data analyses were supported in part by the Cancer Center Support Grant (NCI Grant P30 CA016672).
[a] Department of Plastic Surgery, The University of Texas MD Anderson Cancer Center, 1400 Pressler Street, Unit 1488, Houston, TX 77030, USA; [b] Department of Hematopathology, The University of Texas MD Anderson Cancer Center, 1515 Holcombe Boulevard, Unit 0072, Houston, TX 77030, USA
* Corresponding author.
E-mail address: mwclemens@mdanderson.org

Clin Plastic Surg 42 (2015) 605–613
http://dx.doi.org/10.1016/j.cps.2015.06.006
0094-1298/15/$ – see front matter

malignant degeneration of a breast implant capsule. Several evolving concepts have helped define diagnostic tools, therapeutic strategies, and outcomes of BI-ALCL and are the focus of this article.

LYMPHOMA BACKGROUND

Lymphoma is a cancer of the immune system developing from lymphocytes and is the most common malignancy of the blood.[3] Lymphoma broadly includes Hodgkin lymphoma, non-Hodgkin lymphoma (NHL), multiple myeloma, and immunoproliferative diseases. In the United States, Approximately 65,000 cases of NHL were diagnosed in 2010.[4] Stein and colleagues[5] first described ALCL in 1985 as a novel type of NHL characterized by large anaplastic lymphoid cells that express the cell-surface protein CD30. Estimated incidence of T-cell NHL diagnoses in the United States in 2014 was 7000 to 10,000.[6] ALCL represents approximately 2% to 3% of all NHLs and approximately 20% of all T-cell lymphomas.[7]

ALCL was added as a distinct entity to the Kiel classification in 1988 and to the Revised European American Lymphoma Classification in 1994.[8] The World Health Organization (WHO) classification of lymphomas recognized the disease in 2001 and further delineated variants in their updated 2008 classification.[9,10] NHL prognosis is predicted using the International Prognostic Index (IPI) based on the presence of recognized risk factors, such as the Ann Arbor staging system, age, elevated serum lactate dehydrogenase, performance status, and number of extranodal sites of disease.[11] Clinicopathologic subtypes of ALCL include a spectrum of disease from the more aggressive systemic ALCL down to lymphoproliferative disorders, such as the relatively indolent skin-limited primary cutaneous ALCL (5-year OS >90%–95%) and benign lymphomatoid papulosis.[12] Multiple sites of disease, frequent lymphadenopathy, and metastatic spread characterize systemic ALCL. Systemic ALCL is classified by either the expression or absence of the anaplastic lymphoma kinase (ALK) tyrosine kinase receptor gene translocation. A 2;5 translocation involving the 2p23 and the 5q35 chromosome creates an oncogenic fusion protein of the ALK gene and the nucleophosmin gene.[13] ALK-positive ALCL accounts for approximately 50% to 80% of all ALCLs and occurs most commonly in men (male/female ratio: 6.5:1) under the age of 30 and has a 5-year OS by IPI point value of 0/1: 90%, 2: 68%, 3:33%, and 4/5: 23%.[5] In contrast, ALK-negative ALCL is an immunophenotypically and cytogenetically heterogeneous group and has a 5-year OS by IPI points 0/1: 74%, 2: 62%, 3:31%, and 4/5: 13%. Standard first-line chemotherapy is cyclophosphamide, hydroxydaunorubicin, vincristine, and prednisone (CHOP); and refractory disease is treated with ifosfamide, carboplatin, and etoposide (ICE) or etoposide, methylprednisone, cytarabine, and cisplatin (ESHAP).[14] When treated with chemotherapy, ALK-positive ALCL has a higher 5-year overall survival (OS) rate than systemic ALK-negative ALCL (58% vs 34%, respectively).[15,16] As a percentage of all T-cell lymphomas, ALK-positive ALCL is more common in North America than Europe or Asia (16.0% vs 6.4% vs 3.2%, respectively). Systemic ALK-negative ALCL is more common in Europe than North America or Asia (9.4% vs 7.8% vs 2.6%, respectively).[17]

BREAST IMPLANT–ASSOCIATED ANAPLASTIC LARGE CELL LYMPHOMA: A NOVEL VARIANT

BI-ALCL is distinct from primary breast lymphoma (PBL); PBL, in contrast, is a disease of the breast parenchyma, representing 0.04% to 0.5% of breast cancers and 1% to 2% of all lymphomas.[18] PBL is predominantly a B-cell lymphoma (65%–90%).[19,20] BI-ALCL is a purely T-cell lymphoma arising either in the effusion or scar capsule surrounding a breast implant.[21] All reported cases of BI-ALCL are ALK negative and express a CD30 cell-surface protein (**Figs. 1** and **2**). Most cases are diagnosed during implant revision surgery performed for a late-onset (>1 year), persistent seroma and may be associated with symptoms of pain, breast lumps, swelling, or breast asymmetry. The numbers of BI-ALCL cases reported in primary augmentation and reconstruction for breast cancer or prophylaxis are approximately equivalent. BI-ALCL most commonly follows an indolent course with disease regression after adequate surgical ablation alone without systemic therapy, but aggressive exceptions have been reported.[22] No risk factors have been clearly identified for ALCL although many have been theorized, including the presence of a subclinical biofilm, response to particulate from textured implants, a consequence of capsular contracture or repeated capsular trauma (such as with closed capsulotomies), genetic predisposition, or an autoimmune etiology, but these observations have not been confirmed in formal epidemiologic studies.[23] Recent studies have demonstrated a possible pathogenic mechanism of chronic T-cell stimulation with local antigenic drive, ultimately leading to the development of lymphoma.[24] Further research is required to identify modifiable risk factors, susceptible populations, and optimal screening and surveillance modalities.

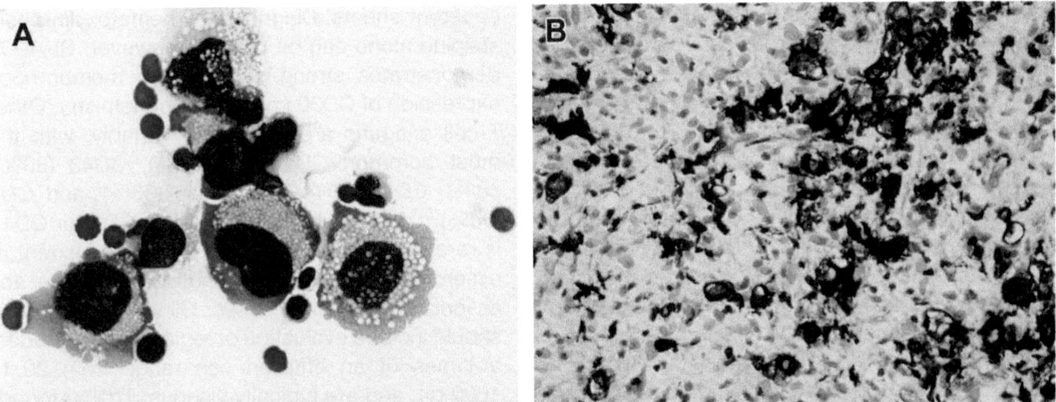

Fig. 1. Hematoxylin-eosin staining of BI-ALCL cells from a malignant effusion demonstrating polymorphic cell shapes with horseshoe-shaped nuclei and nuclear folding (×400 magnification). BI-ALCL cells demonstrate anaplastic large polymorphic cell features, characterized by enlarged horseshoe-shaped nuclei with prominent nucleoli and nuclear folding. Note hematoxylin-eosin staining of BI-ALCL cells at ×400 magnification (*A*). BI-ALCL is characterized by absence of the ALK gene mutation (ALK−) and CD30 staining on immunohistochemistry (*B*).

EPIDEMIOLOGY

Since 1997, approximately 91 patients have been reported either in case reports of BI-ALCL or literature reviews[25–51] (**Fig. 3**). Reporting has benefitted from formal recognition and wider physician education, which has led to an exponential increase in published cases over the past few years. Reliable epidemiologic data for the incidence and prevalence of BI-ALCL has been difficult to determine for the estimated 10 to 11 million women worldwide with breast implants.[52] The FDA database has received approximately 60 reported cases of ALCL in women with breast implants.[42] de Jong and colleagues[53] reported an individually matched case-control study from the Netherlands' nationwide pathology database. The pathology database served a total population of approximately 9 million people. The investigators found a positive association for the development of ALCL in women with breast prostheses compared with those without an implant, with an odds ratio of 18.2 (95% CI, 2.1–156.8). Based on these data, the investigators estimated an incidence of 0.1 to 0.3 per 100,000 BI-ALCL cases for women with prostheses per year. Several prior studies failed to show an association between breast augmentation and risk of lymphoma; however, none was able to review such a large patient population or have sufficient follow-up period.[52,54,55] These studies underscore the difficulty of determining the incidence and prevalence of a rare and recently recognized clinical entity.

DIAGNOSIS AND TREATMENT

Diagnosis of BI-ALCL can be difficult because it remains rare at most medical centers. Two-thirds

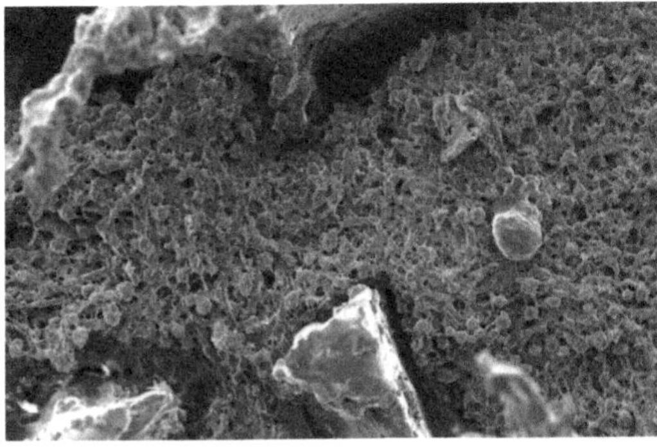

Fig. 2. Scanning electron micrograph at ×300 magnification demonstrating aggregates of lymphoma cells clustered on the surface of a textured silicone implant.

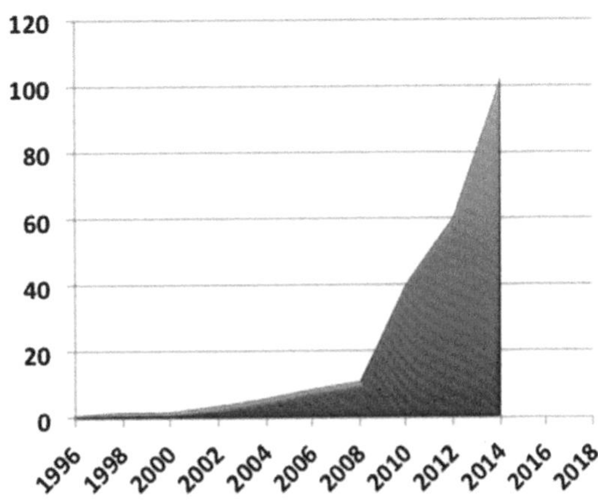

Fig. 3. Timeline of published cases of BI-ALCL.

of BI-ALCL patients present as a malignant effusion associated with the fibrous capsule surrounding an implant occurring on average 9 years after implantation. Any seroma occurring greater than 1 year after implantation not readily explainable by infection or trauma should be considered suspicious for disease[48] (**Fig. 4**). One-third of patients present with a mass that may indicate a more aggressive clinical course. Beatriz and colleagues[56] reviewed 44 BI-ALCL patients with imaging studies and reported on the sensitivity/specificity for detecting an effusion using ultrasound (84%/75%), CT (55%/83%), MRI (82%/33%), and PET (38%/83%). Additionally, the sensitivity/specificity to detect a BI-ALCL mass was reported for ultrasound (46%/100%), CT (50%/100%), MRI (82%/33%), and PET (64%/88%). The sensitivity of mammography was found inferior for BI-ALCL effusion and mass. Ultrasound is used at the authors' institution as a screening tool for suspected cases and in combination with PET for confirmed cases to determine extension and for surveillance of disease.

For suspected patients, any aspiration of periprosthetic fluid should be sent to pathology for cytologic evaluation and include a clinical history with the stated intent to "rule out BI-ALCL." Pathologic evaluation may demonstrate BI-ALCL as individual cells, cell clusters in aggregates, or coherent sheets. Diagnosis by hematoxylin-eosin staining alone can be difficult; however, BI-ALCL demonstrates strong and uniform membranous expression of CD30 immunohistochemistry. Other T-cell antigens are expressed variably, with the most common CD4 (80%–84%), CD43 (80%–88%), CD3 (30%–46%), CD45 (36%), and CD2 (30%).[57] Expression of CD5, CD7, CD8, or CD15 is rare. Ultrasound may help define the extent of a seroma and can be helpful in identifying any associated capsule masses. Clinical examination should include evaluation of regional lymph nodes. Volumes of an effusion can range from 20 to 1000 mL and are typically viscous. The surrounding capsule may be thickened and fibrous or may be completely normal in appearance. If a mass is present, it can protrude into the implant, creating a mass effect distortion on imaging, or the mass may protrude outward into the soft tissue.

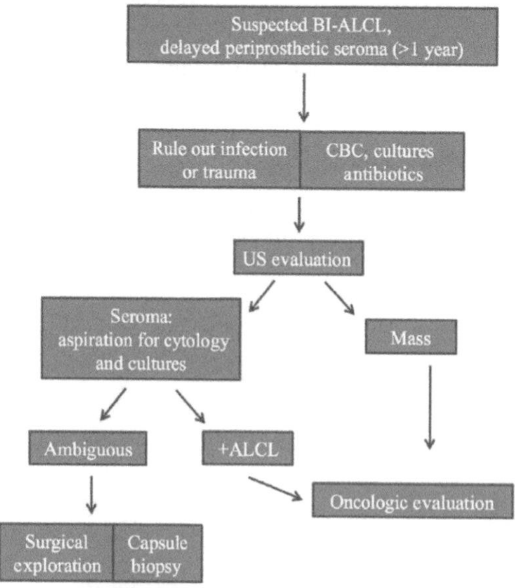

Fig. 4. Approach to a patient with a delayed seroma and suspected BI-ALCL. CBC, complete blood cell count. (*Modified from* Bengtson B, Brody GS, Brown MH, et al. Managing late periprosthetic fluid collections [seroma] in patients with breast implants: a consensus panel recommendation and review of the literature. Plast Reconstr Surg 2011;128(1):1–7.)

Patients with biopsy-proved BI-ALCL must be referred to a lymphoma oncologist. Surgical treatment of BI-ALCL requires complete tumor ablation, which includes removal of the implant, complete removal of any disease mass with negative margins, and total capsulectomy (**Fig. 5**). Because an implant capsule may drain to multiple regional lymph node basins, there does not seem to be a role for sentinel lymph node biopsy in the treatment of BI-ALCL. Fine-needle aspiration of enlarged lymph nodes can yield a false-negative result and, therefore, excisional biopsies should be performed of any suspicious lymph nodes. A surgical oncologist is strongly recommended because incomplete resection and inadequate local surgical control may subject the patient to the need for adjunctive treatments, such as chemotherapy and radiation therapy, whereas complete resection may be definitive treatment in a majority of cases. Surgery should be performed with strict oncologic technique, including use of specimen orientation sutures, placement of surgical clips within the tumor bed, and use of new instruments if performing a contralateral explantation. At this time, the FDA does not recommend screening or prophylactic implant removal for asymptomatic patients or family members. Although not recommended, several BI-ALCL patients have received implant replacement with a smooth implant after definitive treatment, and these patients are closely monitored for any disease sequelae.

CLINICAL CHARACTERISTICS AND OUTCOMES

The clinic-pathologic features of BI-ALCL have been reported in several literature reviews. In

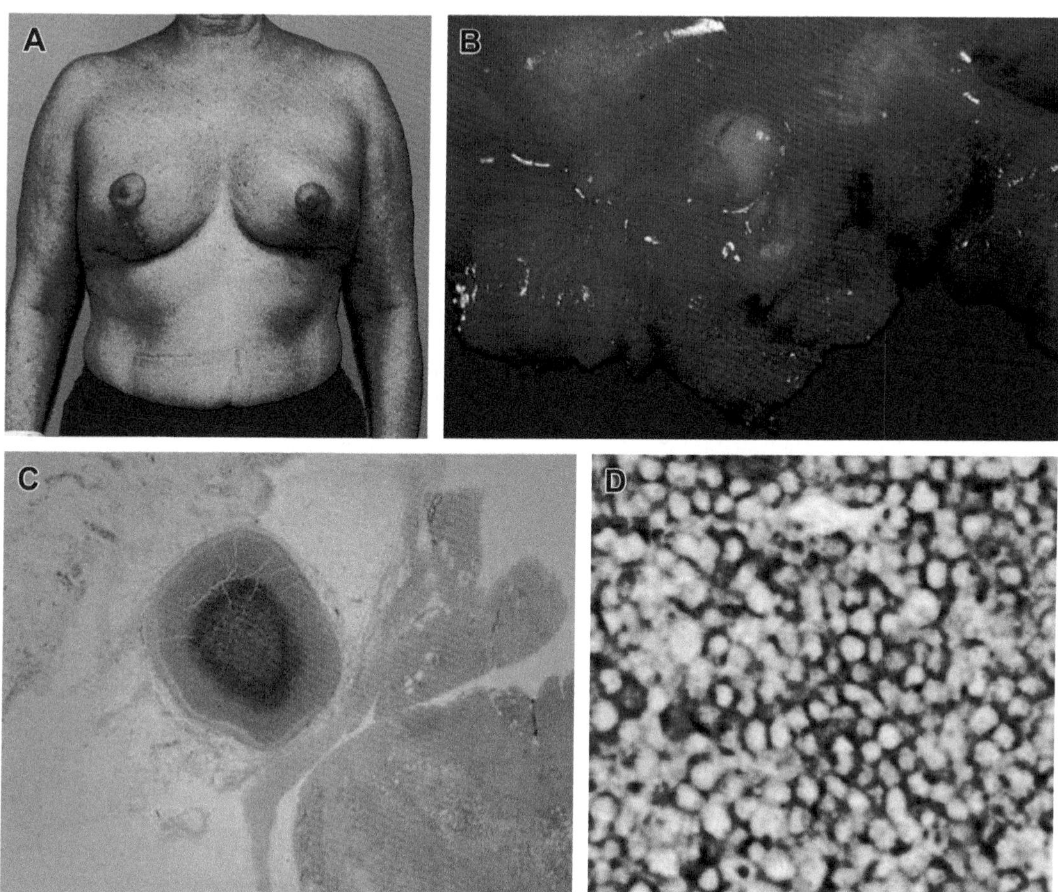

Fig. 5. Patient is a 52-year-old woman who received a cosmetic breast augmentation with textured silicone implants. Twenty years after implantation, she developed an acute swelling of the left breast, which was aspirated multiple times. Patient then received a partial capsulectomy, implant removal, and mastopexy. Postoperative pathology demonstrated BI-ALCL and she was referred to the authors' institution. (*A*) Adequate tumor resection was questionable and, therefore, patient underwent a total capsulectomy with wide local excision of the previous operative site. (*B*) Postoperative pathology again demonstrated persistent BI-ALCL disease now with free margins. (*C, D*) Patient received no further adjunctive treatments and is currently disease-free.

2014, Miranda and colleagues[50] reviewed the long-term follow-up of 60 BI-ALCL patients. The mean age was 52 years (range 28–87 years) with a median of 9 years (range 1–32 years) between implantation and lymphoma diagnosis. Patients presented with either a malignant effusion or seroma (70%) or a distinct mass (30%). The median OS was 12 years (median follow-up, 2 years; range, 0–14 years). A total capsulectomy with implant removal was performed in 93% of patients. OS and progression-free survival (PFS) were similar between patients who received and did not receive chemotherapy (P = .44 and P = .28, respectively). Radiation therapy has also been used for local control of disease, and further research is required to determine specific indications for adjunctive treatments. Patients with a breast mass had a worse OS and PFS (P = .052 and P = .03, respectively). At this time, it is unclear whether the association of mass and worse prognosis indicates a more aggressive variant, more progressed disease, or perhaps a consequence of inadequate surgical ablation of tumor infiltration.

Hart and Lechowicz[58] performed a metanalysis and identified 62 BI-ALCL patients. For patients with available clinical data, the investigators noted rates of 17.3% extracapsular disease and 23.1% with the presence of a mass—39.6% of patients were treated with surgery alone; 9.4% with surgery and radiation; 18.9% with surgery and chemotherapy; 30.2% with surgery, chemotherapy, and radiation; and 1.9% with chemotherapy alone. At a median follow-up of 15 months (3.6–90 months), disease recurrence was 28.3%, of which 73.3% were treated with salvage chemotherapy. BI-ALCL was attributed to 4 patient deaths. Extracapsular disease extension was associated with increased risk for recurrence ($P<.0001$) and patient death ($P = .0008$). This study also found a statistically significant difference in 3- and 5-year survival rates between patients presenting with and without a mass ($P = .0308$ and $P = .0308$, respectively). Although BI-ALCL may follow an indolent course in most patients, reports of disseminated cancer and deaths attributed to the disease emphasizes the importance of timely diagnosis and adequate treatment with appropriate surveillance.

SETTING RESEARCH PRIORITIES

Further research into the development of primary cell lines and biologic models is important to fully elucidate the exact etiology and pathogenesis of BI-ALCL. Lechner and colleagues[33] reported the establishment and characterization of a BI-ALCL model cell line (TLBR-1) as well as heterotransplantation of the disease into immune-compromised mice. Establishment of cell lines from effusion or excisional biopsies will be important to completely characterize the disease and for the identification of potential molecular targets. Future research is warranted to determine if certain patients have a predisposition to the development of the disease and if any modifiable risk factors exist either with the patient or type of implant used. Advances in the treatment of T-cell lymphomas gives promise for BI-ALCL not refractory to surgical therapy alone. Brentuximab vedotin is a novel anti-CD30 monoclonal antibody that has changed the management of systemic ALCL, with a reported objective response rate of 86% and complete remission rate of 59% in relapsed or refractory systemic ALCL.[59,60] Prospective trials of BI-ALCL patients at major referral centers may help delineate chemotherapeutic sensitivity and efficacy of novel agents.

MEDICAL-LEGAL CONSIDERATIONS

After recommendations made by the FDA in 2011, implant manufacturers added language warning of the existence of BI-ALCL to breast implant package inserts within the United States and Canada. Breast implant informed consent examples that include the risk of BI-ALCL were subsequently produced by the American Society of Plastic Surgeons and are available for download from the www.plasticsurgery.org Web site. Patients receiving an implant should be made aware of the existence of BI-ALCL and common presenting symptoms, such as a mass or delayed-presentation (>1 year) seroma/effusion. The future of insurance coverage for screening delayed seromas as well as coverage for complications related to implants continues to evolve and is not guaranteed. When the United States moratorium on silicone implants ended in 2006, the FDA recommended all women with silicone breast implants undergo MRI evaluation for implant failure at 3 years' postimplantation. Because insurance policies do not cover this screening, the suggested study is not widely performed.[61] A similar trend would be concerning if delayed presentation seromas are not routinely sent for pathologic evaluation due to a lack of reimbursement. The WHO is expected to address BI-ALCL in their updated 2015 classification of lymphomas, and formal recognition will facilitate physician awareness and patient education.

REPORTING OF CASES

Many resources exist for oncologists and surgeons treating a BI-ALCL patient. The Plastic Surgery Foundation paired with the American Society of Plastic Surgeons and the FDA to form the Patient Registry and Outcomes for Breast Implants and Anaplastic Large Cell Lymphoma Etiology and Epidemiology (PROFILE). The purpose of PROFILE is to increase the scientific data on BI-ALCL in women with breast implants as well as to support research to characterize BI-ALCL and elucidate the exact role of breast implants in the etiology of the disease. In addition to providing plastic surgeons, oncologists, and patients with information they need about breast implants and treatment of ALCL, confirmed cases in the registry will be available for analytical epidemiologic studies. Treating physicians are encouraged to report confirmed cases to the PROFILE Web site, which can be found at www.thepsf.org.

SUMMARY

Timely diagnosis of BI-ALCL will depend on the millions of women with breast implants having access to heightened surveillance, knowledgeable physicians, and appropriate testing and medical care. BI-ALCL is a rare disease associated with breast implants, although the exact etiology and pathogenesis remain unclear. Accurate diagnosis and complete surgical treatment are important for definitive treatment of patients. Further research is critical for the ideal prevention, diagnosis, and treatment of BI-ALCL.

Editorial Comments by Bradley P. Bengtson, MD

There is a great deal more that we do not know or understand about Breast Implant Associated ALCL than what we do know. It is still unclear if the majority of patients diagnosed represent a true malignancy, but it appears it may be. It is still unclear if it is one entity or multiple. We do not know its true incidence but appears to be somewhere between being struck by lightning and being struck by an asteroid, but may in fact be more common and take years to develop. Dr Clemens and his team at MD Anderson has given us a great deal of information on this rare entity that we do know and how it should be treated. In distinction to nonimplant related ALCL it is always ALK negative and CD30 positive. It is more commonly associated with textured surface implants. It has been reported in pure cases from every implant manufacturer in the US verses exclusively to any one manufacturer. The majority present with a delayed seroma or fluid collection, but some present with a mass associated with the implant capsule. Patients are cured if caught early with total capsulectomy and mass removal. The morbidity and rare mortalities most likely stem from the chemotherapy or radiation treatment in these patients verses the disease itself, so it is very important for hematologists and oncologists to understand that Breast Implant related ALCL has a very indolent course and is a distinct entity from standard forms of ALCL. For the plastic surgeon, if we see a patient with chronic fluid around an implant it should be sent for culture and sensitivity, but also CD30, ALK and cancer cells, particularly if the implant has been in for over 6 years. Plus MRI's should be performed and consideration with involvement of a local surgical oncologist. In the future it will become increasingly important to have one major referral center, or at a minimum, recording referencing center keeping track of these rare cases because of the high degree of multiple reporting and reduplication of patient cases.

REFERENCES

1. U.S. Food and Drug Administration. Anaplastic large cell lymphoma (ALCL) In Women with Breast Implants: preliminary FDA findings and analyses. 2011. Available at: www.fda.gov. Accessed November 20, 2014.
2. Keech JA, Creech BJ. Anaplastic T-cell lymphoma in proximity to a saline-filled breast implant. Plast Reconstr Surg 1997;100(2):554–5.
3. General Information About Adult Non-Hodgkin Lymphoma. National Cancer Institute website, 2014. Available at: http://www.cancer.gov/types/lymphoma/patient/adult-nhl-treatment-pdq. Accessed November 20, 2014.
4. Altekruse SF, Kosary CL, Krapcho M, et al, editors. SEER cancer statistics review, 1975–2007. Bethesda (MD): National Cancer Institute; 2010.
5. Stein H, Mason DY, Gerdes J, et al. The expression of the Hodgkin's disease associated antigen Ki-1 in reactive and neoplastic lymphoid tissue: evidence that Reed-Sternberg cells and histiocytic malignancies are derived from activated lymphoid cells. Blood 1985;66:848–58.
6. SEER Data Fact Sheets: Non-Hodgkin Lymphoma website. Available at: http://seer.cancer.gov/statfacts/html/nhl.html. Accessed November 10, 2014.
7. A clinical evaluation of the International Lymphoma Study Group classification of non-Hodgkin's lymphoma. The non-Hodgkin's Lymphoma Classification Project. Blood 1997;89:3909–15.
8. Willemze R, Jaffe ES, Burg G, et al. WHO-EORTC classification for cutaneous lymphomas. Blood 2005;105(10):3768–85.
9. Delsol G, Ralfkiaer E, Stein H, et al. Anaplastic large cell lymphoma. In: Jaffe ES, Harris NL, Stein H, et al, editors. World Health Organization classification of tumours: pathology and genetics of tumours of haematopoietic and lymphoid tissues. Lyon (France): IARC Press; 2001. p. 230–5.
10. Swerdlow SH, Campo E, Harris NL, et al. WHO classification of tumours of haematopoietic and lymphoid tissues. Lyon (France): IARC Press; 2008.
11. A predictive model for aggressive non-Hodgkin's lymphoma. The international non-Hodgkin's lymphoma prognostic factors Project. N Engl J Med 1993;329(14):987–94.
12. Jacobsen E. Anaplastic large-cell lymphoma, T-/null-cell type. Oncologist 2006;11:831–40.
13. Morris SW, Kirstein MN, Valentine MB, et al. Fusion of a kinase gene, ALK, to a nucleolar protein gene, NPM, in non-Hodgkin's lymphoma. Science 1994; 263:1281–4.
14. Fisher RI, Gaynor ER, Dahlberg S, et al. Comparison of a standard regimen (CHOP) with three intensive chemotherapy regimens for advanced non-Hodgkin's lymphoma. N Engl J Med 1993;328(14):1002–6.
15. Savage KJ, Harris NL, Vose JM, et al. ALK-anaplastic large-cell lymphoma is clinically and immunophenotypically different from both ALK+ ALCL and peripheral T-cell lymphoma, not otherwise specified: report from the International Peripheral T-Cell Lymphoma Project. Blood 2008; 111:5496–504.
16. Savage KJ, Chhanabhai M, Gascoyne RD, et al. Characterization of peripheral T-cell lymphomas in a single North American institution by the WHO classification. Ann Oncol 2004;15:1467–75.

17. Vose J, Armitage J, Weisenburger D. International peripheral T-cell and natural killer/T-cell lymphoma study: pathology findings and clinical outcomes. J Clin Oncol 2008;26:4124–30.
18. Brogi E, Harris NL. Lymphomas of the breast: pathology and clinical behavior. Semin Oncol 1999; 26:357–64.
19. Cao YB, Wang SS, Huang HQ. Primary breast lymphoma–a report of 27 cases with literature review. Ai Zheng 2007;26(1):84–9.
20. Gholam D, Bibeau F, El Weshi A. Primary breast lymphoma. Leuk Lymphoma 2003;44(7):1173–8.
21. Kim B, Roth C, Chung KC, et al. Anaplastic large cell lymphoma and breast implants: a systematic review. Plast Reconstr Surg 2011;127:2141–50.
22. Kim B, Roth C, Young VL, et al. Anaplastic large cell lymphoma and breast implants: results from a structured expert consultation process. Plast Reconstr Surg 2011;128:629–39.
23. Yoshida SH, Swan S, Teuber SS, et al. Silicone breast implants: immunotoxic and epidemiologic issues. Life Sci 1995;56(16):1299–310.
24. Ferreri AJM, Govi S, Pileri SA, et al. Anaplastic large cell lymphoma, ALK-negative. Crit Rev Oncol Hematol 2013;85(2):206–15.
25. Gaudet G, Friedberg JW, Weng A, et al. Breast lymphoma associated with breast implants: two case-reports and a review of the literature. Leuk Lymphoma 2002;43:115–9.
26. Alobeid B, Sevilla DW, El-Tamer MB, et al. Aggressive presentation of breast implant-associated ALK-1 negative anaplastic large cell lymphoma with bilateral axillary lymph node involvement. Leuk Lymphoma 2009;50:831–3.
27. Miranda RN, Lin L, Talwalkar SS, et al. Anaplastic large cell lymphoma involving the breast: a clinicopathologic study of 6 cases and review of the literature. Arch Pathol Lab Med 2009;133:1383–90.
28. Li S, Lee AK. Silicone implant and primary breast ALK1-negative anaplastic large cell lymphoma, fact or fiction? Int J Clin Exp Pathol 2009;3:117–27.
29. Farkash EA, Ferry JA, Harris NL, et al. Rare lymphoid malignancies of the breast: a report of two cases illustrating potential diagnostic pitfalls. J Hematop 2009;2:237–44.
30. Bishara MR, Ross C, Sur M. Primary anaplastic large cell lymphoma of the breast arising in reconstruction mammoplasty capsule of saline filled breast implant after radical mastectomy for breast cancer: an unusual case presentation. Diagn Pathol 2009;4:11.
31. Lazzeri D, Agostini T, Giannotti G, et al. Null-type anaplastic lymphoma kinase-negative anaplastic large cell lymphoma arising in a silicone breast implant capsule. Plast Reconstr Surg 2011;127: 159e–62e.
32. Talwalkar SS, Miranda RN, Valbuena JR, et al. Lymphomas involving the breast: a study of 106 cases comparing localized and disseminated neoplasms. Am J Surg Pathol 2008;32:1299–309.
33. Lechner MG, Lade S, Liebertz DJ, et al. Breast implant-associated, ALK-negative, T-cell, anaplastic, large-cell lymphoma: establishment and characterization of a model cell line (TLBR-1) for this newly emerging clinical entity. Cancer 2011;117:1478–89.
34. Carty MJ, Pribaz JJ, Antin JH, et al. A patient death attributable to implant-related primary anaplastic large cell lymphoma of the breast. Plast Reconstr Surg 2011;128:112e–8e.
35. Aladily TN, Medeiros LJ, Amin MB, et al. Anaplastic large cell lymphoma associated with breast implants: a report of 13 cases. Am J Surg Pathol 2012;36:1000–8.
36. Lazzeri D, Zhang YX, Huemer GM, et al. Capsular contracture as a further presenting symptom of implant-related anaplastic large cell lymphoma. Am J Surg Pathol 2012;36:1735–6 [author reply: 1736–8].
37. Bautista-Quach MA, Nademanee A, Weisenburger DD, et al. Implant-associated primary anaplastic large-cell lymphoma with simultaneous involvement of bilateral breast capsules. Clin Breast Cancer 2013;13:492–5.
38. Farace F, Bulla A, Marongiu F, et al. Anaplastic large cell lymphoma of the breast arising around mammary implant capsule: an Italian report. Aesthetic Plast Surg 2013;37:567–71.
39. Ivaldi C, Perchenet AS, Jallut Y, et al. About two cases of lymphoma in implant capsule: a difficult diagnosis, an unknown pathology. Ann Chir Plast Esthet 2013;58:688–93 [in French].
40. Parthasarathy M, Orrell J, Mortimer C, et al. Chemotherapy-resistant breast implant-associated anaplastic large cell lymphoma. BMJ Case Rep 2013;2013.
41. Thompson PA, Prince HM. Breast implant-associated anaplastic large cell lymphoma: a systematic review of the literature and mini-meta analysis. Curr Hematol Malig Rep 2013;8:196–210.
42. Zakhary JM, Hamidian Jahromi A, Chaudhery S, et al. Anaplastic large cell lymphoma in the setting of textured breast implant: a call for patients and physicians education. J La State Med Soc 2013; 165(1):26–9.
43. Wong AK, Lopategui J, Clancy S, et al. Anaplastic large cell lymphoma associated with a breast implant capsule: a case report and review of the literature. Am J Surg Pathol 2008;32:1265–8.
44. Taylor KO, Webster HR, Prince HM. Anaplastic large cell lymphoma and breast implants: five Australian cases. Plast Reconstr Surg 2012;129:610e–7e.
45. George EV, Pharm J, Houston C, et al. Breast implant-associated ALK-negative anaplastic large cell lymphoma: a case report and discussion of possible pathogenesis. Int J Clin Exp Pathol 2013;6:1631–42.

46. Sorensen K, Murphy J, Lennard A, et al. Anaplastic large cell lymphoma in a reconstructed breast using a silicone implant: a UK case report. J Plast Reconstr Aesthet Surg 2014;67(4):561–3.
47. Smith TJ, Ramsaroop R. Breast implant related Anaplastic Large Cell Lymphoma presenting as late onset peri-implant effusion. Breast 2012;21:102–4.
48. Olack B, Gupta R, Brooks GS. Anaplastic large cell lymphoma arising in a saline breast implant capsule after tissue expander breast reconstruction. Ann Plast Surg 2007;59:56–7.
49. Newman MK, Zemmel NJ, Bandak AZ, et al. Primary breast lymphoma in a patient with silicone breast implants: a case report and review of the literature. J Plast Reconstr Aesthet Surg 2008;61:822–5.
50. Miranda RN, Aladily TN, Prince HM, et al. Breast implant-associated anaplastic large-cell lymphoma: long-term follow-up of 60 patients. J Clin Oncol 2014;32:114–20.
51. Hart AM, Lechowicz MJ, Peters KK, et al. Breast implant-associated anaplastic large cell lymphoma: report of 2 cases and review of the literature. Aesthet Surg J 2014;34(6):884–94.
52. Lipworth L, Tarone RE, McLaughlin JK. Breast implants and lymphoma risk: a review of the epidemiologic evidence through 2008. Plast Reconstr Surg 2009;123(3):790–3.
53. de Jong D, Vasmel WL, de Boer JP, et al. Anaplastic large-cell lymphoma in women with breast implants. JAMA 2008;300(17):2030–5.
54. Largent J, Oefelein M, Kaplan HM, et al. Risk of lymphoma in women with breast implants: analysis of clinical studies. Eur J Cancer Prev 2012; 21:274–80.
55. Brinton LA. The relationship of silicone breast implants and cancer at other sites. Plast Reconstr Surg 2007;120(7 Suppl 1):94S–102S.
56. Beatriz EA, Miranda RN, Rauch GM, et al. Breast implant-associated anaplastic large cell lymphoma: sensitivity, specificity and findings of imaging studies in 44 patients. Breast Cancer Res Treat 2014;147(1):1–14.
57. Taylor CR, Siddiqi IN, Brody GS. Anaplastic large cell lymphoma occurring in association with breast implants: review of pathologic and immunohistochemical features in 103 cases. Appl Immunohistochem Mol Morphol 2013;21(1):13–20.
58. Hart A, Lechowicz MJ. Breast implant-associated anaplastic large cell lymphoma: treatment experience in 53 patients. Blood 2013;122:884–94.
59. Younes A, Bartlett NL, Leonard JP, et al. Brentuximab vedotin forrelapsed CD30 positive lymphomas. N Engl J Med 2010;363:1812–21.
60. Pro B, Advani R, Brice P, et al. Brentuximab vedotin (SGN-35) in patients with relapsed or refractory systemic anaplastic large-cell lymphoma: results of a phase II study. J Clin Oncol 2012;30:2190–6.
61. Chung KC, Malay S, Shauver MJ. Economic analysis of screening strategies for rupture of silicone gel breast implants. Plast Reconstr Surg 2012;130(1):225–37.

Index

Note: Page numbers of article titles are in **boldface** type.

Clin Plastic Surg 42 (2015) 615–617
http://dx.doi.org/10.1016/S0094-1298(15)00093-0

C

E

F

United States Postal Service

Statement of Ownership, Management, and Circulation (All Periodicals Publications Except Requestor Publications)

1. Publication Title: Clinics in Plastic Surgery
2. Publication Number: 0 0 6 - 5 3 0
3. Filing Date: 9/18/15
4. Issue Frequency: Jan, Apr, Jul, Oct
5. Number of Issues Published Annually: 4
6. Annual Subscription Price: $490.00
7. Complete Mailing Address of Known Office of Publication (*Not printer*) (*Street, city, county, state, and ZIP+4®*)
   Elsevier Inc.
   360 Park Avenue South
   New York, NY 10010-1710
   Contact Person: Stephen R. Bushing
   Telephone (Include area code): 215-239-3688
8. Complete Mailing Address of Headquarters or General Business Office of Publisher (*Not printer*)
   Elsevier Inc., 360 Park Avenue South, New York, NY 10010-1710
9. Full Names and Complete Mailing Addresses of Publisher, Editor, and Managing Editor (*Do not leave blank*)

Publisher (*Name and complete mailing address*)
Linda Belfus, Elsevier Inc., 1600 John F. Kennedy Blvd., Ste. 1800, Philadelphia, PA 19103-2899

Editor (*Name and complete mailing address*)
Jessica McCool, Elsevier, Inc., 1600 John F. Kennedy Blvd. Suite 1800, Philadelphia, PA 19103-2899

Managing Editor (*Name and complete mailing address*)
Adrianne Brigido, Elsevier, Inc., 1600 John F. Kennedy Blvd. Suite 1800, Philadelphia, PA 19103-2899

10. Owner (*Do not leave blank. If the publication is owned by a corporation, give the name and address of the corporation immediately followed by the names and addresses of all stockholders owning or holding 1 percent or more of the total amount of stock. If not owned by a corporation, give the names and addresses of the individual owners. If owned by a partnership or other unincorporated firm, give its name and address as well as those of each individual owner. If the publication is published by a nonprofit organization, give its name and address.*)

Full Name	Complete Mailing Address
Wholly owned subsidiary of	1600 John F. Kennedy Blvd, Ste. 1800
Reed/Elsevier, US holdings	Philadelphia, PA 19103-2899

11. Known Bondholders, Mortgagees, and Other Security Holders Owning or Holding 1 Percent or More of Total Amount of Bonds, Mortgages, or Other Securities. If none, check box → ☐ None

Full Name	Complete Mailing Address
N/A	

12. Tax Status (*For completion by nonprofit organizations authorized to mail at nonprofit rates*) (*Check one*)
The purpose, function, and nonprofit status of this organization and the exempt status for federal income tax purposes:
☐ Has Not Changed During Preceding 12 Months
☐ Has Changed During Preceding 12 Months (*Publisher must submit explanation of change with this statement*)

13. Publication Title: Clinics in Plastic Surgery
14. Issue Date for Circulation Data Below: July 2015

PS Form **3526**, July 2014 (Page 1 of 3 (Instructions Page 3)) PSN 7530-01-000-9931 **PRIVACY NOTICE**: See our Privacy policy in www.usps.com

15. Extent and Nature of Circulation		Average No. Copies Each Issue During Preceding 12 Months	No. Copies of Single Issue Published Nearest to Filing Date
a. Total Number of Copies (*Net press run*)		991	737
b. Legitimate Paid and Or Requested Distribution (By Mail and Outside the Mail)	(1) Mailed Outside County Paid/Requested Mail Subscriptions stated on PS Form 3541. (*Include paid distribution above nominal rate, advertiser's proof copies and exchange copies*)	416	308
	(2) Mailed In-County Paid/Requested Mail Subscriptions stated on PS Form 3541. (*Include paid distribution above nominal rate, advertiser's proof copies and exchange copies*)		
	(3) Paid Distribution Outside the Mails Including Sales Through Dealers And Carriers, Street Vendors, Counter Sales, and Other Paid Distribution Outside USPS®	186	192
	(4) Paid Distribution by Other Classes of Mail Through the USPS (e.g. First-Class Mail®)		
c. Total Paid and or Requested Circulation (*Sum of 15b (1), (2), (3), and (4)*)		602	500
d. Free or Nominal Rate Distribution (By Mail and Outside the Mail)	(1) Free or Nominal Rate Outside-County Copies included on PS Form 3541	82	76
	(2) Free or Nominal Rate in-County Copies included on PS Form 3541		
	(3) Free or Nominal Rate Copies mailed at Other classes Through the USPS (e.g. First-Class Mail®)		
	(4) Free or Nominal Rate Distribution Outside the Mail (*Carriers or Other means*)		
e. Total Nonrequested Distribution (Sum of 15d (1), (2), (3) and (4)		82	76
f. Total Distribution (Sum of 15c and 15e)		684	576
g. Copies not Distributed (See instructions to publishers #4 (page #3))		307	161
h. Total (Sum of 15f and g)		991	737
i. Percent Paid and/or Requested Circulation (15c divided by 15f times 100)		88.01%	86.81%

* If you are claiming electronic copies go to line 16 on page 3. If you are not claiming Electronic copies, skip to line 17 on page 3

16. Electronic Copy Circulation	***Average No. Copies Each Issue During Preceding 12 Months***	***No. Copies of Single Issue Published Nearest to Filing Date***
a. Paid Electronic Copies		
b. Total paid Print Copies (Line 15c) + Paid Electronic copies (Line 16a)		
c. Total Print Distribution (Line 15f) + Paid Electronic Copies (Line 16a)		
d. Percent Paid (Both Print & Electronic copies) (16b divided by 16c X 100)		
I certify that 50% of all my distributed copies (electronic and print) are paid above a nominal price		

17. Publication of Statement of Ownership
If the publication is a general publication, publication of this statement is required. Will be printed in the ***October 2015*** *issue of this publication.*

18. Signature and Title of Editor, Publisher, Business Manager, or Owner
Stephen R. Bushing
Stephen R. Bushing – Inventory Distribution Coordinator
Date: September 18, 2015

I certify that all information furnished on this form is true and complete. I understand that anyone who furnishes false or misleading information on this form or who omits material or information requested on the form may be subject to criminal sanctions (including fines and imprisonment) and/or civil sanctions (including civil penalties).

PS Form 3526, July 2014 (Page 3 of 3)

Printed and bound by CPI Group (UK) Ltd, Croydon, CR0 4YY

03/10/2024

01040382-0001